AF498444

Samuel Hahnemann, John Ellis, J. G. Millingen...

Doctrine of Homeopathy – The Art of Healing

e-artnow 2020

Samuel Hahnemann, John Ellis, J. G. Millingen…

Doctrine of Homeopathy – The Art of Healing

Organon of Medicine, Of the Homoeopathic Doctrines, Homoeopathy as a Science…

Translator: William Boericke

e-artnow, 2020
Contact: info@e-artnow.org

ISBN 978-80-273-0842-2

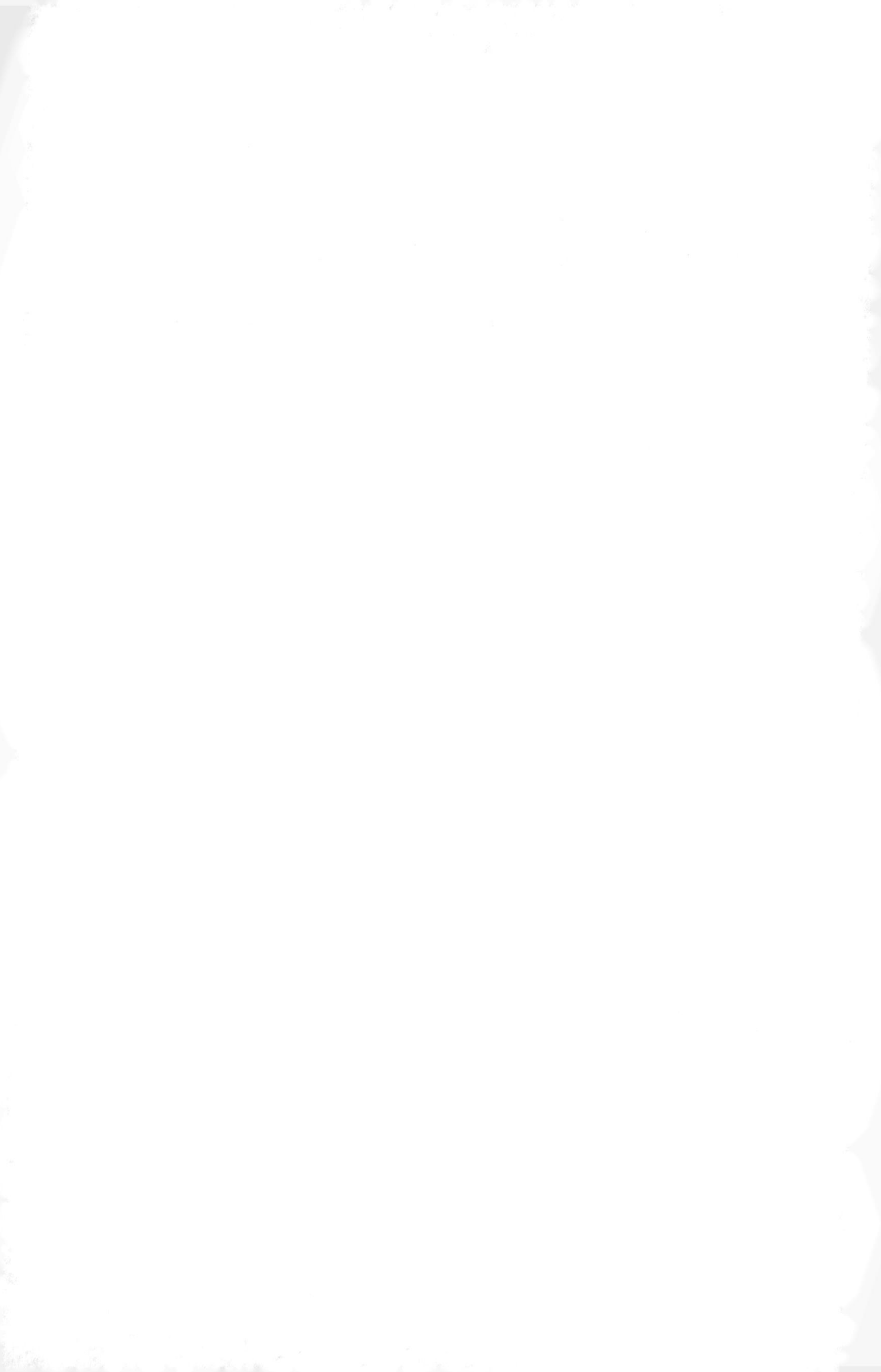

Authors

Samuel Hahnemann
John Ellis
J. G. Millingen
Edward Bayard

Contents

ORGANON OF MEDICINE
by Samuel Hahnemann

AUTHORS PREFACE

Medicine as commonly practised (allopathy) knows no treatment except to draw from diseases the injurious materials which are assumed to be their cause. The blood of the patient is made to flow mercilessly by bleedings, leeches, cuppings, scarifications, to diminish an assumed plethora which never exists as in well women a few days before their menses, an accumulation of blood the loss of which is of no appreciable consequence, while the loss of blood with merely assumed plethora destroys life. Medicine as commonly practised seeks to evacuate the contents of the stomach and sweep the intestines clear by the materials assumed to originate diseases.

In order to give a general notion of the treatment of diseases pursued by the old school of medicine (allopathy) it may be observed that it presupposes the existence sometimes of excess of blood (plethora – which is never present), sometimes of morbid matters and acridities; hence it taps off the life's blood and exerts itself either to clear away the imaginary disease-matter or to conduct it elsewhere (by emetics, purgatives, sialogogues, diaphoretics, diuretics, drawing plasters, setons, issues, etc.), in the vain belief that the disease will thereby be weakened and materially eradicated; in place of which the patient's sufferings are thereby increased, and by such and other painful appliances the forces and nutritious juices indispensable to the curative process are abstracted from the organism. It assails the body with large doses of powerful medicines, often repeated in rapid succession for a long time, whose long-enduring, not infrequently frightful effects it knows not, and which it, purposely it would almost seem, makes unrecognisable by the commingling of several such unknown substances in one prescription, and by their long-continued employment it develops in the body new and often ineradicable medicinal diseases. Whenever it can, it employs, in order to keep in favor with its patient,[1] remedies that immediately suppress and hide the morbid symptoms by opposition (contraria contrariis) for a short time (palliatives), but that leave the cause for these symptoms (the disease itself) strengthened and aggravated. It considers affections on the exterior of the body as purely local and existing there independently, and vainly supposes that it has cured them when it has driven them away by means of external remedies, so that the internal affection is thereby compelled to break out on a nobler and more important part. When it knows not what else to do for the disease which will not yield or which grows worse, the old school of medicine undertakes to change it into something else, it knows not what, by means of an alterative, for example, by the life-undermining calornel, corrosive sublimate and other mercurial preparations in large doses.

It seems that the unhallowed principal business of the old school of medicine (allopathy) is to render incurable if not fatal the majority of diseases, those made chronic through ignorance by continually weakening and tormenting the already debilitated patient by the further addition of new destructive drug diseases. When this pernicious practice has become a habit and one is rendered insensible to the admonitions of conscience, this becomes a very easy business indeed.

And yet for all these mischievous operations the ordinary physician of the old school can assign his reasons, which, however, rest only on foregone conclusions of his books and teachers, and on the authority of this or that distinguished physician of the old school. Even the most opposite and the most senseless modes of treatment find there their defence, their authority – let their disastrous effects speak ever so loudly against them. It is only under the old physician who has been at last gradually convinced, after many years of misdeeds, of the mischievous nature of hi so-called art, and who no longer treats even the severest diseases with anything stronger than plantain water mixed with strawberry syrup (i.e., with nothing), that the smallest number are injured and die.

This non-healing art, which for many centuries has been firmly established in full possession of the power to dispose of the life and death of patients according to its own good will and pleasure, and in that period has shortened the lives of ten times as many human beings as the most destructive wars, and rendered many millions of patients more diseased and wretched than they were originally – this allopathy, I have, in the introduction to the former editions of this book, considered more in detail. Now I shall consider only its exact opposite, the true healing art, discovered by me and now somewhat more perfected. Examples are given to prove that striking cures performed in former times were always due to remedies basically homoeopathic and found by the physician accidentally and contrary to the then prevailing methods of therapeutics.

As regards the latter (homoeopathy) it is quite otherwise. It can easily convince every reflecting person that the diseases of man are not caused by any substance, any acridity, that is to say, any disease-matter, but that they are solely spirit-like (dynamic) derangements of the spirit-like power (the vital principle) that animates the human body. Homoeopathy knows that a cure can only take place by the reaction of the vital force against the rightly chosen remedy that has been ingested, and that the cure will be certain and rapid in proportion to the strength with which the vital force still prevails in the patient. Hence homoeopathy avoids everything in the slightest degree enfeebling,[2] and as much as possible every excitation of pain, for pain also diminishes the strength, and hence it employs for the cure ONLY those medicines whose power for altering and deranging (dynamically) the health it knows accurately, and from these it selects one whose pathogenetic power (its medicinal disease) is capable of removing the natural disease in question by similarity (simila similibus), and this it administers to the patient in simple form, but in rare and minute doses so small that, without occasioning pain or weakening, they just suffice to remove the natural malady whence this result: that without weakening, injuring or torturing him in the very least, the natural disease is extinguished, and the patient, even whilst he is getting better, gains in strength and thus is cured – an apparently easy but actually troublesome and difficult business, and one requiring much thought, but which restores the patient without suffering in a short time to perfect health, – and thus it is a salutary and blessed business.

Thus homoeopathy is a perfectly simple system of medicine, remaining always fixed in its principles as in its practice, which, like the doctrine whereon it is based, if rightly apprehended will be found to be complete (and therefore serviceable). What is clearly pure in doctrine and practice should be self-evident, and all backward sliding to the pernicious routinism of the old school that is as much its antithesis as night is to day, should cease to vaunt itself with the honorable name of Homoeopathy.

Samuel Hahnemann

Paris, 1842

INTRODUCTION.

Review of the therapeutics, allopathy and palliative treatment that have hitherto been practiced in the old school of medicine.

As long as men have existed they have been liable, individually or collectively, to diseases from physical or moral causes. In a rude state of nature but few remedial agents were required, as the simple mode of living admitted of but few diseases; with the civilization of mankind in the state, on the contrary, the occasions of diseases and the necessity for medical aid increased, in equal proportion. But ever since that time (soon after Hippocrates, therefore, for 2500 years) men have occupied themselves with the treatment of the ever increasing multiplicity of diseases, who, led astray by their vanity, sought by reasoning and guessing to excogitate the mode of furnishing this aid. Innumerable and dissimilar ideas respecting the nature of diseases and their remedies sprang from so many dissimilar brains, and the theoretical views these gave rise to the so-called systems, each of which was at variance with the rest and self-contradictory. Each of these subtile expositions at first threw the readers into stupefied amazement at the incomprehensible wisdom contained in it, and attracted to the system-monger a number of followers, who re-echoed his unnatural sophistry, to none of whom, however, was it of the slightest use in enabling them to cure better, until a new system, often diametrically opposed to the first, thrust that aside, and in its turn gained a short-lived renown. None of them, however. was in consonance with nature and experience; they were mere theoretical webs, woven by cunning intellects out of pretended consequences, which could not be made use of in practice, in the treatment at the sick-bed, on account of their excessive subtilty and repugnance to nature, and only served for empty disputations.

Simultaneously, but quite independent of all these theories, there sprung up a mode of treatment with mixtures of unknown medicinal substances for forms of disease arbitrarily set up, and directed towards some material object completely at variance with nature and experience, hence, as may be supposed, with a bad result – such is old medicine, allopathy as it is termed.

Without disparaging the services which many physicians have rendered to the sciences auxiliary to medicine, to natural philosophy and chemistry, to natural history in its various branches, and to that of man in particular, to anthropology, physiology and anatomy, etc., I shall occupy myself here with the practical part of medicine only, with the healing art itself, in order to show how it is that diseases have hitherto been so imperfectly treated. Far beneath my notice is that mechanical routine of treating precious human life according to the prescription manuals, the continual publication of which shows, alas! how frequently they are still used. I pass it by unnoticed, as a despicable practice of the lowest class of ordinary practitioners. I speak merely of the medical art as hitherto practiced, which, pluming itself on its antiquity, imagines itself to possess a scientific character.

The partisans of the old school of medicine flattered themselves that they could justly claim for it alone the title of 'rational medicine', because they alone sought for and strove to remove the cause of disease, and followed the method employed by nature in diseases.

Tolle causam! they cried incessantly. But they went no further than this empty exclamation. They only fancied that they could discover the cause of disease; they did not discover it, however, as it is not perceptible and not discoverable. For as far the greatest number of diseases are of dynamic (spiritual) origin and dynamic (spiritual) nature, their cause is therefore not perceptible to the senses; so they exerted themselves to imagine one, and from a survey of the parts of the normal, inanimate human body (anatomy), compared with the visible changes of the same internal parts in persons who had died of diseases (pathological anatomy), as also from what they could deduce from a comparison of the phenomena and functions in healthy life (physiology) with their endless alterations in the innumerable morbid states (pathology, semeiotics), to draw conclusions relative to the invisible process whereby the changes which take place in the inwardbeing of man in diseases are affected – a dim picture of the imagination, which theoretical medicine regarded as its prima causa morbi;1 and thus it was at one and the same time the proximate cause of the disease, and the internal essence of the disease, the disease itself – although, as sound human reason teaches us, the cause of a thing or of an event, can never be at the same time the thing or the event itself. How could they then, without deceiving themselves, consider this imperceptible internal essence as the object to be treated, and prescribe for it medicines whose curative powers were likewise generally unknown to them, and even give several such unknown medicines mixed together in what are termed prescriptions?

1. It would have been much more consonant with sound human reason and with the nature of things, had they, in order to be able to cure a disease, regarded the originating cause as the causa morbi, and endeavored to discover that, and thus been enabled successfully to employ the mode of treatment which had shown itself useful in maladies having the same exciting cause, in those also of a similar origin, as, for example, the same mercury is efficacious in an ulcer of the glans after impure coitus, as in all previous venereal chancres – if, I say, they had discovered the exciting cause of all other (non-venereal) chronic diseases to be an infection at one period or another with the itch miasm (psora), and had found for all these a common method of treatment, regard being had for the peculiarities of each individual case, whereby all and each of these chronic diseases might have been cured, then might they with justice have boasted that in the treatment of chronic diseases they had in view the only available and useful causa morborum chronicorum (non venereorum), and with this as a basis they might have treated such diseases with the best results. But during these many centuries they were unable to cure the millions of chronic diseases, because they knew not their origin in the psoric miasm (which was first discovered and afterwards provided with a suitable plan of treatment byhomoeopathy), and yet they vaunted that they alone kept in view the prima causa of these diseases in their treatment, and that they alone treated rationally, although they had not the slightest conception of the only useful knowledge of their psoric origin and consequently they bungled the treatment of all chronic diseases!

But this sublime problem, the discovery, namely, a priori, of an internal invisible cause of disease, resolved itself, at least with the more astute physicians of the old school, into a search, under the guidance of the symptoms it is true, for what might be supposed to be the probable general character of the case of disease before them;2 whether it was spasm, or debility, or paralysis, or fever, or inflammation, or induration, or obstruction of this or that part, or excess of blood (plethora), deficiency or excess of oxygen, carbon, hydrogen or nitrogen in the juices, exaltation or depression of the functions of the arterial, venous or capillary system, change in the relative proportion of the factors of sensibility, irritability or reproduction., – conjectures that have been dignified by the followers of the old school with the title of causal indication, and considered to be the only possible rationality in medicine; but which were assumptions, too fallacious and hypothetical to prove of any practical utility – incapable, even had they been well grounded, of indicating the most appropriate remedy for a case of disease; flattering indeed, to the vanity of the learned theorist, but usually leading astray when used as guides to practice, and wherein there was evidenced more of ostentation than of an earnest search for the curative indication.

2. Every physician who treats disease according to such general character however he may affect to claim the name of homoeopathist, is and ever will remain in fact a generalising allopath, for without the most minute individualisation, homoeopathy is not conceivable.

And how often has it happened that, for example, spasm or paralysis seemed to be in one part of the organism, while in another part inflammation was apparently present!

Or, on the other hand, whence are the certain remedies for each of these pretended general characters to be derived? Those that would certainly be of benefit could be none other than the specific medicines, that is, those whose action is homogeneous3 to the morbid irritation; whose employment, however, is denounced and forbidden4 by the old school as highly injurious, because observation has shown that in consequence of the receptivity for homogeneous irritation being so highly increased in diseases, such medicines in the usual large doses are dangerous to life. The old school never dreamt of smaller, and of extremely small doses. Accordingly no attempt was made to cure, in the direct (the most natural) way, by means of homogeneous, specific medicines; nor could it be done, as the effects of most of medicines were, and continued to remain, unknown, and even had they been known it would have been impossible to hit on the right medicine with such generalizing views as were entertained.

3. Now termed Homoeopathic.

4. "Where experience showed the curative power of homoeopathically acting remedies, whose mode of action could not be explained, the difficulty was avoided by calling them specific, and further investigation was stifled by this actually unmeaning word. The homogeneous excitant remedies, the specific (homoeopathic), medicines, however, had long previously been prohibited as of very injurious influence". – Rau, On the Value of the homoeopathic Method of Treatment, Heidelberg, 1824, pp. 101, 102.

However, perceiving that it was more consistent with reason to seek for another path, a straight one if possible, rather than to take circuitous courses, the old school of medicine believed it might cure diseases in a direct manner by the removal of the (imaginary) material cause of disease – for to physicians of the ordinary school, while investigating and forming a judgment upon a disease, and not less while seeking for the curative indication, it was next to impossible to divest themselves of these materialistic ideas, and to regard the nature of the spiritual-corporeal organism as such a highly potentialized entity, that its sensational and functional vital changes, which are called diseases, must be produced and effected chiefly, if not solely, by dynamic (spiritual) influences, and could not be effected in any other way.

The old school regarded all those matters which were altered by the disease, those abnormal matters that occurred in congestions, as well as those that were excreted, as disease-producers, or at least on account of their supposed reacting power, as disease maintainers, and this latter notion prevails to this day.

Hence they dreamed of effecting causal cures by endeavoring to remove these imaginary and presumed material causes of the disease. Hence their assiduous evacuation of the bile by vomiting in bilious fevers;5 their emetics in cases of so-called stomach derangenments;6 their diligent purging away of the mucus, the lumbrici and the ascarides in children who are pale-faced and who suffer from ravenous appetite, bellyache, and enlarged abdomen7; their venesections in cases of haemorrhage;8 and more especially all their varieties of blood-lettings,9 their main remedy in inflammations, which they now, following the example of a well-known bloodthirsty Parisian physician (as a flock of sheep follow the bellwether even into the butcher's slaughter-house), imagine to encounter in almost every morbidly affected part of the body, and feel themselves, bound to remove by the application of often a fatal number of leeches. They believe that by so doing they obey the true casual indications, and treat disease in a rational manner. The adherents of the old school, moreover, believe that by putting a ligature on polypi, by cutting out, or artificially exciting suppuration by means of local irritants in indolent glandular swellings, by enucleating encysted tumors (steatoma and meliceria) by their operations for aneurysm and lacrymal and anal fistula, by removing with the knife scirrhous tumors of the breast, by amputating a limb affected with necrosis, etc., they cure the patient radically, and that their treatment is directed against the cause of the disease; and they also think, when they employ their repellent remedies, dry up old running ulcers in the legs with astringent applications of oxide of lead copper or zinc (aided always by the simultaneous administration of purgatives, which merely debilitate, but have no effect on the fundamental dyscrasia), cauterize chancres, destroy condylomata locally, drive off itch from the skin with ointments of sulphur, oxide of lead, mercury or zinc, suppress ophthalmiae with solutions of lead or zinc, and drive away tearing pains from the limbs by means of opodeldoc, hartshorn liniment or fumigations with cinnabar or amber; in every case they think they have removed the affection, conquered the disease, and pursued a rational treatment directed towards the cause. But what is the result! The metastatic affections that sooner or later, but inevitably appear, caused by this mode of treatment (but which they pretend are entirely new diseases), which are always worse than the original malady, sufficiently prove their error, and might and should open their eyes to the deeper-seated, immaterial nature of the disease, and its dynamic (spirit-like) origin, which can only be removed by dynamic means.

5. The estimable Hofrath Dr. Fau (loc. cit., p.176) at a time when not properly conversant with homowopathy, by firmly convince the dynamic cause of these fevers, cured them without employing ayn evacuation remedy, by means of one or two small doses of homoeopathic remedies, two very remarkable cases of wich he relates in his book.

6. In a case of sudden derangement of the stomach, with constant disgusting eructations with the taste of the vitiated food, generally accompanied by depression of spirits, cold hands and feet, etc., the ordinary physician has hitherto been in the habit of attacking only the degenerated contents of the stomach; a powerful emetic should clean it out completely. This object was generally attained by tartar emetic, with or without ipecacuanha. Does the patient, however, immediately after this become well, brisk and cheerful? Oh, no! Such a derangement of the stomach is usually of dynamic origin, caused by mental disturbance (grief, fright, vexation), a chill, over-exertion of the mund or body immediately after eating, often after even a moderate meal. Those two remedies are not suitable for removing this dynamic derangement, and just as little is the revolutionary vomiting they produce. Moreover, tartar emetic and ipecacuanha, from their other peculiar pathogenetic powers, prove of further injury to the patient's health, and derange the biliary secretion; so that if the patient be not very robust, he must feel ill for several days from the effects of this pretended causal treatment, notwithstanding all this violent expulsion of the whole contents of the stomach. If the patient, however, in place of taking such violent and always (a) hurtful evacuant drugs, smell only a single time at a globule the size of a mustard seed, moistened with highly diluted pulsatillajuice, whereby the derangement of his health in general and of his stomach in particular will certainly be removed, in two hours he is quite well; and if the eructation recur once more, it consists of tasteless and inodorous air; the contents of the stomach cease to be vitiated, and at the next meal he has regained his full usual appetite; he is quite well and lively. This is true causal medication; the former is only an imaginary one and has an injurious efect on the patient.

Even a stomach overloaded with indigestible food never requires a medicinal emetic. In such a case nature is competent to rid herself of the excess in the best way through the oesophagus, by means of nausea, sickness and spontaneous vomiting, assisted, it may be, by mechanical irritation of the palate and fauces, and by this means the accessory medicinal effects of the emetic drugs are avoided; a small quantity of coffee expedites the passage downwards of what remains in the stomach.

But if, after excessive overloading of the stomach, the irritability of the stomach is not sufficient to promote spontaneous vomiting, or is lost altogether, so that the tendency thereto is extinguished, while there are at the same time great pains in the epigastrium, in such a paralyzed state of the stomach, an emetic medicine would only have the effect of producing a dangerous or fatal inflammation of the intestines; where a small quantity of strong infusion of coffee, frequently administered, would dynamically exalt the sunken irritability of the stomach, and put it in a condition to expel its contents, be they ever so great, either upwards or downwards. So here also the pretended causal treatment is out of place.

Even the acrid gastric acid, to eructations of which patients with chronic diseases are not infrequently subject, may be today violently evacuated by means of an emetic, with great suffering, and yet all in vain, for tomorrow or some days later it is replaced by similar acrid gastric acid, and then usually in larger quantities; whereas it goes away by itself when its dynamic cause is removed by a very small dose of a high dilution of sulphuric acid, or still better, if it is of frequent recurrence, by the employment of minutest doses of antipsoric remedies corresponding in similarity to the rest of the symptoms also. And of a similar character are many of the pretended causal cures of the old-school physicians, whose main effort it is, by means of tedious operations, troublesome to themselves and injurious to their patients, to clear away the material product of the dynamic derangement; whereas if they perceived the dynamic source of the affection, and annihilated it and its products homoeopathically, they would thereby effect a rational cure.

7. Conditions dependent solely on a psoric taint, and easily curable by mild (dynamic) antipsoric remedies without emetics or purgatives.

8. Notwithstanding that almost all morbid haemorrhages depend on a dynamic derangement of the vital force (state of health), yet the old-school physicians consider their cause to be excess of blood, and cannot refrain from bleeding in order to draw off the supposed superabundance of this vital fluid; the palpable evil consequences of which procedure, however, such as prostration of the strength, and the tendeny or actual transition, to the typhoid state they ascribe to the malignancy of the disease, which they are then often unable to overcome – in fine, they imagine, even when the patient does not recover, that their treatment has been in conformity with their axiom, causam tolle, and that, according to their mode of speaking, they have done everything in their power for the patient, let the result be what it may.

9. Although there probably never was a drop of blood too much in the living human body, yet the old-school practitioners consider an imaginary excess of blood as the main material cause of all haemorrhages and inflammations, which they must remove and drain off by venesections, cupping and leeches. This they hold to be a rational mode of treatment, causal medication. In general inflammatory fevers, in acute pleurisy, they even regard the coagulable lymph in the blood – the buffy coat, as it is termed – as the materia peccans, which they endeavor to get rid of, if possible, by repeated venesections, notwithstanding that this coat often becomes more consistent and thicker at every repetition of the bloodletting. They thus often bleed the patient nearly to death, when the inflammatory fever will not subside, in order to remove this buffy coat or the imaginary plethora, without suspecting tbat the inflammatory blood is only the product of the acute fever, of the morbid, immaterial (dynamic) inflammatory irritation, and that the latter is the sole cause of the great disturbance in the vascular systan, and may be removed by the smallest dose of a homogeneous (homoeopathic) medicine, as, for instance, by a small globule of the decillion-fold dilution of aconite juice, with abstinence from vegetable acids, so that the most violent pleuritic fever, with all its alarming concomitants, is changed into health and cured, without the least abstraction of blood and without any antiphlogistic remedy, in a few – at the most in twenty-four – hours (a small quantity of blood drawn from a vein by the way of experiment then shows no traces of buffy coat); whereas another patient similarly affected, and treated on the rational principles of the old school, if, after repeated bleedings, with great difficulty and unspeakable sufferings he escape for the nonce with life, he often has still many months to drag through before he can support his emaciated body on his legs, if in the mean time (as often happens from such maltreatment) he be not carried off by typhoid fever, leucophlegmasia or pulmonary phthisis.
Anyone who has felt the tranquil pulse of a man an hour before the occurrence of the rigor that always precedes an attack of acute pleurisy, will not be able to restrain his amazement if told two hours later, after the hot stage has commenced, that the enormous plethora present urgently requires repeated venesections, and will naturally inquire by what magic power could the pounds of blood that must now be drawn off have been conjured into the blood-vessels of this man within these two hours, which but two hours previously he had felt beating in such a tranquil manner. Not a single drachm more of blood can now be circulating in those vessels than existed when he was in good health, not yet two hours ago!

Accordingly the allopathic physician with his venesections draws from the patient laboring under acute fever no oppressive superabundance of blood, as that cannot possibly be present; he only robs him of what is indispensable to life and recovery, the normal quantity of blood and consequently of strength – a great loss which no physician's power can replace! – and yet he vainly imagines that he has conducted the treatment in conformity to his (misunderstood) axiom, causam tolle; whereas it is impossible that the causa morbi in this case can be an excess of blood, which is not present; but the sole true causa morbi was a morbid, dynamical, inflammatory irritation of the circulatory system, as is proved by the rapid and permanent cure of this and every similar case of general inflammatory fever by one or two inconceivably minute doses of aconite juice, which removes such an irritation homoeopathically.

The old school errs equally in the treatment of local inflammations with its topical blood-lettings, more especially with the quantities of leeches which are now applied according to the maniacal principles of Broussais. The palliative amelioration that at first ensues from the treatment is far from being crowned by a rapid and perfect cure; on the contrary, the weak and ailing state of the parts thus treated (frequently also of the whole body), which always remains, sufficiently shows the error that is committed in attributing the local inflammation to a local plethora, and how sad are the consequences of such abstractions of blood; whereas this purely dynamic, apparently local, inflammatory irritation, can be rapidly and permanently removed by an equally small dose of aconite, or, according to circumstances, of belladonna, and the whole disease annihilated and cured, without such unjustifiable shedding of blood.

A favorite idea of the ordinary school of medicine, until recent (would that I could not say the most recent) times, was that of morbific matters (and acridities) in diseases, excessively subtile though they might be thought to be, which must be expelled from the blood-vessels and lymphathics, through the exhalents, skin, urinary apparatus or salivary glands, through the tracheal and bronchial glands in the form of expectoration, from the stomach and bowels by vomiting and purging, in order that the body might be freed from the material cause that produced the disease, and a radical causal treatment be thus carried out.

By cutting holes in the diseased body, which were converted into chronic ulcers kept up for years by the introduction of foreign substances (issues, setons), they sought to draw off the materia peccans from the (always only dynamically) diseased body, just as one lets a dirty fluid run out of a barrel through the tap-hole. By means also of perpetual fly-blisters and the application of mezereum, they thought to draw away the bad humors and to cleanse the diseased body from all morbific matters – but they only weakened it, so as generally to render it incurable, by all these senseless unnatural processes.

I admit that it was more convenient for the weakness of humanity to assume that, in the diseases they were called on to cure, there existed some morbific material of which the mind might form a conception (more particularly as the patients readily lent themselves to such a notion), because in that case the practitioner had nothing further to care about than to procure a good supply of remedies for purifying the blood and humors, exciting diuresis and diaphoresis, promoting expectoration, and scouring out the stomach and bowels. Hence, in all the works on Materia Medica, from Dioscorides down to the latest books on this subject, there is almost nothing said about the special peculiar action of individual medicines; but, besides on account of their supposed utility in various nosological names of diseases, it is merely stated whether they are diuretic, diaphoretic, expectorant or emmenagogue, and more particularly whether they produce evacuation of the stomach and bowels upwards or downwards; because all the aspirations and efforts of the practitioner have ever been chiefly directed to cause the expulsion of a material morbific matter, and of sundry (fictitious) acridities, which it was imagined were the cause of diseases.

These were, however, all idle dreams, unfounded assumptions and hypotheses, cunningly devised for the convenience of therapeutics, as it was expected the easiest way of performing a cure would be to remove the material morbific matters (si modo essent!).

But the essential nature of diseases and their cure will not adapt themselves to such fantasies, nor to the convenience of medical men; to humor such stupid baseless hypotheses diseases will not cease to be (spiritual) dynamic derangements of our spirit-like vital principle in sensations and functions, that is to say, immaterial derangements of our state of health.

The causes of our maladies cannot be material, since the least foreign material substance,10 however mild it may appear to us, if introduced into our blood-vessels, is promptly ejected by the vital force, as though it were a poison; or when this does not happen, death ensues. If even the minutes splinter penetrates a sensitive part of our organism, the vital principle everywhere present in our body never rests until it is removed by pain, fever, suppuration or gangrene. And can it be supposed that in a case of cutaneous disease of twenty years standing, for instance, this indefatigably active vital principle will quietly endure the presence of such an injurious foreign, material exanthematous substance, such as a herpetic, a scrofulous, a gouty acridity, etc., in the fluids of the body? Did any nosologist ever see with corporeal eyes such a morbific matter, to warrant him in speaking so confidently about it, and in founding a system of medical treatment upon it? Has any one ever succeeded in displaying to view the matter of gout or the poison of scrofula ?

10. Life was endangered by injecting a little pure water into a vein. (Vide Mullen, quoted by Birch in the History of the Royal Society.)

Atmospheric air injected into the blood-vessels caused death. (Vide J. M. Voigt, Magazin fur den neuesten Zustand der Naturkunde, i, iii, p. 25.

Even the mildest fluids introduced into the veins endangered life. (Vide Autenreith, Physiologie, ii, Ã› 784.)

Even when the application of a material substance to the skin, or to a wound, has propagated diseases by infection, who can prove (what is so often maintained in works on pathology) that some material portion of this substance has penetrated into our fluids or been absorbed?11 The most careful and prompt washing of the genitals does not protect the system from infection with the venereal chancrous disease. The slightest breath of air emanating from the body of a person affected with smallpox will suffice to produce this horrible disease in a healthy child.

11. A girl in Glasgow, eight years of age, having been bit by a mad dog, the surgeon immediately cut the piece clean out, and yet thirty-six days afterwards she was seized with hydrophobia, which killed her in two days. (Med. Comment. of Edinb., Dec. 2, vol. ii, 1793.)

What ponderable quantity of material substance could have been absorbed into the fluids, in order to devdop, in the first of these instances, a tedious dyscrasia (syphilis), which when uncured is only extinguished with the remotest period of life, with death; in the last, a disease (smallpox) accompanied by almost general suppuration,12 and often rapidly fatal? In these and all similar cases is it possible to entertain the idea of a material morbific matter being introduced into the blood? A letter written in the sick-room at a great distance has often communicated the same contagious disease to the person who read it. In this instance, can the notion of a material morbific matter having penetrated into the fluids be admitted? But what need is there of all such proofs? How often has it happened

that an irritating word has brought on a dangerous bilious fever; a superstitious prediction of death has caused the fatal catastrophe at the very time announced; the abrupt communication of sad or excessively joyful news has occasioned sudden death? In these cases, where is the material morbific principle that entered in substance into the body, there to produce and keep up the disease, and without the material expulsion and ejection of which a radical cure were impossible?

12. In order to account for the large quantity of putrid exerementitious matter and foetid discharge often met with in diseases, and to be able to represent them as the material substance that excites and keeps up disease – although, when infection occurs, nothing perceptible in the shape of miasm, nothing material, could have penetrated into the body – recourse was had to

the hypothesis, that the matter of infection, be it ever so minute, acts in the body like a ferment, bringing the fluids into a like state of corruption, and thus changing them into a similar morbific ferment which constantly increases with the disease and keeps it up. But by what all-potent and all-wise purifying draughts will you purge and cleanse the human fluids from this ever reproductive ferment, from this mass of imaginary morbific matter, and that so perfectly, that there shall not remain a particle of such morbific ferment, which, according to this hypothesis, must ever again, as at first, transform and corrupt the fluids to new morbific matter? Were that so it would evidently be impossible to cure these diseases in your way! – See how all hypotheses, be they ever so ingeniously framed, lead to the most palpable absurdities when they are not founded on truth! – The most deeply rooted syphilis may be cured, after the removal of the psora with which it is often complicated, by one or two small doses of the decillionfiold diluted and potentised solution of mercury, whereby the general syphilitic taint of the fluids is forever (dynamically) annihilated and removed.

The champions of this clumsy doctrine of morbific matters ought to be ashamed that they have so inconsiderately overlooked and failed to appreciate the spiritual nature of life, and the spiritual dynamic power of the exciting causes of diseases, and that they have thereby degraded themselves into mere scavenger-doctors, who, in their efforts to expel from the diseased body morbific matters that never existed, in place of curing, destroy life.

Are, then, the foul, often disgusting excretions which occur in diseases the actual matter that produces and keeps them up?13 Are they not rather always exeretory products of the disease itself, that is, of the life which is only dynamically deranged and disordered?

13. Were this the case, the most inveterate coryza should be certainly and rapidly cured by merely blowing and wiping the nose carefully.

With such false and materialistic views concerning the origin and essential nature of diseases, it was certainly not to be wondered at that in all ages the main endeavor of the most obscure, as well as of the most distinguished practitioners, and even of the inventors of the sublimest medical systems, was always only to separate and expel an imaginary morbific matter, and the indication most frequently laid down was to break up and put in motion this morbific matter, to effect its expulsion by salivation, expectoration, diaphoresis and diuresis, to purify the blood frotn (acridities and impurities) morbific matters, which never existed, by means of the intelligence of sundry obedient decoctions of root and plants; to draw off mechanically the imaginary matter of disease by setons,

by issues, by portions of the skin kept open and discharging by means of perpetual blisters or mezereum bark, but chiefly to expel and purge away the materia peccans, or the injurious matters as they were termed, through the intestines, by means of laxative and purgative medicines, which, in order to give them a more profound meaning and a more prepossessing appearance, were fondly denominated dissolvents and mild aperients – all so many arrangements for the expulsion of inimical morbific matters, which never could be, and never were instrumental in the production and maintenance of the diseases of the human organism, animated as it is by a spiritual principle – of diseases which never were anything else than spiritual dynamic derangements of the life altered in its sensations and functions.

Let it be granted now, what cannot be doubted, that no diseases – if they do not result from the introduction of perfectly indigestible or otherwise injurious substances into the stomach, or into other orifices or cavities of the body, or from foreign bodies penetrating. the skin, etc. – that no disease, in a word, is caused by any material substance, but that every one is only and always a peculiar, virtual, dynamic derangement of the health; how injudicious, in that case, must not a method of treatment directed towards the expulsion14 of that imaginary material substance appear to every rational man, since no good, but only monstrous harm, can result from its employment in the principal diseases of mankind, namely, those of a chronic character!

14. There is a semblance of necessity in the expulsion by purgatives of worms, in so-called vermicular diseases. But even this semblance is false. A few lumbric; may be found in some children; in many there exist ascarides. But the presence of these is always dependent on a general taint of the constitution (the psoric), joined to an unhealthy mode of living. Let the latter be improved, and the former cured homoeopathically, which is most easily effected at this age, and none of the worms remain, and children cured in this manner are never troubled with them more; whereas after mere purgatives, even when combined with cina seeds, they soon reappear in quantities.

"But the tapeworm", methinks I hear some one exclaim, "every effort should be made to expel that monster, which was created for the torment of mankind".

Yes, sometimes it is expelled; but at the cost ot what after-sufferings, and with what danger to life! I should not like to have on my conscience the deaths of so many hundreds of human beings as have fallen sacrifices to the horribly violent purgatives, directed against the tapeworm, or the many years of indisposition of those who have escaped being purged to death. And how often does it happen that after all this health-and-life-destroying purgative treatment, frequently continued for several years, the animal is not expelled, or if so, that it is again produced!

What if there is not the slightest necessity for all these violent, cruel, and dangerous efforts to expel and kill the wormThe various species of tapeworm are only found along with the psoric taint, and always disappear when that is cured. But even before the cure is accomplished, they live – the patient enjoying tolerable health the while – not exactly in the intestines, but in the residue of the food, the excrement of the bowels, as in their proper element, quite quietly, and without causing the least disturbance, and find in the excrement what suffices for their nourishment; they then do not touch the walls of the intestine, and are perfectly harmless. But if the patient happens to be affected with an acute disease of any kind, then the contents of the bowels become intolerable to the animal; it twists about, comes in contact with, and irritates the sensitive walls of the intestines, causing a peculiar kind of spasmodic colic, which increases materially the sufferings of the patient. (So also the foetus in the womb becomes restless, turns about and kicks, only when the mother is ill; but when she is well; it swims quiet in its proper fluid without causing her any suffering.)

It is worthy of remark, that the morbid symptoms of patients suffering from tapeworm are generally of such a kind, that they are rapidly relieved (homoeopathically) by the smallest dose of tincture of male-fern root;[3] so that the ill-health of the patient, which causes this parasitic animal to be restless, is thereby for the time removed; the tapeworm then feels at ease, and lives on quietly in the excrement of the bowels, without particularly distressing the patient or his intestines, until the antipsoric treatment is so far advanced that the worm, after the eradication of the psora, finds the contents of the bowels no longer suitable for its support, and therefore spontaneously disappears, for ever from the now cured patient, without the least purgative medicine.

In short, the degenerated substances and impurities that appear in diseases are, undeniably, nothing more than products of the disease of the abnormally deranged organism, which are expelled by the latter, often violently enough – often much too violently – without requiring the aid of the evacuating art, and fresh products are always developed as long as it labors under that disease. These matters the true physician regards as actual symptoms of the disease, and they aid him to discover the nature of the disease, and to form an accurate portrait of it, so as to enable him to cure it with a similar medicinal morbific agent.

But the more modern adherents of the old school do not wish it to be supposed, that in their treatment they aim at the expulsion of material morbific substances. They allege that their multifarious evacuant processes are a mode of treatment by derivation, wherein they follow the example of nature which, in her efforts to assist the diseased organism, resolves fever by perspiration and diuresis pleurisy by epistaxis, sweat and mucous expectoration – other diseases by vomiting, diarrhaea and bleeding from the anus, articular pains by suppurating ulcers on the legs, cynanche tonsillaris by salivation, etc., or removes them by metastases and abscesses which she develops in parts at a distance from the seat of the disease.

Hence they thought the best thing to do was to imitate nature, by also going to work in the treatment of most diseases in a circuitous manner like the diseased vital force when left to itself and thus in an indirect manner,15 by means of stronger heterogeneous irritants applied to organs remote from the seat of disease, and totally dissimilar to the affected tissues, they produce evacuations, and generally kept them up, in order to draw, as it were, the disease thither.

15. In place of extinguishing the disease rapidly, without exhaustion of the strength and without going about the bush, with homogeneous, dynamic medicinal agents acting directly on the diseased points of the organism, as homoeopathy does.

This derivation, as it is called, was and continues to be one of the principal modes of treatment of the old school of medicine.

In this imitation of the self-aiding operation of nature, as some call it, they endeavored to excite, by force, new symptoms in the tissues that are least diseased and best able to bear the medicinal disease, which should draw away16 the primary disease under the semblance of crises and under the form of excretions, in order to admit of a gradual lysis by the curative powers of nature.17

16. Just as if anything immaterial could be drawn away! So that here too was the notion of a substance and a morbific matter, excessively subtile though it might be supposed to be!

17. It is only the slighter and acute diseases that tend, when the natural period of their course has expired, to terminate quietly in resolution, as it is called, with or without the employment of not very aggressive allopathic remedies; the vital force, having regained its powers, then gradually substitutes the normal condition for the derangement of the health that has now ceased to exist. But in severe acute and in chronic diseases which constitute by far the greater portion of all human ailments, crude nature and the old school are equally powerless; in these, neither the vital force, with its self-aiding faculty, nor allopathy in imitation of it, can affect a lysis, but at the most a mere temporary truce, during which the enemy fortifies himself, in order, sooner or later, to recommence the attack with still greater violence.

This they accomplished by means of diaphoretic and diuretic remedies, blood-lettings, setons and issues, but chiefly by irritant drugs to cause evacuation of the alimentary canal, sometimes upwards by means of emetics, sometimes (and this was the favorite plan) downwards by means of purgatives, which were termed aperient and dissolvent18 remedies.

18. An expression which likewise betrays that they imagined and presupposed a morbific substance, which had to be dissolved and expelled.

To assist this derivative method they employed the allied treatment by counter-irritants; woolen garments to the bare skin, foot-baths, nauseants, inflicting on the stomach and bowels the pangs of hunger (the hunger-treatment), substances to cause pain, inflammation, and suppuration in near or distant parts as the application of horseradish, mustard plasters, cantharides, blisters, mezereum setons, issues, tartar-emetic ointment, moxa, actual cautery, acupuncture, etc.; here also following the example of crude unassisted nature, which endeavors to free herself from the dynamic disease (in the case of a chronic disease, unavailingly) by exciting pain in distant parts of the body, by metastases and abscesses, by eruptions and suppurating ulcers.

It was evidently no rational principle, but merely imitation, with the view of making practice easy that seduced the old school into those unhelpful and injurious indirect modes of treatment, the derivative as well as the counter-irritant; that led them to this inefficacious, debilitating and hurtful practice of apparently ameliorating diseases for a short time, or removing them in such a manner that another and a worse disease was roused up to occupy the place of the first. Such a destructive plan cannot certainly be termed curing.

They merely followed the example of crude instinctive nature in her efforts, which are barely19 successful even in the slighter cases of acute disease; they merely imitated the unreasoning life-preserving power when left to itself in diseases, which entirely dependent as it is upon the organic laws of the body, is only capable of acting in conformity with these laws and is not guided by reason and reflection – they copied nature, which cannot, like an intelligent surgeon, bring together the gaping lips of a wound and by their union effect a cure; which knows not how to straighten and adjust the broken ends of a bone lying far apart and exuding much (often an excess of) new osseous matter; which cannot put a ligature on a wounded artery, but in its energy causes the patient to bleed to death; which does not understand how to replace a dislocated shoulder, but by the swelling it occasions round about it soon presents an obstacle to reduction; which in order to remove a foreign body from the cornea, destroys the whole eye by suppuration; which, with all its efforts can only liberate a strangulated hernia by gangrene of the bowel and death; and which, by the metaschematisms it produces in dynamic diseases, often renders them much worse than they were originally. But more, this irrational vital force receives into our body without hesitation, the greatest plagues of our terrestrial existence, the spark that kindles the countless diseases beneath which tortured mankind has groaned for hundreds and thousands of year, the chronic miasms – psora, syphilis, sycosis – not one of which can it diminish in the slightest degree far less expel single-handed from the organism; on the contrary, it allows them to rankle therein until often after a long life of misery, death at last closes the eyes of the sufferer.

19.. In the ordinary school of medicine, the efforts made by nature for the relief of the organism in diseases where no medicine was given, were regarded as models of treatment worthy of imitation. But this was a great error. The pitiable and highly imperfect efforts of the vital force to relieve itself in acute diseases is a spectacle that should excite our compassion, and command the aid of all the powers of our rational mind, to terminate the self-inflictedtorture by a real cure. If nature is unable to cure homoeopathically a disease already existing in the organism, by the production of another fresh malady similar to it (□ 43-46), which very rarely lies in her power (□ 50), and if to the organism alone is left the task of overcoming, by its own forces without external aid, a disease newly contracted (in cases of chronic miasms its power of resistance is quite inefficacious), we then witness nought but painful, often dangerous, efforts of nature to save the individual at whatever cost, which often terminate in extinction of the earthly existence, in death.

Little as we mortals know of the operations that take place in the interior economy in health – which must be hidden from us as certainly as they are patent to the eye of the all-seeing Creator and Preserver of his creatures – just as little can we perceive the operations that go on in the interior in disturbed conditions of life, in diseases. The internal operations in diseases are manifested only by the visible changes, the sufferings and the symptoms, whereby alone our life betrays the inward disturbance; so that in no given case can we ascertain which of the morbid symptoms are caused by the primary action of the morbific agent, which by the reaction of the vital force for its own relief. Both are inextricably mixed up together before our eyes, and only present to us an outwardly reflected picture of the entire internal malady, for the fruitless efforts of unassisted vitality to terminate the sufferings are themselves sufferings of the whole organism. Hence, even in those evacuations termed crises, which nature generally produces at the termination of diseases which run a rapid course, there is frequently more of suffering than of efficacious relief.

What the vital force does in these so-called crises, and how it does it, remains a mystery to us, like all the internal operations of the organic vital economy. One thing, however, is certain: that in all these efforts more or less of the affected parts are sacrificed and destroyed in order to save the rest. These self-aiding operations of the vital force for the removal of an acute disease, performed only in obedience to the laws of organic life and not guided by the reflection of an intellect, are mostly but a species of allopathy; in order to relieve the primarily affected organ by a crisis, an increased, often violent, activity is excited in the excretory organs, to draw away the disease from the former to the latter; there ensue vomitings, purgings, diuresis, diaphoresis, abscesses, etc., in order, by this irritation of distant parts, to effect a sort of derivation from the primarily diseased part, and the dynamically affected nervous power seems to unload itself in the material product.

It is only by the destruction and sacrifice of a portion of the organism itself that unaided nature can save the patient in acute diseases, and, if death do not ensue, restore, though only slowly and imperfectly, the harmony of life – health.

The great weakness of the parts which had been exposed to the disease, and even of the whole body, the emaciation, etc., remaining after spontaneous cures, are convincing proofs of this.

In short, the whole operation of the self-aiding power of the organism when attacked by diseases displays to the observer nothing but suffering – nothing that he could or ought to imitate if he wishes to cure disease in a truly artistic manner.

In such an important affair as that of healing, which demands so much intelligence, reflection and judgment, how could the old school, which arrogates to itself the title of rational, choose as its best instructor, as its guide to be blindly followed, the unintelligent vital force, inconsiderately copy its indirect and revolutionary operations in diseases, imagining these to be the non plus ultra, the best conceivable, when that greatest gift of God, reflective reason and unfettered judgment, was given us to enable us infinitely to surpass it in salutary help to suffering humanity?

When the old school practitioners, thoughtlessly imitating the crude, senseless, automatic vital energy with their counter-irritant and derivative methods of treatment – by far their most usual plans – attack innocent parts and organs of the body, either inflicting on them excruciating pains, or as is most frequently done, compelling them to perform evacuations whereby strength and fluids are wasted, their object is to direct the morbid vital action in the primarily affected parts away to those artificially attacked, and thus to effect the cure of the natural disease indirectly, by the production of a disease much greater in intensity and of quite a different kind, in the healthy parts of the body, consequently by a circuitous way, at the cost of much loss of strength, and usually of great suffering to the patient.20

20. Daily experience shows the sad effects of this manoeuvre in chronic diseases. Anything but a cure is effected. Who would ever call that a victory if, in place of attacking the enemy in front in a hand-to-hand fight, and by his destruction terminating at once his hostile assaults, we should, in a cowardly manner and behind his back, lay an embargo on everything, cut off his supplies, burn down everything for a great way round him? By so doing we would at length deprive him of all courage to resist, but our object is not gained, the enemy is far from being destroyed, – he is still there, and when he can again procure provisions and supplies, he once more rears his head, more exasperated than before – the enemy, I repeat, is far from being destroyed, but the poor innocent country is so completely ruined that it will be long before it can recover itself. In like manner acts allopathy in chronic diseases, when, by its indirect attacks on innocent parts at a distance from the seat of the disease, instead of effecting a cure, it destroys the organism. Such is the result of its hurtful operations!

The disease, if it be acute, and consequently naturally of but short duration, may certainly disappear, even during these heterogeneous attacks on distant and dissimilar parts – but it is not cured. There is nothing that can merit the honorable name of cure in this revolutionary treatment, which has no direct, immediate, pathological relation to the tissues primarily affected. Often indeed, without these serious attacks on the rest of the organism, would the acute disease have ceased of itself, sooner most likely, with fewer subsequent sufferings and less sacrifice of strength. But neither the mode of operation of the crude natural forces, nor the allopathic copy of that, can for a moment be compared to the dynamic (homoeopathic) treatment, which sustains the strength, while it extinguishes the disease in a direct and rapid manner.

In far the greatest number of cases of disease, however – I mean those of a chronic nature – these perturbing, debilitating, indirect modes of treatment of the old school are scarcely ever of the slightest use. They suspend for a few days only, some troublesome symptom or other, which, however, returns when the system has become accustomed to the distant irritation, and the disease recurs worse than before, because by the antagonistic pains21 and the injudicious evacuations the vital powers have been depressed.

21. What good results have ever ensued from those foetid artificial ulcers, so much in vogue, called issues? If even during the first week or two, whilst they still cause pain, they appear somewhat to check by antagonism a chronic disease, yer by and by, when the body has become accustomed to the pain, they have no other effect than that of weakening the patient and giving still greater scope to the chronic affection. Or does anyone imagine, in this nineteenth century, that they serve as an outlet for the escape of the materia peccans? It almost appears as if this were the case!

Whilst most physicians of the old school, imitating in a general manner the efforts of crude, unaided nature for its own relief, carried out in their practice these derivations of merely hypothetical utility, just as they judged expedient (guided by some imaginary indication), others, aiming at a higher object, undertook designedly to promote the efforts of the vital force to aid itself by evacuations and antagonistic metatases, as seen in diseases, and by way of lending it a helping hand, to increase still more these derivations and evacuations; and they believed that by this hurtful procedure they were acting duce natura, and might justly claim the title of minister naturae.

As the evacuations effected by the natural powers of the patient in chronic diseases are not infrequently the precursors of alleviations – though only of a temporary character – of troublesome symptoms, violent pains, paralyses, spasms, etc., so the old school imagined these derivations to be the true way of curing diseases, and endeavored to promote, maintain and even increase such evacuations. But they did not perceive that all these evacuations and excretions (pseudo-crises) produced by nature when left to herself were, in chronic diseases, only palliative, transient alleviations which, far from contributing to a real cure, on the contrary, rather aggravate the original, internal dyscrasia, by the waste of strength and juices they occasioned. No one ever saw a chronic patient recover his health permanently by such efforts of crude nature, nor any chronic disease cured by such evacuations effected by the organism.22 On the contrary, in such cases the original dyscrasia is always perceptibly aggravated, after alleviations, whose duration always becomes shorter and shorter; the bad attacks recur more frequently and more severely in spite of the continuation of the evacuations. In like manner, on the occurrence of symptoms excited by an internal chronic affection that threaten to destroy life, when nature left to its own resources, cannot help herself in any other way than by the production of external local symptoms, in order to avert the danger from parts indispensable to life and direct it to tissues of less vital importance (metastasis), these operations of the energetic but unintelligent, unreasoding and improvident vital force conduce to anything but genuine relief or recovery; they only silence in a palliative manner, for a short time, the dangerous internal affection at the cost of a large portion of the humours and of the strength, without diminishing the original disease by a hair's breadth; they can, at the most, only retard the fatal termination which is inevitable without true homoeopathic treatment.

22. Equally inefficacious are those produced artificially.

The allopathy of the old school not only greatly overrated these efforts of the crude automatic power of nature, but completely misjudged them, falsely considered them to be truly curative, and endeavored to increase and promote them, vainly imagining that thereby they might perhaps succeed in annihilating and radically curing the whole disease. When, in chronic diseases, the vital force seemed to silence this or that troublesome symptom of the internal affection by the production, for example, of some humid cutaneous eruption, then the servant of the crude power of nature (minister naturae) applied to the discharging surface a cantharides plaster or an exutory (mezereum), in order, duce natura, to draw still more moisture from the skin, and thus to promote and to assist natures object – the cure (by the removal of the morbific matter from the body?); but when the effect of the remedy was too violent, the eczema already of long standing, and the system too irritable, he increased the external affection to a great degree without the slightest advantage, to the origirial disease, and aggravated the pains, which deprived the patient of sleep and depressed his strength (and sometimes even developed a malignant febrile erysipelas); or if the effect upon the local affection (still recent, perhaps) was of milder character, he thereby repelled from its seat, by a species of ill-applied external homoeopathy, the local symptom which had been established by nature on the skin for the relief of the internal disease, thus renewing the more dangerous internal malady, and by this repulsion of the local symptom compelling the vital force to effect a transference of a worse form of morbid action to other and more important parts, the patient became affected with dangerous ophthalmia, or deafness, or spasms of the stomach, or epileptic convulsions, or attacks of asthma or apoplexy, or mental derangement, etc., in place of the repelled local disease.23

23. Natural effects of the repulsion of these local symptoms – effects that are often regarded by the allopathic physiclan as fresh diseases of quite a different kind.

When the diseased natural force propelled blood into the veins of the rectum or anus (blind h¾morrhoids), the minister natura, under the same delusive idea of assisting the vital force in its curative efforts, applied leeches, often in large numbers, in order to give an outlet to the blood there – with but brief, often scarcely noteworthy, relief, but thereby weakening the body and occasioning still greater congestions in those parts, without the slightest diminution of the original disease.

In almost all cases in which the diseased vital force endeavored to subdue the violence of a dangerous internal malady by evacuating blood by means of vomiting, coughing, etc., the old school physician, duce natura, made haste to assist these supposed salutary efforts of nature, and performed a copious venesection, which was invariably productive of injurious consequences and palpable weakening of the body. In cases of frequently occurring chronic nausea, he produced, with the view of furthering the intentions of nature, copious evacuations of the stomach, by means of powerful emetics – never with a good result, often with bad, not infrequently danger-ous and even fatal consequences.

The vital force, in order to relieve the internal malady, sometimes produces indolent enlarge-ments of the external glands, and he thinks to forward the intentions of nature, in his assumed character of her servant, when, by the use of all sorts of heating embrocations and plasters, he causes them to inflame, so that, when the abscess is ripe, he may incise it and let out the bad morbific matter (?)

Experience has shown, hundreds of times, that lasting evil almost invariably results from such a plan.

And having often noticed slight amelioration of the severe symptoms of chronic diseases to result from spontaneous night sweats or frequent liquid stools, he imagines himself bound to obey these hints of nature (duce natura), and to promote them, by instituting and maintaining a complete course of sweating treatment or by the employment of so-called gentle laxatives for years, in order to promote and increase these efforts of nature (of the vital force of the unintelligent organism), which he thinks tend to the cure of the whole chronic affection, and thus to free the patient more speedily and certainly from his disease (the matter of his disease?).

But he thereby always produces quite the contrary result: aggravation of the original disease.

In conformity with this preconseived by unfounded idea, the old school physician goes on thus promoting24 the efforts of the diseased and and increasing those derivations and evacu-ations in the patient which never lead to the desired end, but are always disastrous, without being aware that all the local affections, evacuations, and seemingly derivative efforts, set up and continued by the unintelligent vital force when left to its own resources, for the relief of the original chronic disease, are actually the disease itself, the phenomena of the whole disease, for the totality of which, properly speaking, the only efficacious remedy, and the one, moreover, that will act in the most direct manner, is a homoeopathic medicine, chosen on account of its similarity of action.

24. In direct opposition to this treatment, the old school not infrequently indulged themselves in the very reverse of this: thus when the efforts of the vital force for the relief of the internal disease by evacuations and the production of local symptoms on the exterior of the body became troublesome, they capriciously suppressed them by their repercutients and repellents, they subdued chronic pains, sleeplessness and diarrhoea of long standing by doses of opium pushed to a dangerous extent; vomitings by effervescent saline draughts; foetid perspiration of the feet by cold footbaths and astringent applications; eruptions on the skin by preparations of lead and zinc; they checked uterine haemorrhage by injections of vinegar; colliquative perspiration by alum; nocturnal seminal emissions by the free use of camphor; frequent attacks of flushes of heat in the body and face by nitre vegetable acids and sulphuric acid; bleeding of the nose by plugging the nostrils with dossils of lint soaked in alcohol or astringent fluids; they dried up discharging ulcers on the legs, established by the vital power for the relief of great internal suffering with the oxides of lead and zinc, etc

APHORISMS 1 - 100.

1

The physician's high and only mission is to restore the sick to health, to cure, as it is termed.[4]

2

The highest ideal of cure is rapid, gentle and permanent restoration of the health, or removal and annihilation of the disease in its whole extent, in the shortest, most reliable, and most harmless way, on easily comprehensible principles.

3

If the physician clearly perceives what is to be cured in diseases, that is to say, in every individual case of disease (knowledge of disease, indication), if he clearly perceives what is curative in medicines, that is to say, in each individual medicine (knowledge of medical powers), and if he knows how to adapt, according to clearly defined principles, what is curative in medicines to what he has discovered to be undoubtedly morbid in the patient, so that the recovery must ensue – to adapt it, as well in respect to the suitability of the medicine most appropriate according to its mode of action to the case before him (choice of the remedy, the medicine indicated), as also in respect to the exact mode of preparation and quantity of it required (proper dose), and the proper period for repeating the dose; – if, finally, he knows the obstacles to recovery in each case and is aware how to remove them, so that the restoration may be permanent, then he understands how to treat judiciously and rationally, and he is a true practitioner of the healing art .

4

He is likewise a preserver of health if he knows the things that derange health and cause disease, and how to remove them from persons in health.

5

Useful to the physician in assisting him to cure are the particulars of the most probable exciting cause of the acute disease, as also the most significant points in the whole history of the chronic disease, to enable him to discover its fundamental cause, which is generally due to a chronic miasm. In these investigations, the ascertainable physical constitution of the patient (especially when the disease is chronic), his moral and intellectual character, his occupation, mode of living and habits, his social and domestic relations, his age, sexual function, etc., are to be taken into consideration.

6

The unprejudiced observer – well aware of the futility of transcendental speculations which can receive no confirmation from experience – be his powers of penetration ever so great, takes note of nothing in every individual disease, except the changes in the health of the body and of the mind (morbid phenomena, accidents, symptoms) which can be perceived externally by means of the senses; that is to say, he notices only the deviations from the former healthy state of the now diseased individual, which are felt by the patient himself, remarked by those around him and observed by the physician. All these perceptible signs represent the disease in its whole extent, that is, together they form the true and only conceivable portrait of the disease.[5]

Is not, then, that which is cognizable by the senses in diseases through the phenomena it displays, the disease itself in the eyes of the physician, since he never can see the spiritual being that produces the disease, the vital force? nor is it necessary that he should see it, but only that he should ascertain its morbid actions, in order that he may thereby be enabled to cure the disease. What else will the old school search for in the hidden interior of the organism, as a prima causa morbi, whilst they reject as an object of cure and contemptuously despise the sensible and manifest representation of the disease, the symptoms, that so plainly address themselves to us? What else do they wish to cure in disease but these?

7

Now, as in a disease, from which no manifest exciting or maintaining cause (causa occasionalis) has to be removed[6], we can perceive nothing but the morbid symptoms, it must (regard being had to the possibility of a miasm, and attention paid to the accessory circumstances, 5) be the symptoms alone by which the disease demands and points to the remedy suited to relieve it – and, moreover, the totality of these its symptoms, of this outwardly reflected picture of the internal essence of the disease, that is, of the affection of the vital force, must be the principal, or the sole means, whereby the disease can make known what remedy it requires – the only thing that can determine the choice of the most appropriate remedy – and thus, in a word, the totality[7] of the symptoms must be the principal, indeed the only thing the physician has to take note of in every case of disease and to remove by means of his art, in order that it shall be cured and transformed into health.

8

It is not conceivable, not can it be proved by any experience in the world, that, after removal of all the symptoms of the disease and of the entire collection of the perceptible phenomena, there should or could remain anything else besides health, or that the morbid alteration in the interior could remain uneradicated.[8]

9

In the healthy condition of man, the spiritual vital force (autocracy), the dynamis that animates the material body (organism), rules with unbounded sway, and retains all the parts of the organism in admirable, harmonious, vital operation, as regards both sensations and functions, so that our indwelling, reason-gifted mind can freely employ this living, healthy instrument for the higher purpose of our existence.

10

The material organism, without the vital force, is capable of no sensation, no function, no self-preservation[9], it derives all sensation and performs all the functions of life solely by means of the immaterial being (the vital principle) which animates the material organism in health and in disease.

11

When a person falls ill, it is only this spiritual, self acting (automatic) vital force, everywhere present in his organism, that is primarily deranged by the dynamic[10] influence upon it of a morbific agent inimical to life; it is only the vital force, deranged to such an abnormal state, that can furnish the organism with its disagreeable sensations, and incline it to the irregular processes which we call disease; for, as a power invisible in itself, and only cognizable by its effects on the organism, its morbid derangement only makes itself known by the manifestation of disease in the sensations and functions of those parts of the organism exposed to the senses of the observer and physician, that is, by morbid symptoms, and in no other way can it make itself known.[11]

For instance, the dynamic effect of the sick-making influences upon healthy man, as well as the dynamic energy of the medicines upon the principle of life in the restoration of health is nothing else than infection and so not in any way material, not in any way mechanical. Just as the energy of a magnet attracting a piece of iron or steel is not material, not mechanical. One sees that the piece of iron is attracted by one pole of the magnet, but how it is done is not seen. This invisible energy of the magnet does not require mechanical (material) auxiliary means, hook or lever, to attract the iron. The magnet draws to itself and this acts upon the piece of iron or upon a steel needle by means of a purely immaterial invisible, conceptual, inherent energy, that is, dynamically, and communicates to the steel needle the magnetic energy equally invisibly (dynamically). The steel needle becomes itself magnetic, even at a distance when the magnet does not touch it, and magnetises other steel needles with the same magnetic property (dynamically) with which it had been endowered previously by the magnetic rod, just as a child with small-pox or measles communicates to a near, untouched healthy child in an invisible manner (dynamically) the small-pox or measles, that is, infects it at a distance without anything material from the infective child going or capable of going to the one to be infected. A purely specific conceptual influence communicated to the near child small-pox or measles in the same way as the magnet communicated to the near needle the magnetic property.

In a similar way, the effect of medicines upon living man is to be judged. Substances, which are used as medicines, are medicines only in so far as they possess each its own specific energy to alter the well-being of man through dynamic, conceptual influence, by means of the living sensory fibre, upon the conceptual controlling principle of life. The medicinal property of those material substances which we call medicines proper, relates only to their energy to call out alterations in the well-being of animal life. Only upon this conceptual principle of life, depends their medicinal health-altering, conceptual (dynamic) influence. Just as the nearness of a magnetic pole can communicate only magnetic energy to the steel (namely, by a kind of infection) but cannot communicate other properties (for instance, more hardness or ductility, etc.). And thus every special medicinal substance alters through a kind of infection, that well-being of man in a peculiar manner exclusively its own and not in a manner peculiar to another medicine, as certainly as the nearness of the child ill with small-pox will communicate to a healthy child only small-pox and not measles. These medicines act upon our well-being wholly without communication of material parts of the medicinal substances, thus dynamically, as if through infection. Far more healing energy is expressed in a case in point by the smallest dose of the best dynamized medicines, in which there can be, according to calculation, only so little of material substance that its minuteness cannot be thought and conceived by the best arithmetical mind, than by large doses of the same medicine in substance. That smallest dose can therefore contain almost entirely only the pure, freely-developed, conceptual medicinal energy, and bring about only dynamically such great effects as can never be reached by the crude medicinal substances itself taken in large doses.

It is not in the corporal atoms of these highly dynamized medicines, nor their physical or mathematical surfaces (with which the higher energies of the dynamized medicines are being interpreted but vainly as still sufficiently material) that the medicinal energy is found. More likely, there lies invisible in the moistened globule or in its solution, an unveiled, liberated, specific, medicinal force contained in the medicinal substance which acts dynamically by contact with the living animal fibre upon the whole organism (without communicating to it anything material however highly attenuated) and acts more strongly the more free and more immaterial the energy has become through the dynamization.

Is it then so utterly impossible for our age celebrated for its wealth in clear thinkers to think of dynamic energy as something non-corporeal, since we see daily phenomena which cannot be explained in any other manner? If one looks upon something nauseous and becomes inclined to vomit, did a material emetic come into his stomach which compels him to this anti-peristaltic movement? Was it not solely the dynamic effect of the nauseating aspect upon his imagination? And if one raises his arm, does it occur through a material visible instrument? a lever? Is it not solely the conceptual dynamic energy of his will which raises it?

12

It is the morbidly affected vital energy alone that produces disease[12], so that the morbid phenomena perceptible to our senses express at the same time all the internal change, that is to say, the whole morbid derangement of the internal dynamis; in a word, they reveal the whole disease; consequently, also, the disappearance under treatment of all the morbid phenomena and of all the morbid alterations that differ from the healthy vital operations, certainly affects and necessarily implies the restoration of the integrity of the vital force and, therefore, the recovered health of the whole organism.

13

Therefore disease (that does not come within the province of manual surgery) considered, as it is by the allopathists, as a thing separate from the living whole, from the organism and its animating vital force, and hidden in the interior, be it ever so subtle a character, is an absurdity, that could only be imagined by minds of a materialistic stamp, and has for thousands of years given to the prevailing system of medicine all those pernicious impulses that have made it a truly mischievous (non-healing) art.

14

There is, in the interior of man, nothing morbid that is curable and no invisible morbid alteration that is curable which does not make itself known to the accurately observing physicians by means of morbid signs and symptoms – an arrangement in perfect conformity with the infinite goodness of the all-wise Preserver of human life.

15

The affection of the morbidly deranged, spirit-like dynamis (vital force) that animates our body in the invisible interior, and the totality of the outwardly cognizable symptoms produced by it in the organism and representing the existing malady, constitute a whole; they are one and the same. The organism is indeed the material instrument of the life, but it is not conceivable without the animation imparted to it by the instinctively perceiving and regulating dynamis, just as the vital force is not conceivable without the organism, consequently the two together constitute a unity, although in thought our mind separates this unity into two distinct conceptions for the sake of easy comprehension.

16

Our vital force, as a spirit-like dynamis, cannot be attacked and affected by injurious influences on the healthy organism caused by the external inimical forces that disturb the harmonious play of life, otherwise than in a spirit-like (dynamic) way, and in like manner, all such morbid derangements (diseases) cannot be removed from it by the physician in any other way than by the spirit-like (dynamic[13], virtual) alterative powers of the serviceable medicines acting upon our spirit-like vital force, which perceives them through the medium of the sentient faculty of the nerves everywhere present in the organism, so that it is only by their dynamic action on the vital force that remedies are able to re-establish and do actually re-establish health and vital harmony, after the changes in the health of the patient cognizable by our senses (the totality of the symptoms) have revealed the disease to the carefully observing and investigating physician as fully as was requisite in order to enable him to cure it.

17

Now, as in the cure effected by the removal of the whole of the perceptible signs and symptoms of the disease the internal alteration of the vital principle to which the disease is due – consequently the whole of the disease – is at the same time removed,[14] it follows that the physician has only to remove the whole of the symptoms in order, at the same time, to abrogate and annihilate the internal change, that is to say, the morbid derangement of the vital force – consequently the totality of the disease, the disease itself.[15] But when the disease is annihilated the health is restored, and this is the highest, the sole aim of the physician who knows the true object of his mission, which consists not in learned – sounding prating, but in giving aid to the sick.

18

From this indubitable truth, that besides the totality of the symptoms with consideration of the accompanying modalities (5) nothing can by any means be discovered in disease wherewith they could express their need of aid, it follows undeniably that the sum of all the symptoms and conditions in each individual case of disease must be the sole indication, the sole guide to direct us in the choice of a remedy.

19

Now, as diseases are nothing more than alterations in the state of health of the healthy individual which express themselves by morbid signs, and the cure is also only possible by a change to the healthy condition of the state of health of the diseased individual, it is very evident that medicines could never cure disease if they did not possess the power of altering man's state of health which depends on sensations and functions; indeed, that their curative power must be owing solely to this power they possess of altering man's state of health.

20

This spirit-like power to alter man's state of health (and hence to cure diseases) which lies hidden in the inner nature of medicines can in itself never be discovered by us by a mere effort of reason; it is only by experience of the phenomena it displays when acting on the state of health of man that we can become clearly cognizant of it.

21

Now, as it is undeniable that the curative principle in medicines is not in itself perceptible, and as in pure experiments with medicines conducted by the most accurate observers, nothing can be observed that can constitute them medicines or remedies except that power of causing distinct alterations in the state of health of the human body, and particularly in that of the healthy individual, and of exciting in him various definite morbid symptoms; so it follows that when medicines act as remedies, they can only bring their curative property into play by means of this their power of altering man's state of health by the production of peculiar symptoms; and that, therefore, we have only to rely on the morbid phenomena which the medicines produce in the healthy body as the sole possible revelation of their in-dwelling curative power, in order to learn what disease-producing power, and at the same time what disease-curing power, each individual medicine possesses.

22

But as nothing is to be observed in diseases that must be removed in order to change them into health besides the totality of their signs and symptoms, and likewise medicines can show nothing curative besides their tendency to produce morbid symptoms in healthy persons and to remove them in diseased persons; it follows, on the one hand, that medicines only become remedies and capable of annihilating disease, because the medicinal substance, by exciting certain effects and symptoms, that is to say, by producing a certain artificial morbid state, removes and abrogates the symptoms already present, to wit, the natural morbid state we wish to cure. On the other hand, it follows that, for the totality of the symptoms of the disease to be cured, a medicine must be sought which (according as experience shall prove whether the morbid symptoms are most readily, certainly, and permanently removed and changed into health by similar or opposite medicinal symptoms[16]) have the greatest tendency to produce similar or opposite symptoms.

For the purpose of cure, the morbidly depressed vital energy possesses so little ability worthy of imitation since all changes and symptoms produced by it in the organism are the disease itself. What intelligent physician would want to imitate it with the intention to heal if he did not thereby sacrifice his patient?

23

All pure experience, however, and all accurate research convince us that persistent symptoms of disease are far from being removed and annihilated by opposite symptoms of medicines (as in the antipathic, enantiopathic or palliative method), that, on the contrary, after transient, apparent alleviation, they break forth again, only with increased intensity, and become manifestly aggravated (see 58 – 62 and 69).

24

There remains, therefore, no other mode of employing medicines in diseases that promises to be of service besides the homoeopathic, by means of which we seek, for the totality of the symptoms of the case of disease, a medicine which among all medicines (whose pathogenetic effects are known from having been tested in healthy individuals) has the power and the tendency to produce an artificial morbid state most similar to that of the case of disease in question.

25

Now, however, in all careful trials, pure experience,[17] the sole and infallible oracle of the healing art, teaches us that actually that medicine which, in its action on the healthy human body, has demonstrated its power of producing the greatest number of symptoms similar to those observable in the case of disease under treatment, does also, in doses of suitable potency and attenuation, rapidly, radically and permanently remove the totality of the symptoms of this morbid state, that is to say (6 – 16), the whole disease present, and change it into health; and that all medicines cure, without exception, those diseases whose symptoms most nearly resemble their own, and leave none of them uncured.

26

This depends on the following homoeopathic law of nature which was sometimes, indeed, vaguely surmised but not hitherto fully recognized, and to which is due every real cure that has ever taken place:
A weaker dynamic affection is permanently extinguished in the living organism by a stronger one, if the latter (whilst differing in kind) is very similar to the former in its manifestations.[18]

27

The curative power of medicines, therefore, depends on their symptoms, similar to the disease but superior to it in strength (12 – 26), so that each individual case of disease is most surely, radically, rapidly and permanently annihilated and removed only by a medicine capable of producing (in the human system) in the most similar and complete manner the totality of its symptoms, which at the same time are stronger than the disease.

28

As this natural law of cure manifests itself in every pure experiment and every true observation in the world, the fact is consequently established; it matters little what may be scientific explanation of how it takes place; and I do not attach much importance to the attempts made to explain it. But the following view seems to commend itself as the most probable one, as it is founded on premises derived from experience.

29

As every disease (not entirely surgical) consists only in a special, morbid, dynamic alteration of our vital energy (of the principle of life) manifested in sensation and motion, so in every homoeopathic cure this principle of life dynamically altered by natural disease is seized through the administration of medicinal potency selected exactly according to symptom-similarity by a somewhat stronger, similar artificial disease-manifestation. By this the feeling of the natural (weaker) dynamic disease-manifestation ceases and disappears. This disease-manifestation no longer exists for the principle of life which is now occupied and governed merely by the stronger, artificial disease-manifestation. This artificial disease-manifestation has soon spent its force and leaves the patient free from disease, cured. The dynamis, thus freed, can now continue to carry life on in health. This most highly probable process rests upon the following propositions.

30

The human body appears to admit of being much more powerfully affected in its health by medicines (partly because we have the regulation of the dose in our own power) than by natural morbid stimuli – for natural diseases are cured and overcome by suitable medicines.[19]

31

The inimical forces, partly psychical, partly physical, to which our terrestrial existence is exposed, which are termed morbific noxious agents, do not possess the power of morbidly deranging the health of man unconditionally[20]; but we are made ill by them only when our organism is sufficiently disposed and susceptible to attack of the morbific cause that may be present, and to be altered in its health, deranged and made to undergo abnormal sensations and functions – hence they do not produce disease in every one nor at all times.

32

But it is quite otherwise with the artificial morbific agents which we term medicines. Every real medicine, namely, acts at all times, under all circumstances, on every living human being, and produces in him its peculiar symptoms (distinctly perceptible, if the dose be large enough), so that evidently every living human organism is liable to be affected, and, as it were, inoculated with the medicinal disease at all times, and absolutely (unconditionally), which, as before said, is by no means the case with the natural diseases.

33

In accordance with this fact, it is undeniably shown by all experience[21] that the living organism is much more disposed and has a greater liability to be acted on, and to have its health deranged by medicinal powers, than by morbific noxious agents and infectious miasms, or, in order words, that the morbific noxious agents possess a power of morbidly deranging man's health that is subordinate and conditional, often very conditional; whilst medicinal agents have an absolute unconditional power, greatly superior to the former.

34

The greater strength of the artificial diseases producible by medicines is, however, not the sole cause of their power to cure natural disease. In order that they may effect a cure, it is before all things requisite that they should be capable of producing in the human body an artificial disease as similar as possible to the disease to be cured, which, with somewhat increased power, transforms to a very similar morbid state the instinctive life principle, which in itself is incapable of any reflection or act of memory. It not only obscures, but extinguishes and thereby annihilates the derangement caused by the natural disease. This is so true, that no previously existing disease can be cured, even by Nature herself, by the accession of a new dissimilar disease, be it ever so strong, and just as little can it be cured by medical treatment with drugs which are incapable of producing a similar morbid condition in the healthy body.

35

In order to illustrate this, we shall consider in three different cases, as well what happens in nature when two dissimilar natural diseases meet to in one person, as also the result of the ordinary medical treatment of diseases with unsuitable allopathic drugs, which are incapable of producing an artificial morbid condition similar to the disease to be cured, whereby it will appear that even Nature herself is unable to remove a dissimilar disease already present by one that is unhomoeopathic, even though it be stronger, and just as little is the unhomoeopathic employment of even the strongest medicines ever capable of curing any disease whatsoever.

36

I. If the two dissimilar diseases meeting together in the human being be of equal strength, or still more if the older one be the stronger, the new disease will be repelled by the old one from the body and not allowed to affect it. A patient suffering from a severe chronic disease will not be infected by a moderate autumnal dysentery or other epidemic disease. The plague of the Levant, according to Larry,[22] does not break out where scurvy is prevalent, and persons suffering from eczema are not infected by it. Rachitis, Jenner alleges, prevents vaccination from taking effect. Those suffering from pulmonary consumption are not liable to be attacked by epidemic fevers of a not very violent character, according to Von Hildenbrand.

37

So, also under ordinary medical treatment, an old chronic disease remains uncured and unaltered if it is treated according to the common allopathic method, that is to say, with medicines that are incapable of producing in healthy individuals a state of health similar to the disease, even though the treatment should last for years and is not of too violent character.[23] This is daily witnessed in practice, it is therefore unnecessary to give any illustrative examples.

38

II. Or the new dissimilar disease is the stronger. In this case the disease under which the patient originally labored, being the weaker, will be kept back and suspended by the accession of the stronger one, until the latter shall have run its course or been cured, and then the old one reappears uncured. Two children affected with a kind of epilepsy remained free from epileptic attacks after infection with ringworm (tinea) but as soon as the eruption on the head was gone the epilepsy returned just as before, as Tulpius[24] observed. The itch, as Schopf[25] saw, disappeared on the occurrence of the scurvy, but after the cure of the latter it again broke out. So, also the pulmonary phthisis remained stationary when the patient was attacked by a violent typhus, but went on again after the latter had run its course.[26] If mania occur in a consumptive patient, the phthisis with all its symptoms is removed by the former; but if that go off, the phthisis returns immediately and proves fatal.[27] When measles and smallpox are prevalent at the same time, and both attack the same child, the measles that had already broken out is generally checked by the smallpox that came somewhat later; nor does the measles resume its course until after the cure of the smallpox; but it not infrequently happens that the inoculated smallpox is suspended for four days by the supervention of the measles, as observed by Manget,[28] after the desquamation of which the smallpox completes its course. Even when the inoculation of the smallpox had taken effect for six days, and the measles then broke out, the inflammation of the inoculation remained stationary and the smallpox did not ensue until the measles had completed its regular course of seven days.[29] In an epidemic of measles, that disease attacked many individuals on the fourth or fifth day after the inoculation of smallpox and prevented the development of the smallpox until it had completed its own course, whereupon the smallpox appeared and proceeded regularly to its termination.[30] The true, smooth, erysipelatous-looking scarlatina of Sydenham, with sore throat, was checked on the fourth day by the eruption of cow-pox, which ran its regular course, and not till it was ended did the scarlatina again establish itself; but on another occasion, as both diseases seem to be of equal strength, the cow-pox was suspended on the eighth day by the supervention of the true, smooth scarlatina of Sydenham,[31] and the red areola of the former disappeared until the scarlatina was gone, wherein the cow-pox immediately resumed its course, and went on its regular termination.[32] The measles suspended the cow-pox; on the eighth day, when the cow-pox had nearly attained its climax, the measles broke out; the cow-pox now remained stationary, and did not resume and complete its course until the desquamation of the measles, had taken place, so that on the sixteenth day it presented the appearance it otherwise would have shown on the tenth day, as Kortum[33] observed.

Even after the measles had broken out the cow-pox inoculation took effect, but did not run its course until these measles had disappeared, as Kortum likewise witnessed.[34]

I myself saw the mumps (angina parotidea) immediately disappear when the cow-pox inoculation had taken effect and had nearly attained its height; it was not until the complete termination of the cow-pox and the disappearance of its red areola that this febrile tumefaction of the parotid and submaxillary glands, that is caused by a peculiar miasm, reappeared and ran its regular course of seven days.

And thus it is with all dissimilar disease; the stronger suspends the weaker (when they do not complicate one another, which is seldom the case with acute disease), but they never cure one another.

39

Now the adherents of the ordinary school of medicine saw all this for so many centuries; they saw that Nature herself cannot cure any disease by the accession of another, be it ever so strong, if the new disease be dissimilar to that already present in the body. What shall we think of them, that they nevertheless went on treating chronic disease with allopathic remedies, namely, with medicines and prescriptions capable of producing God knows what morbid state – almost invariably, however, one dissimilar to the disease to be cured? And even though physicians did not hitherto observe nature attentively, the miserable results of their treatment should have taught them that they were pursuing an inappropriate, a false path. Did they not perceive when they employed, as was their custom, and aggressive allopathic treatment in a chronic disease, that thereby they only created an artificial disease dissimilar to the original one, which, as long as it was kept up, merely held in abeyance, merely suppressed, merely suspended the original disease, which latter, however, always returned, and must return, as soon as the diminished strength of the patient no longer admitted of a continuance of the allopathic attacks on the life? Thus the itch exanthema certainly disappears very soon from the skin under the employment of violent purgatives, frequently repeated; but when the patient can no longer stand the factitious (dissimilar) disease of the bowels, and can take no more purgatives, then either the cutaneous eruption breaks out as before, or the internal psora displays itself in some bad symptom, and the patient, in addition to his undiminished original disease, has to endure the misery of a painful ruined digestion and impaired strength to boot. So, also, when the ordinary physicians keep up artificial ulcerations of the skin and issues on the exterior of the body, with the view of thereby eradicating a chronic disease, they can NEVER cure them by that means, as such artificial cutaneous ulcers are quite alien and allopathic to the internal affection; but inasmuch as the irritation produced by several tissues is at least sometimes a stronger (dissimilar) disease than the indwelling malady, the latter is thereby sometimes silenced and suspended for a week or two. But it is only suspended, and that for a very short time, while the patient's powers are gradually worn out. Epilepsy, suppressed for many years by means of issues, invariably recurred, and in an aggravated form, when they were allowed to heal up, as Pechlin[35] and others testify. But purgatives for itch, and issues for epilepsy, cannot be more heterogeneous, more dissimilar deranging agents – cannot be more allopathic, more exhausting modes of treatment – than are the customary prescriptions, composed of unknown ingredients, used in ordinary practice for the other nameless, innumerable forms of disease. These likewise do nothing but debilitate, and only suppress or suspend the malady for a short time without being able to cure it, and when used for a long time always add a new morbid state to the old disease.

40

III. Or the new disease, after having long acted on the organism, at length joins the old one that is dissimilar to it, and forms with it a complex disease, so that each of them occupies a particular locality in the organism, namely, the organs peculiarly adapted for it, and, as it were, only the place specially belonging to it, while it leaves the rest to the other disease that is dissimilar to it. Thus a syphilitic patient may become psoric, and vice versa. As two disease dissimilar to each other, they cannot remove, cannot cure one another. At first the venereal symptoms are kept in abeyance and suspended when the psoric eruption begins to appear; in course of time, however (as the syphilis is at least as strong as the psora), the two join together,[36] that is, each involves those parts of the organism only which are most adapted for it, and the patient is thereby rendered more diseased and more difficult to cure.

When two dissimilar acute infectious diseases meet, as, for example, smallpox and measles, the one usually suspends the other, as has been before observed; yet there have also been severe epidemics of this kind, where, in rare cases, two dissimilar acute diseases occurred simultaneously in one and the same body, and for a short time combined, as it were, with each other. During an epidemic, in which smallpox and measles were prevalent at the same time, among three hundred cases (in which these diseases avoided or suspended one another, and measles attacked patients twenty days after the smallpox broke out, the smallpox, however, from seventeen to eighteen days after the appearance of the measles, so that the first disease had previously completed its regular course) there was yet one single case in which P. Russell[37] met with both these dissimilar diseases in one person at the same time. Rainey[38] witnessed the simultaneous occurrence of smallpox and measles in two girls. J. Maurice[39], in his whole practice, only observed two such cases. Similar cases are to be found in Ettmuller's[40] works, and in the writings of a few others.

Zencker[41] saw cow-pox run its regular course along with measles and along with purpura.

The cow-pox went on its course undisturbed during a mercurial treatment for syphilis, as Jenner saw.

41

Much more frequent than the natural diseases associating with and complicating one another in the same body are the morbid complication resulting from the art of the ordinary practitioner, which the inappropriate medical treatment (the allopathic method) is apt to produce by the long-continued employment of unsuitable drugs. To the natural disease, which it is proposed to cure, there are then added, by the constant repetition of the unsuitable medical agent, the new, often very tedious, morbid conditions corresponding to the nature of this agent; these gradually coalesce with and complicate the chronic malady which is dissimilar to them (which they were unable to cure by similarity of action, that is, homoeopathically), adding to the old disease a new, dissimilar, artificial malady of a chronic nature, and thus give the patient a double in place of a single disease, that is to say, render him much worse and more difficult to cure, often quite incurable. Many of the cases for which advice is asked in medical journals, as also the records of other cases in medical writings, attest the truth of this. Of a similar character are the frequent cases in which the venereal chancrous disease, complicated especially with psora or with the venereal chancrous disease, complicated especially with psora or with dyscrasia of condylomatous gonorrhoea, is not cured by long-continued or frequently repeated treatment with large doses of unsuitable mercurial preparations, but assumes its place in the organism beside the chronic mercurial affection1 that has been in the meantime gradually developed, and thus along with it often forms a hideous monster of complicated disease (under the general name of masked venereal disease), which then, when not quite incurable, can only be transformed into health with the greatest difficulty.

42

Nature herself permits, as has been stated, in some cases, the simultaneous occurrence of two (indeed, of three) natural disease in one and the same body. This complication, however, it must be remarked, happens only in the case of two dissimilar disease, which according to the eternal laws of nature do not remove, do not annihilate and cannot cure one another, but, as it seems, both (or all three) remain, as it were, separate in the organism, and each takes possession of the parts and systems peculiarly appropriate to it, which, on account of the want of resemblance of these maladies to each other, can very well happen without disparagement to the unity of life.

43

Totally different, however, is the result when two similar disease meet together in the organism, that is to say, when to the disease already present a stronger similar one is added. In such cases we see how a cure can be effected by the operations of nature, and we get a lesson as to how man ought to cure.

44

Similar diseases can neither (as is asserted of dissimilar disease in I) repel one another, nor (as has been shown of dissimilar disease in II) suspend on another, so that the old one shall return after the new one has run its course; and just as little can two similar disease (as has been demonstrated in III respecting dissimilar affections) exist beside each other in the same organism, or together form a double complex disease.

45

No! Two diseases, differing, it is true, in kind[42] but very similar in their phenomena and effects and in the sufferings and symptoms they severally produce, invariably annihilate one another whenever they meet together in the organism; the stronger disease namely, annihilates the weaker, and that for this simple reason, because the stronger morbific power when it invades the system, by reason of its similarity of action involves precisely the same part of the organism that were previously affected by the weaker morbid irritation, which, consequently, can no longer act on these parts, but is extinguished[43], or (in other words), the new similar but stronger morbific potency controls the feelings of the patient and hence the life principle on account of its peculiarity, can no longer feel the weaker similar which becomes extinguished – exists no longer – for it was never anything material, but a dynamic – spirit-like – (conceptual) affection. The life principle henceforth is affected only and this but temporarily by the new, similar but stronger morbific potency.

46

Many examples might be adduced of disease which, in the course of nature, have been homoeopathically cured by other diseases presenting similar symptoms, were it not necessary, as our object is to speak about something determinate and indubitable, to confine our attention solely to those (few) disease which are invariably the same, arise from a fixed miasm, and hence merit a distinct name.

Among these the smallpox, so dreaded on account of the great number of its serious symptoms, occupies a prominent position, and it has removed and cured a number of maladies with similar symptoms.

How frequently does smallpox produce violent ophthalmia, sometimes even causing blindness! And see! By its inoculation Dezoteux[44] cured a chronic ophthalmia permanently, and Leroy[45] another.

An amaurosis of two years' duration, consequent on suppressed scald head, was perfectly cured by it, according to Klein.[46]

How often does smallpox cause deafness and dyspnoea! And both these chronic diseases it removed on reaching its acme, as J. Fr. Closs[47] observed.

Swelling of the testicle, even of a very severe character, is a frequent symptom of small-pox, and on this account it was enabled, as Klein[48] observed, to cure, by virtue of similarity, a large hard swelling of the left testicle, consequently on a bruise. And another observer[49] saw a similar swelling of the testicle cured by it.

Among the troublesome symptoms of small-pox is a dysenteric state of the bowels; and it subdued, as Fr. Wendt[50] observed, a case of dysentery, as a similar morbific agent.

Smallpox coming on after vaccination, as well on account of its greater strength as its great similarity, at once removes entirely the cow-pox homoeopathically, and does not permit it to come to maturity; but, on the other hand, the cow-pox when near maturity does, on account of its great similarity, homoeopathically diminish very much the supervening smallpox and make it much milder[51], as Muhry[52] and many others testify.

The inoculated cow-pox, whose lymph, besides the protective matter, contains the contagion of a general cutaneous eruption of another nature, consisting of usually small, dry (rarely large, pustular) pimples, resting on a small red areola, frequently conjoined with round red cutaneous spots and often accompanied by the most violent itching, which rash appears in not a few children several days before, more frequently, however, after the red areola of the cow-pock, and goes off in a few days, leaving behind small, red, hard spots on the skin; – the inoculated cow-pox, I say, after it has taken, cures perfectly and permanently, in a homoeopathic manner, by the similarity of this accessory miasm, analogous cutaneous eruptions of children, often of very long standing and of a very troublesome character, as a number of observers assert.[53]

The cow-pox, a peculiar symptom of which is to cause tumefaction of the arm[54], cured, after it broke out, a swollen half-paralyzed arm.[55]

The fever accompanying cow-pox, which occurs at the time of the production of the red areola, cured homoeopathically intermittent fever in two individuals, as the younger Hardege[56] reports, confirming what J. Hunter[57] had already observed, that two fevers (similar diseases) cannot co-exist in the same body.

The measles bear a strong resemblance in the character of its fever and cough to the whooping-cough, and hence it was that Bosquillon[58] noticed, in an epidemic where both these affections prevailed, that many children who then took measles remained free from whooping-cough during that epidemic. They would all have been protected from, and rendered incapable of being infected by, the whooping-cough in that and all subsequent epidemics, by the measles, if the whooping-cough were not a disease that has only a partial similarity to the measles, that is to say, if it had also a cutaneous eruption similar to what the latter possesses. As it is, however, the measles can but preserve a large number from whooping-cough homoeopathically, and that only in the epidemic prevailing at the time.

If, however, the measles come in contact with a disease resembling it in its chief symptom, the eruption, it can indisputably remove, and effect a homoeopathic cure of the latter. Thus a chronic herpetic eruption was entirely and permanently (homoeopathically) cured[59] by the breaking out of the measles, as Kortum[60] observed. An excessively burning miliary rash on the face, neck, and arms, that had lasted six years, and was aggravated by every change of weather, on the invasion of measles assumed the form of a swelling of the surface of the skin; after the measles had run its course the exanthema was cured, and returned no more.[61]

47

Nothing could teach the physician in a plainer and more convincing manner than the above what kind of artificial morbific agent (medicine) he ought to choose in order to cure in a sure, rapid and permanent manner, conformably with the process that takes place in nature.

48

Neither in the course of nature, as we see from all the above examples, nor by the physician's art, can an existing affection or malady in any one instance be removed by a dissimilar morbific agent, be it ever so strong, but solely by one that is similar in symptoms and is somewhat stronger, according to eternal, irrevocable laws of nature, which have not hitherto been recognized.

49

We should have been able to meet with many more real, natural homoeopathic cures of this kind if, on the one hand, the attention of observers had been more directed to them, and, on the other hand, if nature had not been so deficient in helpful homoeopathic diseases.

50

Mighty Nature herself has, as we see, at her command, as instruments for effecting homoeopathic cures, little besides the miasmatic diseases of constant character, (the itch) measles and smallpox[62], morbific agents which[63], as remedies, are either more dangerous to life and more to be dreaded than the disease they are to cure, they themselves require curing, in order to be eradicated in their turn – both circumstances that make their employment, as homoeopathic remedies, difficult, uncertain and dangerous. And how few diseases are there to which man is subject that find their similar remedy in smallpox, measles or itch! Hence, in the course of nature, very few maladies can be cured by these uncertain and hazardous homoeopathic remedies, and the cure by their instrumentality is also attended with danger and much difficulty, for this reason that the doses of these morbific powers cannot be diminished according to circumstances, as doses of medicine can; but the patient afflicted with an analogous malady of long standing must be subjected to the entire dangerous and tedious disease, to the entire disease of smallpox, measles (or itch), which in its turn has to be cured. And yet, as is seen, we can point to some striking homoeopathic cures effected by this lucky concurrence, all so many incontrovertible proofs of the great, the sole therapeutic law of nature that obtains in them: Cure by symptoms similarity!

51

This therapeutic law is rendered obvious to all intelligent minds by these instances, and they are amply sufficient for this end. But, on the other hand, see what advantages man has over crude Nature in her happy-go-lucky operations. How many thousands more of homoeopathic morbific agents has not man at his disposal for the relief of his suffering fellow-creatures in the medicinal substances universally distributed throughout creation! In them he has producers of disease of all possible varieties of action, for all the innumerable, for all conceivable and inconceivable natural diseases, to which they can render homoeopathic aid – morbific agents (medicinal substances), whose power, when their remedial employment is completed, being overcome by the vital force, disappears spontaneously without requiring a second course of treatment for its extirpation, like the itch – artificial morbific agents, which the physician can attenuate, subdivide and potentize almost to an infinite extent, and the dose of which he can diminish to such a degree that they shall remain only slightly stronger than the similar natural disease they are employed to cure; so that in this incomparable method of cure, there is no necessity for any violent attack upon the organism for the eradication of even an inveterate disease of old standing; the cure by this method takes place by only a gentle, imperceptible and yet often rapid transition from the tormenting natural disease to the desired state of permanent health.

52

There are but two principle methods of cure: the one based only on accurate observation of nature, on careful experimentation and pure experience, the homoeopathic (before we never designedly used) and a second which does not do this, the heteropathic or allopathic. Each opposes the other, and only he who does not know either can hold the delusion that they can ever approach each other or even become united, or to make himself so ridiculous as to practice at one time homoeopathically at another allopathically, according to the pleasure of the patient; a practice which may be called criminal treason against divine homoeopathy.

53

The true mild cures take place only according to the homoeopathic method, which, as we have found (7-25) by experience and deduction, is unquestionably the proper one by which through art the quickest, most certain and most permanent cures are obtained since this healing art rests upon an eternal infallible law of nature.

The pure homoeopathic healing art is the only correct method, the one possible to human art, the straightest way to cure, as certain as that there is but one straight line between two given points.

54

The allopathic method of treatment utilized many things against disease, but usually only improper ones (alloea) and ruled for ages in different forms called systems. Every one of these, following each other from time to time and differing greatly each from the other, honored itself with the name of Rational Medicine[64].

Every builder of such a system cherished the haughty estimation of himself that he was able to penetrate into the inner nature of life of the healthy as well as of the sick and clearly to recognize it and accordingly gave the prescription which noxious matter[65] should be banished from the sick man, and how to banish it in order to restore him to health, all this according to empty assumptions and arbitrary suppositions without honestly questioning nature and listening without prejudice to the voice of experience. Diseases were held to be conditions that reappeared pretty much in the same manner. Most systems gave, therefore, names to their imagined disease pictures and classified them, every system differently. To medicines were ascribed actions which were supposed to cure these abnormal conditions. (Hence the numerous text books on Materia Medica.[66])

55

Soon, however, the public became convinced that the sufferings of the sick increased and heightened with the introduction of every one of these systems and methods of cure if followed exactly. Long ago these allopathic physicians would have been left had it not been for the palliative relief obtained at times from empirically discovered remedies whose almost instantaneous flattering action is apparent to the patient and this to some extent served to keep up their credit.

56

By means of this palliative (antipathic, enantiopathic) method, introduced according to Galen's teaching "Contraria contrariis" for seventeen centuries, the physicians hitherto could hope to win confidence while they deluded with almost instantaneous amelioration. But how fundamentally unhelpful and hurtful this method of treatment is (in diseases not running a rapid course) we shall see in what follows. It is certainly the only one of the modes of treatment adopted by the allopaths that had any manifest relation to a portion of the sufferings caused by the natural disease; but what kind of relation? Of a truth the very one (the exact contrary of the right one) that ought carefully to be avoided if we would not delude and make a mockery of the patient affected with a chronic disease[67].

To attempt to cure by means of the very same morbific potency (per Idem) contradicts all normal human understanding and hence all experience. Those who first brought Isopathy to notice, probably thought of the benefit which mankind received from cowpox vaccination by which the vaccinated individual is protected against future cowpox infection and as it were cured in advance. But both, cowpox and smallpox are only similar, in no way the same disease. In many respects they differ, namely in the more rapid course and mildness of cowpox and especially in this, that is never contagious to man by more nearness. Universal vaccination put an end to all epidemics of that deadly fearful smallpox to such an extent that the present generation does no longer possess a clear conception of the former frightful smallpox plague.

Moreover, in this way, undoubtedly, certain diseases peculiar to animals may give us remedies and thus happily enlarge our stock of homoeopathic remedies.

But to use a human morbific matter (a Psorin taken from the itch in man) as a remedy for the same itch or for evils arisen therefrom is – ?

Nothing can result from this but trouble and aggravation of the disease.

57

In order to carry into practice this antipathic method, the ordinary physician gives, for a single troublesome symptom from among the many other symptoms of the disease which he passes by unheeded, a medicine concerning which it is known that it produces the exact opposite of the morbid symptom sought to be subdued, from which, agreeably to the fifteen – centuries – old traditional rule of the antiquated medical school (contraria contrariis) he can expect the speediest (palliative) relief. He gives large doses of opium for pains of all sorts, because this drug soon benumbs the sensibility, and administers the same remedy for diarrhoeas, because it speedily puts a stop to the peristaltic motion of the intestinal canal and makes it insensible; and also for sleeplessness, because opium rapidly produces a stupefied, comatose sleep; he gives purgatives when the patient has suffered long from constipation and costiveness; he causes the burnt hand to be plunged into cold water, which, from its low degree of temperature, seems instantaneously to remove the burning pain, as if by magic; he puts the patient who complains of chilliness and deficiency of vital heat into warm baths, which warm him immediately; he makes him who is suffering from prolonged debility drink wine, whereby he is instantly enlivened and refreshed; and in like manner he employs other opposite (antipathic) remedial means, but he has very few besides those just mentioned, as it is only of very few substances that some peculiar (primary) action is known to the ordinary medical school.

58

If, in estimating the value of this mode of employing medicines, we should even pass over the circumstance that it is an extremely faulty symptomatic treatment (v. note to 7), wherein the practitioner devotes his attention in a merely one-sided manner to a single symptom , consequently to only a small part of the whole, whereby relief for the totality of the disease, which is what the patient desires, cannot evidently be expected, – we must, on the other hand, demand of experience if, in one single case where such antipathic employment of medicine was made use of in a chronic or persisting affection, after the transient amelioration there did not ensue an increased aggravation of the symptom which was subdued at first in a palliative manner, an aggravation, indeed, of the whole disease? And every attentive observer will agree that, after such short antipathic amelioration, aggravation follows in every case without exception, although the ordinary physician is in the habit of giving his patient another explanation of this subsequent aggravation, and ascribes it to malignancy of the original disease, now for the first time showing itself, or to the occurrence of quite a new disease[68].

59

Important symptoms of persistent diseases have never yet been treated with such palliative, antagonistic remedies, without the opposite state, a relapse – indeed, a palpable aggravation of the malady – occurring a few hours afterwards. For a persistent tendency to sleepiness during the day the physician prescribed coffee, whose primary action is to enliven; and when it had exhausted its action the day – somnolence increased; – for frequent waking at night he gave in the evening, without heeding the other symptoms of the disease, opium, which by virtue of its primary action produced the same night (stupefied, dull) sleep, but the subsequent nights were still more sleepless than before; – to chronic diarrhoeas he opposed, without regarding the other morbid signs, the same opium, whose primary action is to constipate the bowels, and after a transient stoppage of the diarrhoea it subsequently became all the worse; – violent and frequently recurring pains of all kinds he could suppress with opium for but a short time; they then always returned in greater, often intolerable severity, or some much worse affection came in their stead. For nocturnal cough of long standing the ordinary physician knew no better than to administer opium, whose primary action is to suppress every irritation; the cough would then perhaps cease the first night, but during the subsequent nights it would be still more severe, and if it were again and again suppressed by this palliative in increased doses, fever and nocturnal perspiration were added to the disease; – weakness of the bladder, with consequent retention of urine, was sought to be conquered by the antipathic work of cantharides to stimulate the urinary passages whereby evacuation of the urine was certainly at first effected but thereafter the bladder becomes less capable of stimulation and less able to contract, and paralysis of the bladder is imminent; – with large doses of purgative drugs and laxative salts, which excite the bowels to frequent evacuation, it was sought to remove a chronic tendency to constipation, but in the secondary action the bowels became still more confined; – the ordinary physician seeks to remove chronic debility by the administration of wine, which, however, stimulates only in its primary action, and hence the forces sink all the lower in the secondary its primary action, and hence the forces sink all the lower in the secondary action; – by bitter substances and heating condiments he tries to strengthen and warm the chronically weak and cold stomach, but in the secondary action of these palliatives, which are stimulating in their primary action only, the stomach becomes yet more inactive; – long standing deficiency of vital heat and chilly disposition ought surely to yield to prescriptions of warm baths, but still more weak, cold, and chilly do the patients subsequently become; – severely burnt parts feel instantaneous alleviation from the application of cold water, but the burning pain afterwards increases to an incredible degree, and the inflammation spreads and rises to a still greater height;[69] – by means of the sternutatory remedies that provoke a secretion of mucus, coryza with stoppage of the nose of long standing is sought to be removed, but it escapes observation that the disease is aggravated all the more by these antagonistic remedies (in their secondary action), and the nose becomes still more stopped; – by electricity and galvanism, with in their primary action greatly stimulate muscular action, chronically weak and almost paralytic limbs were soon excited to more active movements, but the consequence (the secondary action) was complete deadening of all muscular irritability and complete paralysis; – by venesections it was attempted to remove chronic determination of blood to the head, but they were always followed by greater congestion; – ordinary medical practitioners know nothing better with which to treat the paralytic torpor of the corporeal and mental organs, conjoined with unconsciousness, which prevails in many kinds of typhus, than with large doses of valerian, because this is one of the most powerful medicinal agents for causing animation and increasing the motor faculty; in their ignorance, however, they knew not that this action is only a primary action, and that the organism, after that is passed, most certainly falls back, in the secondary (antagonistic) action, into still greater stupor and immobility, that is to say, into paralysis of the mental and corporeal organs (and death); they did not see, that the very diseases they supplied most plentifully with valerian, which is in such cases an oppositely acting, antipathic remedy, most infallibly terminated fatally. The old school physician rejoices[70] that he is able to reduce for several hours the velocity of the small rapid pulse in cachectic patients with the very first dose of uncombined purple foxglove (which in its primary action makes the pulse slower); its rapidity, however, soon returns; repeated, and now increased doses effect an ever smaller diminution of its rapidity, and at length none at all – indeed – in the secondary action the pulse becomes uncountable; sleep, appetite and strength depart, and a speedy death is invariably the result, or else insanity ensues. How often, in one word, the disease is aggravated, or something even worse is effected by the secondary action of such antagonistic (antipathic) remedies, the old school with its false theories does not perceive, but experience teaches it in a terrible manner.

60

If these ill-effects are produced, as may very naturally be expected from the antipathic employment of medicines, the ordinary physician imagines he can get over the difficulty by giving, at each renewed aggravation, a stronger dose of the remedy, whereby an equally transient suppression[71] is effected; and as there then is a still greater necessity for giving ever – increasing quantities of the palliative there ensues either another more serious disease or frequently even danger to life and death itself, but never a cure of a disease of considerable or of long standing.

Being able to heal disease with mild innocent remedies and thus establish health, Brousseau found the easier way to quiet the sufferings of patients more and more at the cost of their life and at last to extinguish life wholly – a method of treatment that, alas, seemed sufficient to his contemporaries. In the degree that the patient retains his strength will his ailments be apparent and the more intensely will he feel his pains. He moans and groans and cries out and calls for help more and more vociferously so that the physician cannot come any too soon to give relief. Brousseau needed only to depress the vital force, to lessen it more and more and behold, the more frequently the patient was bled, the more leeches and cupping glasses sucked out the vital fluid (for the innocent irreplaceable blood was according to him responsible for almost all ailments). In the same proportion the patient lost strength to feel pain or to express his aggravated condition by violent complaint and gestures. The patient appears more quiet in proportion as he grows weaker, the bystanders rejoice in his apparent improvement, ready to return to the same measures on the renewal of his sufferings – be they spasms, suffocation, fears or pain, for they had so beautifully quieted him before and gave promise of further ease. In disease of long duration and when the patient retained some strength, he was deprived of food, put on a "hunger diet," in order to depress life so much more successfully and inhibit the restless states. The debilitated patient feels unable to protest against further similar measures of blood-letting leeches, vesication, warm baths and so forth to refuse their employment. That death must follow such frequently repeated reduction and exhaustion of the vital energy is not noticed by the patient, already robbed of all consciousness, and the relatives, blinded by the improvements even of the last sufferings of the patient by means of blood letting and warm baths, cannot understand and are surprised when the patient quietly slips away.

"But God knows the patient on his bed of sickness was not treated with violence, for the prick of a small lancet is not really painful and the gum Arabic solution (Eau de Gourme, almost the only medicine that Brousseau used) was mild in taste and without apparent action – the bite of the leeches insignificant and the blood letting by the physician done quietly while the luke warm baths could only soothe, hence the disease from the very start must have been fatal, so that the patient, notwithstanding all efforts of the physician, had to leave the earth." In this way the relatives, and especially the heirs of the dear departed, consoled themselves.

The physicians in Europe and elsewhere accepted this convenient treatment of all disease according to a single rule, since it saved them from all further thinking (the most laborious of all work under the sun). They only had to take care "to assuage the pangs of conscience and console themselves that they were not the originators of this system and this method of treatment, that all the other thousands of Brousseauists did the same and that possibly everything would cease with death anyway as was taught by their master." In this way many thousand physicians were miserably misled to shed (with cold heart) the warm blood of their patients that were capable of cure and thereby rob millions of men gradually of their life, according to Brousseau's method, more than fell on Napoleon's battlefields. Was it perhaps necessary by the disposition of God for that system of Brousseau which destroyed medically the life of curable patients to precede homoeopathy in order to open the eyes of the world to the only true science and art of medicine, homoeopathy, in which curable patients find health and new life when this most difficult of all arts is practised by an indefatigable discriminating physician in a pure and conscientious manner?

61

Had physicians been capable of reflecting on the sad results of the antagonistic employment of medicines, they had long since discovered the grand truth, THAT THE TRUE RADICAL HEALING ART MUST BE FOUND IN THE EXACT OPPOSITE OF SUCH AN ANTI-PATHIC TREATMENT OF THE SYMPTOMS OF DISEASE; they would have become convinced, that as a medicinal action antagonistic to the symptoms of the disease (an antipathically employed medicine) is followed by only transient relief, and after that is passed, by invariable aggravation, the converse of that procedure, the homoeopathic employment of medicines according to similarity of symptoms, must effect a permanent and perfect cure, if at the same time the opposite of their large doses, the most minute doses, are exhibited. But neither the obvious aggravation that ensued from their antipathic treatment, nor the fact that no physician ever effected a permanent cure of disease of considerable or of long standing unless some homoeopathic medicinal agent was accidentally a chief ingredient in his prescription, nor yet the circumstances that all the rapid and perfect cures that nature ever performed (46), were always effected by the supervention upon the old disease of one of a similar character, ever taught them, during such a long series of centuries, this truth, the knowledge of which can alone conduce to the benefit of the sick.

62

But on what this pernicious result of the palliative, antipathic treatment and the efficacy of the reverse, the homoeopathic treatment, depend, is explained by the following facts, deduced from manifold observations, which no one before me perceived, though they are so very palpable and so very evident, and are of such infinite importance to the healing art.

63

Every agent that acts upon the vitality, every medicine, deranges more or less the vital force, and causes a certain alteration in the health of the individual for a longer or a shorter period. This is termed primary action. Although a product of the medicinal and vital powers conjointly, it is principally due to the former power. To its action our vital force endeavors to oppose its own energy. This resistant action is a property, is indeed an automatic action of our life-preserving power, which goes by the name of secondary action or counteraction.

64

During the primary action of the artificial morbific agents (medicines) on our healthy body, as seen in the following examples, our vital force seems to conduct itself merely in a passive (receptive) manners, and appears, so to say, compelled to permit the impressions of the artificial power acting from without to take place in it and thereby after its state of health; it then, however, appears to rouse itself again, as it were, and to develop (A) the exact opposite condition of health (counteraction, secondary action) to this effect (primary action) produced upon it, if there be such an opposite, and that in as great a degree as was the effect (primary action) of the artificial morbific agent on it, and proportionate to its own energy; – or (B) if there be not in nature a state exactly the opposite of the primary action, it appears to endeavor to indifferentiate itself, that is, to make its superior power available in the extinction of the change wrought in it from without (by the medicine), in the place of which it substitutes its normal state (secondary action, curative action).

65

Examples of (A) are familiar to all. A hand bathed in hot water is at first much warmer than the other hand that has not been so treated (primary action); but when it is withdrawn from the hot water and again thoroughly dried, it becomes in a short time cold, and at length much colder than the other (secondary action). A person heated by violent exercise (primary action) is afterwards affected with chilliness and shivering (secondary action). To one who was yesterday heated by drinking much wine (primary action), today every breath of air feels too cold (counteraction of the organism, secondary action). An arm that has been kept long in very cold water is at first much paler and colder (primary action) than the other; but removed from the cold water and dried, it subsequently becomes not only warmer than the other, but even hot, red and inflamed (secondary action, reaction of the vital force). Excessive vivacity follows the use of strong coffee (primary action), but sluggishness and drowsiness remain for a long time afterwards (reaction, secondary action), if this be not always again removed for a short time by imbibing fresh supplies of coffee (palliative). After the profound stupefied sleep caused by opium (primary action), the following night will be all the more sleepless (reaction, secondary action). After the constipation produced by opium (primary action), diarrhoea ensues (secondary action); and after purgation with medicines that irritate the bowels, constipation of several days' duration ensues (secondary action). And in like manner it always happens, after the primary action of a medicine that produces in large doses a great change in the health of a healthy person, that its exact opposite, when, as has been observed, there is actually such a thing, is produced in the secondary action by our vital force.

66

An obvious antagonistic secondary action, however, is, as may readily be conceived, not to be noticed from the action of quite minute homoeopathic doses of the deranging agents on the healthy body. A small dose of every one of them certainly produces a primary action that is perceptible to a sufficiently attentive; but the living organism employs against it only so much reaction (secondary action) as is necessary for the restoration of the normal condition.

67

These incontrovertible truths, which spontaneously offer themselves to our notice and experience, explain to us the beneficial action that takes place under homoeopathic treatment; while, on the other hand, they demonstrate the perversity of the antipathic and palliative treatment of diseases with antagonistically acting medicines.[72]

68

In homoeopathic cures they show us that from the uncommonly small doses of medicine (275 – 287) required in this method of treatment, which are just sufficient, by the similarity of their symptoms, to overpower and remove from the sensation of the life principle the similar natural disease there certainly remains, after the destruction of the latter, at first a certain amount of medicinal disease alone in the organism, but, on account of the extraordinary minuteness of the dose, it is so transient, so slight, and disappears so rapidly of its own accord, that the vital force has no need to employ, against this small artificial derangement of its health, any more considerable reaction than will suffice to elevate its present state of health up to the healthy point – that is, than will suffice to effect complete recovery, for which after the extinction of the previous morbid derangement but little effort is required (64, B).

69

In the antipathic (palliative) mode of treatment, however precisely the reverse of this takes place. The medicinal symptom which the physician opposes to the disease symptom (for example, the insensibility and stupefaction caused by opium in its primary action to acute pain) is certainly not alien, not allopathic of the latter; there is a manifest relation of the medicinal symptom to the disease symptom, but it is the reverse of what should be; it is here intended that the annihilation of the disease symptom shall be effected by an opposite medicinal symptom, which is nevertheless impossible. No doubt the antipathically chosen medicine touches precisely the same diseased point in the organism as the homoeopathic medicine chosen on account of the similar affection it produces; but the former covers the opposite symptom of the disease only as an opposite, and makes it unobservable to our life principle for a short time only, so that in the first period of the action of the antagonistic palliative the vital force perceives nothing disagreeable from either if the two (neither from the disease symptom nor from the medicinal symptom), as they seem both to have mutually removed and dynamically neutralized one another as it were (for example, the stupefying power of opium does this to the pain). In the first minutes the vital force feels quite well, and perceives neither the stupefaction of the opium nor the pain of the disease. But as the antagonistic medicinal symptom cannot (as in the homoeopathic treatment) occupy the place of the morbid derangement present in the organism in the sensation of the life principle as a similar, stronger (artificial) disease, and cannot, therefore, like a homoeopathic medicine, affect the vital force with a similar artificial disease, so as to be able to step into the place of the original natural morbid derangement, the palliative medicine must, as a thing totally differing from, and the opposite of the disease derangement, leave the latter uneradicated; it renders it, as before said, by a semblance of dynamic neutralization,[73] at first unfelt by the vital force, but, like every medicinal disease, it is soon spontaneously extinguished, and not only leaves the disease behind, just as it was, but compels the vital force (as it must, like all palliatives, be given in large doses in order to effect the apparent removal) to produce an opposite condition (63,64) to this palliative medicine, the reverse of the medicinal action, consequently the analogue of the still present, undestroyed, natural morbid derangement, which is necessarily strengthened and increased[74] by this addition (reaction against the palliative) produced by the vital force. The disease symptom (this single part of the disease) consequently becomes worse after the term of the action of the palliative has expired; worse in proportion to the magnitude of the dose of the palliative. Accordingly (to keep to the same example) the larger the dose of opium given to allay the pain, so much the more does the pain increase beyond its original intensity as soon as the opium has exhausted its action.[75]

70

From what has been already adduced we cannot fail to draw the following inferences:

That everything of a really morbid character and which ought to be cured that the physician can discover in diseases consists solely of the sufferings of the patient, and the sensible alterations in his health, in a word, solely of the totality of the symptoms, by means of which the disease demands the medicine requisite for its relief; while, on the other hand, every internal cause attributed to it, every occult quality or imaginary material morbific principle, is nothing but an idle dream;

That this derangement of the state of health, which we term disease, can only be converted into health by another revolution effected in the state of health by means of medicines, whose sole curative power, consequently, can only consist in altering man's state of health – that is to say, in a peculiar excitation of morbid symptoms, and is learned with most distinctness and purity by testing them on the healthy body;

That, according to all experience, a natural disease can never be cured by medicines that possess the power of producing in the healthy individual an alien morbid state (dissimilar morbid symptoms) differing from that of the disease to be cured (never, therefore, by an allopathic mode of treatment), and that even in nature no cure ever takes place in which an inherent disease is removed, annihilated and cured by the addition of another disease dissimilar to it, be the new one ever so strong;

That, moreover, all experience proves that, by means of medicines which have a tendency to produce in the healthy individual an artificial morbid symptom, antagonistic to the single symptom of disease sought to be cured, the cure of a long-standing affection will never be effected, but merely a very transientalleviation, always follows by its aggravation; and that, in a word, this antipathic and merely palliative treatment in long-standing diseases of a serious character is absolutely inefficacious;

That, however, the third and only other possible mode of treatment (the homoeopathic), in which there is employed for the totality of the symptoms of a natural disease a medicine capable of producing the most similar symptoms possible in the healthy individual, given in suitable dose, is the only efficacious remedial method whereby diseases, which are purely dynamic deranging irritations of the vital force, are overpowered, and being thus easily, perfectly and permanently extinguished, must necessarily cease to exist. This is brought about by means of the stronger similar deranging irritation of the homoeopathic medicine in the sensation of the life principle. – and for this mode of procedure we have the example of unfettered Nature herself, when to an old disease there is added a new one similar to the first, whereby the new one is rapidly and forever annihilated and cured.

71

As it is now no longer a matter of doubt that the diseases of mankind consist merely of groups of certain symptoms, and may be annihilated and transformed into health by medicinal substances, but only by such as are capable of artificially producing similar morbid symptoms (and such is the process in all genuine cures), hence the operation of curing is comprised in the three following points:

I. How is the physician to ascertain what is necessary to be known in order to cure the disease?

II. How is he to gain a knowledge of the instruments adapted for the cure of the natural disease, the pathogenetic powers of the medicines?

III. What is the most suitable method of employing these artificial morbific agents (medicines) for the cure of natural disease?

72

With respect to the first point, the following will serve as a general preliminary view. The disease to which man is liable are either rapid morbid processes of the abnormally deranged vital force, which have a tendency to finish their course more or less quickly, but always in a moderate time – these are termed acute diseases; – or they are diseases of such a character that, with small, often imperceptible beginnings, dynamically derange the living organism, each in its own peculiar manner, and cause it gradually to deviate from the healthy condition, in such a way that the automatic life energy, called vital force, whose office is to preserve the health, only opposes to them at the commencement and during their progress imperfect, unsuitable, useless resistance, but is unable of itself to extinguish them, but must helplessly suffer (them to spread and) itself to be ever more and more abnormally deranged, until at length the organism is destroyed; these are termed chronic diseases. They are caused by infection with a chronic miasm.

73

As regards acute diseases, they are either of such a kind as attack human beings individually, the exciting cause being injurious influences to which they were particularly exposed. Excesses in food, or an insufficient supply of it, severe physical impression, chills, over heatings, dissipation, strains, etc., or physical irritations, mental emotions, and the like, are exciting causes of such acute febrile affections; in reality, however, they are generally only a transient explosion of latent psora, which spontaneously returns to its dormant state if the acute diseases were not of too violent a character and were soon quelled. Or they are of such a kind as attack several persons at the same time, here and there (sporadically), by means of meteoric or telluric influences and injurious agents, the susceptibility for being morbidly affected by which is possessed by only a few persons at one time. Allied to these are those diseases in which many persons are attacked with very similar sufferings from the same cause (epidemically); these diseases generally become infectious (contagious) when they prevail among thickly congregated masses of human beings. Thence arise fevers[76], in each instance of a peculiar nature, and, because the cases of disease have an identical origin, they set up in all those they affect an identical morbid process, which when left to itself terminates in a moderate period of time in death or recovery. The calamities of war, inundations and famine are not infrequently their exciting causes and producers – sometimes they are peculiar acute miasms which recur in the same manner (hence known by some traditional name), which either attack persons but once in a lifetime, as the smallpox, measles, whooping-cough, the ancient, smooth, bright red scarlet fever[77] of Sydenham, the mumps, etc., or such as recur frequently in pretty much the same manner, the plague of the Levant, the yellow fever of the sea-coast, the Asiatic cholera, etc.

74

Among chronic diseases we must still, alas!, reckon those so commonly met with, artificially produced in allopathic treatment by the prolonged use of violent heroic medicines in large and increasing doses, by the abuse of calomel, corrosive sublimate, mercurial ointment, nitrate of silver, iodine and its ointments, opium, valerian, cinchona bark and quinine, foxglove, prussic acid, sulphur and sulphuric acid, perennial purgatives[78], venesections, shedding streams of blood, leeches, issues, setons, etc., whereby the vital energy is sometimes weakened to an unmerciful extent, sometimes, if it do not succumb, gradually abnormally deranged (by each substance in a peculiar manner) in such a way that, in order to maintain life against these inimical and destructive attacks, it must produce a revolution in the organism, and either deprive some part of its irritability and sensibility, or exalt these to an excessive degree, cause dilatation or contraction, relaxation or induration or even total destruction of certain parts, and develop faulty organic alterations here and there in the interior or the exterior (cripple the body internally or externally), in order to preserve the organism from complete destruction of the life by the ever – renewed, hostile assaults of such destructive forces.[79]

75

These inroads on human health effected by the allopathic non-healing art (more particularly in recent times) are of all chronic diseases the most deplorable, the most incurable; and I regret to add that it is apparently impossible to discover or to hit upon any remedies for their cure when they have reached any considerable height.

76

Only for natural diseases has the beneficent Deity granted us, in Homoeopathy, the means of affording relief; but those devastations and maimings of the human organism exteriorly and interiorly, effected by years, frequently, of the unsparing exercise of a false art,[80] with its hurtful drugs and treatment, must be remedied by the vital force itself (appropriate aid being given for the eradication of any chronic miasm that may happen to be lurking in the background), if it has not already been too much weakened by such mischievous acts, and can devote several years to this huge operation undisturbed. A human healing art, for the restoration to the normal state of those innumerable abnormal conditions so often produced by the allopathic non-healing art, there is not and cannot be.

77

Those diseases are inappropriately named chronic, which persons incur who expose them-selves continually to avoidable noxious influences, who are in the habit of indulging in injurious liquors or aliments, are addicted to dissipation of many kinds which undermine the health, who undergo prolonged abstinence from things that are necessary for the support of life, who reside in unhealthy localities, especially marshy districts, who are housed in cellars or other confined dwellings, who are deprived of exercise or of open air, who ruin their health by overexertion of body or mind, who live in a constant state of worry, etc. These states of ill-health, which persons bring upon themselves, disappear spontaneously, provided no chronic miasm lurks in the body, under an improved mode of living, and they cannot be called chronic diseases.

78

The true natural chronic diseases are those that arise from a chronic miasm, which when left to themselves, and unchecked by the employment of those remedies that are specific for them, always go on increasing and growing worse, notwithstanding the best mental and cor-poreal regimen, and torment the patient to the end of his life with ever aggravated sufferings. These, excepting those produced by medical malpractice (74), are the most numerous and great-est scourges of the human race; for the most robust constitution, the best regulated mode of living and the most vigorous energy of the vital force are insufficient for their eradication.[81]

Hitherto syphilis alone has been to some extent known as such a chronic miasmatic disease, which when uncured ceases only with the termination of life. Sycosis (the condylomatous disease), equally ineradicable by the vital force without proper medicinal treatment, was not recognized as a chronic miasmatic disease of a peculiar character, which it nevertheless undoubtedly is, and physicians imagined they had cured it when they had destroyed the growths upon the skin, but the persisting dyscrasia occasioned by it escaped their observation.

Incalculably greater and more important than the two chronic miasms just named, however, is the chronic miasm of psora, which, while those two reveal their specific internal dyscrasia, the one by the venereal chancre, the other by the cauliflower-like growths, does also, after the completion of the internal infection of the whole organism, announce by a peculiar cutaneous eruption, sometimes consisting only of a few vesicles accompanied by intolerable voluptuous tickling itching (and a peculiar odor), the monstrous internal chronic miasm – the psora, the only real fundamental cause and producer of all the other numerous, I may say innumerable, forms of disease[82], which, under the names of nervous debility, hysteria, hypochondriasis, mania, melancholia, imbecility, madness, epilepsy and convulsions of all sorts, softening of the bones (rachitis), scoliosis and cyphosis, caries, cancer, fungus nematodes, neoplasms, gout, haemorrhoids, jaundice, cyanosis, dropsy, amenorrhoea, haemorrhage from the stomach, nose, lungs, bladder and womb, of asthma and ulceration of the lungs, of impotence and barrenness, of megrim, deafness, cataract, amaurosis, urinary calculus, paralysis, defects of the senses and pains of thousands of kinds, etc., figure in systematic works on pathology as peculiar, independent diseases.

The fact that this extremely ancient infecting agent has gradually passed, in some hundreds of generations, through many millions of human organisms and has thus attained an incredible development, renders it in some measure conceivable how it can now display such innumerable morbid forms in the great family of mankind, particularly when we consider what a number of circumstances[83] contribute to the production of these great varieties of chronic diseases (secondary symptoms of psora), besides the indescribable diversity of men in respect of their congenital corporeal constitutions, so that it is no wonder if such a variety of injurious agencies, acting from within and from without and sometimes continually, on such a variety of organisms permeated with the psoric miasm, should produce an innumerable variety of defects, injuries, derangements and sufferings, which have hitherto been treated of in the old pathological works[84], under a number of special names, as diseases of an independent character.

From all this it is clear that these useless and misused names of diseases ought to have no influence on the practice of the true physician, who knows that he has to judge of and to cure diseases, not according to the similarity of the name of a single one of their symptoms, but according to the totality of the signs of the individual state of each particular patient, whose affection it is his duty carefully to investigate, but never to give a hypothetical guess at it.

If, however, it is deemed necessary sometimes to make use of names of diseases, in order, when talking about a patient to ordinary persons, to render ourselves intelligible in few words, we ought only to employ them as collective names, and tell them, eg., the patient has a kind of St. Vitus's dance, a kind of dropsy, a kind of typhus, a kind of ague; but (in order to do away once and for all with the mistaken notions these names give rise to) we should never say he has the St. Vitus's dance, the typhus, the dropsy, the ague, as there are certainly no disease of these and similar names of fixed unvarying character.

Although, by the discovery of that great source of chronic diseases, as also by the discovery of the specific homoeopathic remedies for the psora, medicine has advanced some steps nearer to a knowledge of the nature of the majority of diseases it has to cure, yet, for settling the indication in each case of chronic (psoric) disease he is called on to cure, the duty of a careful apprehension of its ascertainable symptoms and characteristics is as indispensable for the homoeopathic physician as it was before that discovery, as no real cure of this or of other diseases can take place without a strict particular treatment (individualization) of each case of disease – only that in this investigation some difference is to be made when the affection is an acute and rapidly developed disease, and when it is a chronic one; seeing that, in acute disease, the chief symptoms strike us and become evident to the senses more quickly, and hence much less time is requisite for tracing the picture of the disease and much fewer questions are required to be asked[85], as almost everything is self-evident, than in a chronic disease which has been gradually progressing for several years, in which the symptoms are much more difficult to be ascertained.

83

This individualizing examination of a case of disease, for which I shall only give in this place general directions, of which the practitioner will bear in mind only what is applicable for each individual case, demands of the physician nothing but freedom from prejudice and sound senses, attention in observing and fidelity in tracing the picture of the disease.

84

The patient details the history of his sufferings; those about him tell what they heard him complain of, how he has behaved and what they have noticed in him; the physician sees, hears, and remarks by his other senses what there is of an altered or unusual character about him. He writes down accurately all that the patient and his friends have told him in the very expressions used by them. Keeping silence himself he allows them to say all they have to say, and refrains from interrupting them[86] unless they wander off to other matters. The physician advises them at the beginning of the examination to speak slowly, in order that he may take down in writing the important parts of what the speakers say.

85

He begins a fresh line with every new circumstance mentioned by the patient or his friends, so that the symptoms shall be all ranged separately one below the other. He can thus add to any one, that may at first have been related in too vague a manner, but subsequently more explicitly explained.

86

When the narrators have finished what they would say of their own accord, the physician then reverts to each particular symptom and elicits more precise information respecting it in the following manner; he reads over the symptoms as they were related to him one by one, and about each of them he inquires for further particulars, e.g., at what period did this symptom occur? Was it previous to taking the medicine he had hitherto been using? While taking the medicine? Or only some days after leaving off the medicine? What kind of pain, what sensation exactly, was it that occurred on this spot? Where was the precise spot? Did the pain occur in fits and by itself, at various times? Or was it continued, without intermission? How long did it last? At what time of the day or night, and in what position of the body was it worst, or ceased entirely? What was the exact nature of this or that event or circumstance mentioned – described in plain words?

87

And thus the physician obtains more precise information respecting each particular detail, but without ever framing his questions so as to suggest the answer to the patient[87], so that he shall only have to answer yes or no; else he will be misled to answer in the affirmative or negative something untrue, half true, or not strictly correct, either from indolence or in order to please his interrogator, from which a false picture of the disease and an unsuitable mode of treatment must result.

88

If in these voluntary details nothing has been mentioned respecting several parts or functions of the body or his metal state, the physician asks what more can be told in regard to these parts and these functions, or the state of his disposition or mind[88], but in doing this he only makes use of general expressions, in order that his informants may be obliged to enter into special details concerning them.

89

When the patient (for it is on him we have chiefly to rely for a description of his sensations, except in the case of feigned diseases) has by these details, given of his own accord and in answer to inquiries, furnished the requisite information and traced a tolerably perfect picture of the disease, the physician is at liberty and obliged (if he feels he has not yet gained all the information he needs) to ask more precise, more special questions.[89]

90

When the physician has finished writing down these particulars, he then makes a note of what he himself observes in the patient[90], and ascertains how much of that was peculiar to the patient in his healthy state.

91

The symptoms and feelings of the patient during a previous course of medicine do not furnish the pure picture of the disease; but on the other hand, those symptoms and ailments which he suffered from before the use of the medicines, or after they had been discontinued for several days, give the true fundamental idea of the original form of the disease, and these especially the physician must take note of. When the disease is of a chronic character, and the patient has been taking medicine up to the time he is seen, the physician may with advantage leave him some days quite without medicine, or in the meantime administer something of an unmedicinal nature and defer to a subsequent period the more precise scrutiny of the morbid symptoms, in order to be able to grasp in their purity the permanent uncontaminated symptoms of the old affection and to form a faithful picture of the disease.

92

But if it be a disease of a rapid course, and if its serious character admit of no delay, the physician must content himself with observing the morbid condition, altered though it may be by medicines, if he cannot ascertain what symptoms were present before the employment of the medicines, – in order that he may at least form a just apprehension of the complete picture of the disease in its actual condition, that is to say, of the conjoint malady formed by the medicinal and original diseases, which from the use of inappropriate drugs is generally more serious and dangerous than was the original disease, and hence demands prompt and efficient aid; and by thus tracing out the complete picture of the disease he will be enabled to combat it with a suitable homoeopathic remedy, so that the patient shall not fall a sacrifice to the injurious drugs he was swallowed.

93

If the disease has been brought on a short time or, in the case of a chronic affection, a considerable time previously, by some obvious cause, then the patient – or his friends when questioned privately – will mention it either spontaneously or when carefully interrogated.[91]

94

While inquiring into the state of chronic disease, the particular circumstances of the patient with regard to his ordinary occupations, his usual mode of living and diet, his domestic situation, and so forth, must be well considered and scrutinized, to ascertain what there is in them that may tend to produce or to maintain disease, in order that by their removal the recovery may by prompted.[92]

95

In chronic disease the investigation of the signs of disease above mentioned, and of all others, must be pursued as carefully and circumstantially as possible, and the most minute peculiarities must be attended to, partly because in these diseases they are the most characteristic and least resemble those of acute diseases, and if a cure is to be affected they cannot be too accurately noted; partly because the patients become so used to their long sufferings that they pay little or no heed to the lesser accessory symptoms, which are often very pregnant with meaning (characteristic) – often very useful in determining the choice of the remedy – and regard them almost as a necessary part of their condition, almost as health, the real feeling of which they have well-nigh forgotten in the sometimes fifteen or twenty years of suffering, and they can scarcely bring themselves to believe that these accessory symptoms, these greater or less deviations from the healthy state, can have any connection with their principal malady.

96

Besides this, patients themselves differ so much in their dispositions, that some, especially the so-called hypochondriacs and other persons of great sensitiveness and impatient of suffering, portray their symptoms in too vivid colors and, in order to induce the physician to give them relief, describe their ailments in exaggerated expression.[93]

97

Other individuals of an opposite character, however, partly from indolence, partly from false modesty, partly from a kind of mildness of disposition or weakness of mind, refrain from mentioning a number of their symptoms, describe them in vague terms, or allege some of them to be of no consequence.

98

Now, as certainly as we should listen particularly to the patient's description of his sufferings and sensations, and attach credence especially to his own expressions wherewith he endeavors to make us understand his ailments – because in the mouths of his friends and attendants they are usually altered and erroneously stated, – so certainly, on the other hand, in all diseases, but especially in the chronic ones, the investigation of the true, complete picture and its peculiarities demands especial circumspection, tact, knowledge of human nature, caution in conducting the inquiry and patience in an eminent degree.

99

On the whole, the investigation of acute diseases, or of such as have existed but a short time, is much the easiest for the physician, because all the phenomena and deviations from the health that has been put recently lost are still fresh in the memory of the patient and his friends, still continue to be novel and striking. The physician certainly requires to know everything in such cases also; but he has much less to inquire into; they are for the most part spontaneously detailed to him.

100

In investigating the totality of the symptoms of epidemic and sporadic diseases it is quite immaterial whether or not something similar has ever appeared in the world before under the same or any other name. The novelty or peculiarity of a disease of that kind makes no difference either in the mode of examining or of treating it, as the physician must any way regard to pure picture of every prevailing disease as if it were something new and unknown, and investigate it thoroughly for itself, if he desire to practice medicine in a real and radical manner, never substituting conjecture for actual observation, never taking for granted that the case of disease before him is already wholly or partially known, but always carefully examining it in all its phases; and this mode of procedure is all the more requisite in such cases, as a careful examination will show that every prevailing disease is in many respects a phenomenon of a unique character, differing vastly from all previous epidemics, to which certain names have been falsely applied – with the exception of those epidemics resulting from a contagious principle that always remains the same, such as smallpox, measles, etc.

101

It may easily happen that in the first case of an epidemic disease that presents itself to the physician's notice he does not at once obtain a knowledge of its complete picture, as it is only by a close observation of several cases of every such collective disease that he can become conversant with the totality of its signs and symptoms. The carefully observing physician can, however, from the examination of even the first and second patients, often arrive so nearly at a knowledge of the true state as to have in his mind a characteristic portrait of it, and even to succeed in finding a suitable, homoeopathically adapted remedy for it.

102

In the course of writing down the symptoms of several cases of this kind the sketch of the disease picture becomes ever more and more complete, not more spun out and verbose, but more significant (more characteristic), and including more of the peculiarities of this collective disease; on the one hand, the general symptoms (e.g., loss of appetite, sleeplessness, etc.) become precisely defined as to their peculiarities; and on the other, the more marked and special symptoms which are peculiar to but few diseases and of rarer occurrence, at least in the same combination, become prominent and constitute what is characteristic of this malady.[94] All those affected with the disease prevailing at a given time have certainly contracted it from one and the same source and hence are suffering from the same disease; but the whole extent of such an epidemic disease and the totality of its symptoms (the knowledge whereof, which is essential for enabling us to choose the most suitable homoeopathic remedy for this array of symptoms, is obtained by a complete survey of the morbid picture) cannot be learned from one single patient, but is only to be perfectly deduced (abstracted) and ascertained from the sufferings of several patients of different constitutions.

103

In the same manner as has here been taught relative to the epidemic disease, which are generally of an acute character, the miasmatic chronic maladies, which, as I have shown, always remain the same in their essential nature, especially the psora, must be investigated, as to the whole sphere of their symptoms, in a much more minute manner than has ever been done before, for in them also one patient only exhibits a portion of their symptoms, a second, a third, and so on, present some other symptoms, which also are but a (dissevered, as it were), portion of the totality of the symptoms which constitute the entire extent of this malady, so that the whole array of the symptoms belonging to such a miasmatic, chronic disease, and especially to the psora, can only be ascertained from the observation of very many single patients affected with such a chronic disease, and without a complete survey and collective picture of these symptoms the medicines capable of curing the whole malady homoeopathically (to wit, the antipsorics) cannot be discovered; and these medicines are, at the same time, the true remedies of the several patients suffering from such chronic affections.

104

When the totality of the symptoms that specially mark and distinguish the case of disease or, in other words, when the picture of the disease, whatever be its kind, is once accurately sketched,[95] the most difficult part of the task is accomplished. The physician has then the picture of the disease, especially if it be a chronic one, always before him to guide him in his treatment; he can investigate it in all its parts and can pick out the characteristic symptoms, in order to oppose to these, that is to say, to the whole malady itself, a very similar artificial morbific force, in the shape of a homoeopathically chosen medicinal substance, selected from the lists of symptoms of all the medicines whose pure effects have been ascertained. And when, during the treatment, he wishes to ascertain what has been the effect of the medicine, and what change has taken place in the patient's state, at this fresh examination of the patient he only needs to strike out of the list of the symptoms noted down at the first visit those that have become ameliorated, to mark what still remain, and add any new symptoms that may have supervened.

105

The second point of the business of a true physician related to acquiring a knowledge of the instruments intended for the cure of the natural diseases, investigating the pathogenetic power of the medicines, in order, when called on to cure, to be able to select from among them one, from the list of whose symptoms an artificial disease may be constructed, as similar as possible to the totality of the principal symptoms of the natural disease sought to be cured.

106

The whole pathogenetic effect of the several medicines must be known; that is to say, all the morbid symptoms and alterations in the health that each of them is specially capable of developing in the healthy individual must first have been observed as far as possible, before we can hope to be able to find among them, and to select, suitable homoeopathic remedies for most of the natural disease.

107

If, in order to ascertain this, medicines be given to sick persons only, even though they be administered singly and alone, then little or nothing precise is seen of their true effects, as those peculiar alterations of the health to be expected from the medicine are mixed up with the symptoms of the disease and can seldom be distinctly observed.

108

There is, therefore, no other possible way in which the peculiar effects of medicines on the health of individuals can be accurately ascertained – there is no sure, no more natural way of accomplishing this object, than to administer the several medicines experimentally, in moderate doses, to healthy persons, in order to ascertain what changes, symptoms and signs of their influence each individually produces on the health of the body and of the mind; that is to say, what disease elements they are able and tend to produce[96], since, as has been demonstrated (24-27), all the curative power of medicines lies in this power they possess of changing the state of man's health, and is revealed by observation of the latter.

109

I was the first that opened up this path, which I have pursued with a perseverance that could only arise and be kept up by a perfect conviction of the great truth, fraught with such blessings to humanity, that it is only by the homoeopathic employment of medicines[97] that the certain cure of human maladies is possible.[98]

110

I saw, moreover, that the morbid lesions which previous authors had observed to result from medicinal substances when taken into the stomach of healthy persons, either in large doses given by mistake or in order to produce death in themselves or others, or under other circumstances, accorded very much with my own observations when experimenting with the same substances on myself and other healthy individuals. These authors give details of what occurred as histories of poisoning and as proofs of the pernicious effects of these powerful substances, chiefly in order to warn others from their use; partly also for the sake of exalting their own skill, when, under the use of the remedies they employed to combat these dangerous accidents, health gradually returned; but partly also, when the persons so affected died under their treatment, in order to seek their own justification in the dangerous character of these substances, which they then termed poisons. None of these observers ever dreamed that the symptoms they recorded merely as proofs of the noxious and poisonous character of these substances were sure revelations of the power of these drugs to extinguish curatively similar symptoms occurring in natural disease, that these their pathogenetic phenomena were intimations of their homoeopathic curative action, and that the only possible way to ascertain their medicinal powers is to observe those changes of health medicines are capable of producing in the healthy organism; for the pure, peculiar powers of medicines available for the cure of disease are to be learned neither by any ingenious a priori speculations, nor by the smell, taste or appearance of the drugs, nor by their chemical analysis, nor yet by the employment of several of them at one time in a mixture (prescription) in diseases; it was never suspected that these histories of medicinal diseases would one day furnish the first rudiments of the true, pure materia medica, which from the earliest times until now has consisted solely of false conjectures and fictions of the imagination – that is to say, did not exist at all.[99]

111

The agreement of my observations on the pure effects of medicines with these older ones – although they were recorded without reference to any therapeutic object, – and the very concordance of these accounts with others of the same kind by different authors must easily convince us that medicinal substances act in the morbid changes they produce in the healthy human body according to fixed, eternal laws of nature, and by virtue of these are enabled to produce certain, reliable disease symptoms each according to its own peculiar character.

112

In those older prescriptions of the often dangerous effects of medicines ingested in excessively large doses we notice certain states that were produced, not at the commencement, but towards the termination of these sad events, and which were of an exactly opposite nature to those that first appeared. These symptoms, the very reverse of the primary action (63) or proper action of the medicines on the vital force are the reaction of the vital force of the organism, its secondary action (62-67), of which, however, there is seldom or hardly ever the least trace from experiments with moderate doses on healthy bodies, and from small doses none whatever. In the homoeopathic curative operation the living organism reacts from these only so much as is requisite to raise the health again to the normal healthy state (67).

113

The only exceptions to this are the narcotic medicines. As they, in their primary action, take away sometimes the sensibility and sensation, sometimes the irritability, it frequently happens that in their secondary action , even from moderate experimental doses on healthy bodies, an increased sensibility (and a greater irritability) is observable.

114

With the exception of these narcotic substances, in experiments with moderate doses of medicine on healthy bodies, we observe only their primary action, i.e., those symptoms wherewith the medicine deranges the health of the human being and develops in him a morbid state of longer or shorter duration.

115

Among these symptoms, there occur in the case of some medicines not a few which are partially, or under certain conditions, directly opposite to other symptoms that have previously or subsequently appeared, but which are not therefore to be regarded as actual secondary action or the mere reaction of the vital force, but which only represent the alternating state of the various paroxysms of the primary action; they are termed alternating actions.

116

Some symptoms are produced by the medicines more frequently – that is to say, in many individuals, others more rarely or in few persons, some only in very few healthy bodies.

117

To the latter category belong the so-called idiosyncrasies, by which are meant peculiar corporeal constitutions which, although otherwise healthy, possess a disposition to be brought into a more or less morbid state by certain things which seem to produce no impression and no change in many other individuals.[100] But this inability to make an impression on every one is only apparent. For as two things are required for the production of these as well as all other morbid alterations in the health of man – to wit., the inherent power of the influencing substance, and the capability of the vital force that animates the organism to be influenced by it – the obvious derangements of health in the so-called idiosyncrasies cannot be laid to the account of these peculiar constitutions alone, but they must also be ascribed to these things that produce them, in which must lie the power of making the same impressions on all human bodies, yet in such a manner that but a small number of healthy constitutions have a tendency to allow themselves to be brought into such an obvious morbid condition by them. That these agents do actually make this impression on every healthy body is shown by this, that when employed as remedies they render effectual homoeopathic service[101] to all sick persons for morbid symptoms similar to those they seem to be only capable of producing in so-called idiosyncratic individuals.

118

Every medicine exhibits peculiar actions on the human frame, which are not produced in exactly the same manner by any other medicinal substance of a different kind.[102]

119

As certainly as every species of plant differs in its external form, mode of life and growth, in its taste and smell from every other species and genus of plant, as certainly as every mineral and salt differs from all others, in its external as well as its internal physical and chemical properties (which alone should have sufficed to prevent any confounding of one with another), so certainly do they all differ and diverge among themselves in their pathogenetic – consequently also in their therapeutic – effects.[103] Each of these substances produces alterations in the health of human beings in a peculiar, different, yet determinate manner, so as to preclude the possibility of confounding one with another.[104]

120

Therefore medicines, on which depend man's life and death, disease and health, must be thoroughly and most carefully distinguished from one another, and for this purpose tested by careful, pure experiments on the healthy body for the purpose of ascertaining their powers and real effects, in order to obtain an accurate knowledge of them, and to enable us to avoid any mistake in their employment in diseases, for it is only by correct selection of them that the greatest of all earthly blessings, the health of the body and of the mind, can be rapidly and permanently restored.

121

In proving medicines to ascertain their effects on the healthy body, it must be borne in mind that the strong, heroic substances, as they are termed, are liable even in small doses to produce changes in the health even of robust persons. Those of milder power must be given for these experiments in more considerable quantities; in order to observe the action of the very weakest, however, the subjects of experiment should be persons free from disease, and who are delicate, irritable and sensitive.

122

In these experiments – on which depends the exactitude of the whole medical art, and the weal of all future generations of mankind – no other medicines should be employed except such as are perfectly well known, and of whose purity, genuineness and energy we are thoroughly assured.

123

Each of these medicines must be taken in a perfectly simple, unadulterated form; the indigenous plants in the form of freshly expressed juice, mixed with a little alcohol to prevent it spoiling; exotic vegetable substances, however, in the form of powder, or tincture prepared with alcohol when they were in the fresh state and afterwards mingled with a certain proportion of water; salts and gums, however, should be dissolved in water just before being taken. If the plant can only be procured in its dry state, and if its powers are naturally weak, in that case there may be used for the experiment an infusion of it, made by cutting the herb into small pieces and pouring boiling water on it, so as to extract its medicinal parts; immediately after its preparation it must be swallowed while still warm, as all expressed vegetable juices and all aqueous infusions of herbs, without the addition of spirit, pass rapidly into fermentation and decomposition, whereby all their medicinal properties are lost.

124

For these experiments every medicinal substance must be employed quite alone and perfectly pure, without the admixture of any foreign substance, and without taking anything else of a medicinal nature the same day, nor yet on the subsequent days, nor during all the time we wish to observe the effects of the medicine.

125

During all the time the experiment lasts the diet must be strictly regulated; it should be as much as possible destitute of spices, of a purely nutritious and simple character, green vegetables,[105] roots and all salads and herb soups (which, even when most carefully prepared, possess some disturbing medicinal qualities) should be avoided. The drinks are to be those usually partaken of, as little stimulating as possible.[106]

126

The person who is proving the medicine must be pre-eminently trustworthy and conscientious and during the whole time of the experiment avoid all over-exertion of mind and body, all sorts of dissipation and disturbing passions; he should have no urgent business to distract his attention; he must devote himself to careful self-observation and not be disturbed while so engaged; his body must be in what is for him a good state of health, and he must possess a sufficient amount of intelligence to be able to express and describe his sensations in accurate terms.

127

The medicines must be tested on both males and females, in order also to reveal the alterations of the health they produce in the sexual sphere.

128

The most recent observations have shown that medicinal substances, when taken in their crude state by the experimenter for the purpose of testing their peculiar effects, do not exhibit nearly the full amount of the powers that lie hidden in them which they do when they are taken for the same object in high dilutions potentized by proper trituration and succussion, by which simple operations the powers which in their crude state lay hidden, and, as it were, dormant, are developed and roused into activity to an incredible extent. In this manner we now find it best to investigate the medicinal powers even of such substances as are deemed weak, and the plan we adopt is to give to the experimenter, on an empty stomach, daily from four to six very small globules of the thirtieth potency of such a substance, moistened with a little water or dissolved in more or less water and thoroughly mixed, and let him continue this for several days.

129

If the effects that result from such a dose are but slight, a few more globules may be taken daily, until they become more distinct and stronger and the alterations of the health more conspicuous; for all persons are not effected by a medicine in an equally great degree; on the contrary, there is a vast variety in this respect, so that sometimes an apparently weak individual may by scarcely at all affected by moderate doses of a medicine known to be of a powerful character, while he is strongly enough acted on by others of a much weaker kind. And, on the other hand, there are very robust persons who experience very considerable morbid symptoms from an apparently mild medicine, and only slighter symptoms from stronger drugs. Now, as this cannot be known beforehand, it is advisable to commence in every instance with a small dose of the drug and, where suitable and requisite, to increase the dose more and more from day to day.

130

If, at the very commencement, the first dose administered shall have been sufficiently strong, this advantage is gained, that the experimenter learns the order of succession of the symptoms and can note down accurately the period at which each occurs, which is very useful in leading to a knowledge of the genius of the medicine, for then the order of the primary actions, as also that of the alternating actions, is observed in the most unambiguous manner. A very moderate dose, even, often suffices for the experiment, provided only the experimenter is endowed with sufficiently delicate sensitiveness, and is very attentive to his sensations. The duration of the action of a drug can only be ascertained by a comparison of several experiments.

131

If, however, in order to ascertain anything at all, the same medicine must be given to the same person to test for several successive days in ever increasing doses, we thereby learn, no doubt, the various morbid states this medicine is capable of producing in a general manner, but we do not ascertain their order of succession; and the subsequent dose often removes, curatively, some one or other of the symptoms caused by the previous dose, or develops in its stead an opposite state; such symptoms should be enclosed in brackets, to mark their ambiguity, until subsequent purer experiments show whether they are the reaction of the organism and secondary action or an alternating action of this medicine.

132

But when the object is, without reference to the sequential order of the phenomena and the duration of the action of the drug, only to ascertain the symptoms themselves, especially those of a weak medicinal substance, in that case the preferable course to pursue is to give it for several successive days, increasing the dose every day. In this manner the action of an unknown medicine, even of the mildest nature, will be revealed, especially if tested on sensitive persons.

133

On experiencing any particular sensation from the medicine, it is useful, indeed necessary, in order to determine the exact character of the symptom, to assume various positions while it lasts, and to observe whether, by moving the part affected, by walking in the room or the open air, by standing, sitting or lying the symptom is increased, diminished or removed, and whether it returns on again assuming the position in which it was first observed, – whether it is altered by eating or drinking, or by any other condition, or by speaking, coughing, sneezing or any other action of the body, and at the same time to note at what time of the day or night

it usually occurs in the most marked manner, whereby what is peculiar to and characteristic of
each symptom will become apparent.

134

All external influences, and more especially medicines, possess the property of producing
in the health of the living organism a particular kind of alteration peculiar to themselves; but
all the symptoms peculiar to a medicine do not appear in one person, nor all at once, nor in
the same experiment, but some occur in one person chiefly at one time, others again during
a second or third trail; in another person some other symptoms appear, but in such a manner
that probably some of the phenomena are observed in the fourth, eighth or tenth person which
had already appeared in the second, sixth or ninth person, and so forth; moreover, they may
not recur at the same hour.

135

The whole of the elements of disease a medicine is capable of producing can only be brought
to anything like completeness by numerous observations on suitable persons of both sexes and
of various constitutions. We can only be assured that a medicine has been thoroughly proved in
regard to the morbid states it can produce – that is to say, in regard to its pure powers of altering
the health of man – when subsequent experimenters can notice little of a novel character from
its action, and almost always only the same symptoms as had been already observed by others.

136

Although, as has been said, a medicine, on being proved on healthy subjects, cannot develop
in one person all the alterations of health it is capable of causing, but can only do this when
given to many different individuals, varying in their corporeal and mental constitution, yet the
tendency to excite all these symptoms in every human being exists in it (117), according to
an eternal and immutable law of nature, by virtue of which all its effects, even those that are
but rarely developed in the healthy person, are brought into operation in the case of every
individual if administered to him when he is in a morbid state presenting similar symptoms;
it then, even in the smallest dose, being homoeopathically selected, silently produces in the
patient an artificial state closely resembling the natural disease, which rapidly and permanently
(homoeopathically) frees and cures him of his original malady.

137

The more moderate, within certain limits, the doses of the medicine used for such experiments are – provided we endeavor to facilitate the observation by the selection of a person who
is a lover of truth, temperate in all respects, of delicate feelings, and who can direct the most
minute attention to his sensation – so much the more distinctly are the primary effects developed, and only these, which are most worth knowing, occur without any admixture of secondary
effects or reactions of the vital force. When, however, excessively large doses are used there
occur at the same time not only a number of secondary effects among the symptoms, but the
primary effects developed, and only these, which are most worth knowing, occur without any
admixture of secondary effects or reactions of the vital force. When, however, excessively large
doses are used there occur at the same time not only a number of secondary effects among the
symptoms, but the primary effects also come on in such hurried confusion and with such im-
petuosity that nothing can be accurately observed; let alone the danger attending them, which
no one who has any regard for his fellow-creatures, and who looks on the meanest of mankind
as his brother, will deem an indifferent manner.

138

All the sufferings, accidents and changes of the health of the experimenter during the action
of a medicine (provided the above condition (124-127) essential to a good and pure experiment

are complied with) are solely derived from this medicine, and must be regarded and registered as belonging peculiarly to this medicine, as symptoms of this medicine, even though the experimenter had observed, a considerable time previously, the spontaneous occurrence of similar phenomena in himself. The reappearance of these during the trial of the medicine only shows that this individual is, by virtue of his peculiar constitution, particularly disposed to have such symptoms excited in him. In this case they are the effect of the medicine; the symptoms do not arise spontaneously while the medicine that has been taken is exercising an influence over the health of the whole system, but are produced by the medicine.

139

When the physician does not make the trial of the medicine on himself, but gives it to another person, the latter must note down distinctly the sensations, sufferings, accidents and changes of health he experiences at the time of their occurrence, mentioning the time after the ingestion of the drug when each symptom arose and, if it lasts long, the period of its duration. The physician looks over the report in the presence of the experimenter immediately after the experiment is concluded, or if the trial lasts several days he does this every day, in order, while everything is still fresh in his memory, to question him about the exact nature of every one of these circumstances, and to write down the more precise details so elicited, or to make such alterations as the experimenter may suggest.[107]

140

If the person cannot write, the physician must be informed by him every day of what has occurred to him, and how it took place. What is noted down as authentic information on this point, however, must be chiefly the voluntary narration of the person who makes the experiment, nothing conjectural and as little as possible derived from answers to leading questions should be admitted; everything must be ascertained with the same caution as I have counselled above (84-99) for the investigation of the phenomena and for tracing the picture of natural diseases.

141

But the best provings of the pure effects of simple medicines in altering the human health, and of the artificial diseases and symptoms they are capable of developing in the healthy individual, are those which the healthy, unprejudiced and sensitive physician institutes on himself with all the caution and care here enjoined. He knows with the greatest certainty the things he has experienced in his own person.[108]

142

But how some symptoms[109] of the simple medicine employed for a curative purpose can be distinguished amongst the symptoms of the original malady, even in diseases, especially in those of a chronic character that usually remain unaltered, is a subject appertaining to the higher art of judgement, and must be left exclusively to masters in observation.

143

If we have thus tested on the healthy individual a considerable number of simple medicines and carefully and faithfully registered all the disease elements and symptoms they are capable of developing as artificial disease-producers, then only have we a true materia medica – a collection of real, pure, reliable[110] modes of action of simple medicinal substances, a volume of the book of nature, wherein is recorded a considerable array of the peculiar changes of the health and symptoms ascertained to belong to each of the powerful medicines, as they were revealed to the attention of the observer, in which the likeness of the (homoeopathic) disease elements of many natural diseases to be hereafter cured by them are present, which, in a word, contain artificial morbid states, that furnish for the similar natural morbid states the only true, homoeopathic, that is to say, specific, therapeutic instruments for effecting their certain and permanent cure.

144

From such a materia medica everything that is conjectural, all that is mere assertion or imaginary should be strictly excluded; everything should be the pure language of nature carefully and honestly interrogated.

145

Of a truth, it is only by a very considerable store of medicines accurately known in respect of these their pure modes of action in altering the health of man, that we can be placed in a position to discover a homoeopathic remedy, a suitable artificial (curative) morbific analogue for each of the infinitely numerous morbid states in nature, for every malady in the world.[111] In the meantime, even now – thanks to the truthful character of the symptoms, and to the abundance of disease elements which every one of the powerful medicinal substances has already shown in its action on the healthy body – but few disease remain, for which a tolerably suitable homoeopathic remedy may not be met with among those now proved as to their pure action,[112] which, without much disturbance, restores health in a gentle, sure and permanent manner – infinitely more surely and safely than can be effected by all the general and special therapeutics of the old allopathic medical art with its unknown composite remedies, which do but alter and aggravate but cannot cure chronic diseases, and rather retard than promote recovery from acute diseases and frequently endanger life.

146

The third point of the business of a true physician relates to the judicious employment of the artificial morbific agents (medicines) that have been proved on healthy individuals to ascertain their pure action in order to effect the homoeopathic cure of natural diseases.

147

Whichever of these medicines that have been investigated as to their power of altering man's health we find to contain in the symptoms observed from its use the greatest similarity to the totality of the symptoms of a given natural disease, this medicine will and must be the most suitable, the most certain homoeopathic remedy for the disease; in it is found the specific remedy of this case of disease.

148

The natural disease is never to be considered as a noxious material situated somewhere within the interior or exterior of man (11-13) but as one produced by an inimical spirit-like (conceptual) agency which, like a kind of infection (note to 11) disturbs in its instinctive existence of the spirit-like (conceptual) principle of life within the organism torturing it as an evil spirit and compelling it to produce certain ailments and disorders in the regular course of its life. These are known as symptoms (disease). If, now, the influence of this inimical agency that not only caused but strives to continue this disorder, be taken away as is done when the physician administers an artificial potency, capable of altering the life principle in the most similar manner (a homoeopathic medicine) which exceeds in energy even in the smallest dose the similar natural disease (33, 279), then the influence of the original noxious morbid agent on the life principle is lost during the action of this stronger similar artificial disease. Thence the evil no longer exists for the life principle – it is destroyed. If, as has been said, the selected homoeopathic remedy is administered properly, then the acute natural disease which is to be overruled if recently developed, will disappear imperceptibly in a few hours.

An older, more chronic disease will yield somewhat later together with all traces of discomfort, by the use of several doses of the same more highly potentized remedy or after careful selection[113] of one or another more similar homoeopathic medicine. Health, recovery, follow in imperceptible, often rapid transitions. The life principle is freed again and capable of resuming the life of the organism in health as before and strength returns.

Diseases of long standing (and especially such as are of a complicated character) require for their cure a proportionately longer time. More especially do the chronic medicinal dyscrasia so often produced by allopathic bungling along with the natural disease left uncured by it, require a much longer time for their recovery; often, indeed, are they incurable, in consequence of the shameful robbery of the patient's strength and juices (venesections, purgatives, etc.), on account of long continued use of large doses of violently acting remedies given on the basis of empty, false theories for alleged usefulness in cases of disease appearing similar, also in prescribing unsuitable mineral baths, etc., the principal feat performed by allopathy in its so-called methods of treatment.

150

If a patient complain of one or more trivial symptoms, that have been only observed a short time previously, the physician should not regard this as a fully developed disease but requires serious medical aid. A slight alteration in the diet and regimen will usually suffice to dispel such an indisposition.

151

But if the patient complain of a few violent sufferings, the physician will usually find, on investigation, several other symptoms besides, although of a slighter character, which furnish a complete picture of the disease.

152

The worse of the acute disease is, of so much the more numerous and striking symptoms is it generally composed, but with so much the more certainly may a suitable remedy for it be found, if there be a sufficient number of medicines known, with respect to their positive action, to choose from. Among the lists of symptoms of many medicines it will not be difficult to find one from whose separate disease elements an antitype of curative artificial disease, very like the totality of the symptoms of the natural disease, may be constructed, and such a medicine is the desired remedy.

153

In this search for a homoeopathic specific remedy, that is to say, in this comparison of the collective symptoms of the natural disease with the list of symptoms of known medicines, in order to find among these an artificial morbific agent corresponding by similarity to the disease to be cured, the more striking, singular, uncommon and peculiar (characteristic) signs and symptoms[114] of the case of disease are chiefly and most solely to be kept in view; for it is more particularly these that very similar ones in the list of symptoms of the selected medicine must correspond to, in order to constitute it the most suitable for effecting the cure. The more general and undefined symptoms: loss of appetite, headache, debility, restless sleep, discomfort, and so forth, demand but little attention when of that vague and indefinite character, if they cannot be more accurately described, as symptoms of such a general nature are observed in almost every disease and from almost every drug.

154

If the antitype constructed from the list of symptoms of the most suitable medicine contain those peculiar, uncommon, singular and distinguishing (characteristic) symptoms, which are to be met with in the disease to be cured in the greatest number and in the greatest similarity, this medicine is the most appropriate homoeopathic specific remedy for this morbid state; the disease, if it be not one of very long standing, will generally be removed and extinguished by the first dose of it, without any considerable disturbance.

I say without any considerable disturbance. For in the employment of this most appropriate homoeopathic remedy it is only the symptoms of the medicine that correspond to the symptoms of the disease that are called into play, the former occupying the place of the latter (weaker) in the organism, i.e., in the sensation of the life principle, and thereby annihilating them by overpowering them; but the other symptoms of the homoeopathic medicine, which are often very numerous, being in no way applicable to the case of disease in question, are not called into play at all. The patient, growing hourly better, feels almost nothing of them at all, because the excessively minute dose requisite for homoeopathic use is much too weak to produce the other symptoms of the medicine that are not homoeopathic to the case, in those parts of the body that are free from disease, and consequently can allow only the homoeopathic symptoms to act on the parts of the organism that are already most irritated and excited by the similar symptoms of the disease, in order that the sick life principle may react only to a similar but stronger medicinal disease, whereby the original malady is extinguished.

156

There is, however, almost no homoeopathic medicine, be it ever so suitably chosen, that, especially if it should be given in an insufficiently minute dose, will not produce, in very irritable and sensitive patients, at least one trifling, unusual disturbance, some slight new symptom while its action lasts; for it is next to impossible that medicine and disease should cover one another symptomatically as exactly as two triangles with equal sides and equal angles. But this (in ordinary circumstances) unimportant difference will be easily done away with by the potential activity (energy) of the living organism, and is not perceptible by patients not excessively delicate; the restoration goes forward, notwithstanding, to the goal of perfect recovery, if it be not prevented by the action of heterogeneous medicinal influences upon the patient, by errors of regimen or by excitement of the passions.

157

But though it is certain that a homoeopathically selected remedy does, by reason of its appropriateness and the minuteness of the dose, gently remove and annihilate the acute disease analogous to it, without manifesting its other unhomoeopathic symptoms, that is to say, without the production of new, serious disturbances, yet it usually, immediately after ingestion – for the first hour, or for a few hours – causes a kind of slight aggravation when the dose has not been sufficiently small and (where the dose has been somewhat too large, however, for a considerable number of hours), which has so much resemblance to the original disease that it seems to the patient to be an aggravation of his own disease. But it is, in reality, nothing more than an extremely similar medicinal disease, somewhat exceeding in strength the original affection.

158

This slight homoeopathic aggravation during the first hours – a very good prognostic that the acute disease will most probably yield to the first dose – is quite as it ought to be, as the medicinal disease must naturally be somewhat stronger than the malady to be cured if it is to overpower and extinguish the latter, just as a natural disease can remove and annihilate another one similar to it only when it is stronger than the latter (43 – 48).

159

The smaller the dose of the homoeopathic remedy is in the treatment of acute diseases so much the slighter and shorter is the apparent increase of the disease during the first hours.

160

But as the dose of a homoeopathic remedy can scarcely ever be made so small that it shall not be able to relieve, overpower, indeed completely cure and annihilate the uncomplicated natural disease of not long standing that is analogous to it (249, note), we can understand why a does of an appropriate homoeopathic medicine, not the very smallest possible, does always, during the first hour after its ingestion, produce a perceptible homoeopathic aggravation of this kind.[115]

161

When I here limit the so-called homoeopathic aggravation, or rather the primary action of the homoeopathic medicine that seems to increase somewhat the symptoms of the original disease, to the first or few hours, this is certainly true with respect to diseases of a more acute character and of recent origin, but where medicines of long action have to combat a malady of, considerable or of very long standing, where no such apparent increase of the original disease ought to appear during treatment and it does not so appear if the accurately chosen medicine was given in proper small, gradually higher doses, each somewhat modified with renewed dynamization (247). Such increase of the original symptoms of a chronic disease can appear only at the end of treatment when the cure is almost or quite finished.

162

Sometimes happens, owing to the moderate number of medicines yet known with respect to their true, pure action , that but a portion of the symptoms of the disease under treatment are to be met with in the list of symptoms of the most appropriate medicine, consequently this imperfect medicinal morbific agent must be employed for lack of a more perfect one.

163

In this case we cannot indeed expect from this medicine a complete, untroubled cure; for during its use some symptoms appear which were not previously observable in the disease, accessory symptoms of the not perfectly appropriate remedy. This does by no means prevent a considerable part of the disease (the symptoms of the disease that resemble those of the medicine) from being eradicated by this medicine, thereby establishing a fair commencement of the cure, but still this does not take place without those accessory symptoms, which are, however, always moderate when the dose of the medicine is sufficiently minute.

164

The small number of homoeopathic symptoms present in the best selected medicine is no obstacle to the cure in cases where these few medicinal symptoms are chiefly of an uncommon kind and such as are peculiarly distinctive (characteristic) of the disease; the cure takes place under such circumstances without any particular disturbance.

165

If, however, among the symptoms of the remedy selected, there be none that accurately resemble the distinctive (characteristic), peculiar, uncommon symptoms of the case of disease, and if the remedy correspond to the disease only in the general, vaguely described, indefinite states (nausea, debility, headache, and so forth), and if there be among the known medicines none more homoeopathically appropriate, in that case the physician cannot promise himself any immediate favorable result from the employment of this unhomoeopathic medicine.

166

Such a case is, however, very rare, owing to the increased number of medicines whose pure effects are now known, and the bad effects resulting from it, when they do occur, are diminished whenever a subsequent medicine, of more accurate resemblance, can be selected.

167

Thus if there occur, during the use of this imperfectly homoeopathic remedy first employed, accessory symptoms of some moment, then, in the case of acute diseases, we do not allow

69

this first dose to exhaust its action, nor leave the patient to the full duration of the action of the remedy, but we investigate afresh the morbid state in its now altered condition, and add the remainder of the original symptoms to those newly developed in tracing a new picture of the disease.

168

We shall then be able much more readily to discover, among the known medicines, an analogue to the morbid state before us, a single dose of which, if it do not entirely destroy the disease, will advance it considerably on the way to be cured. And thus we go on, if even this medicine be not quite sufficient to effect the restoration of health, examining again and again the morbid state that still remains, and selecting a homoeopathic medicine as suitable as possible for it, until our object, namely, putting the patient in the possession of perfect health, is accomplished.

169

If, on the first examination of a disease and the first selection of a medicine, we should find that the totality of the symptoms of the disease would not be effectually covered by the disease elements of a single medicine – owing to the insufficient number of known medicines, – but that two medicines contend for the preference in point of appropriateness, one of which is more homoeopathically suitable for one part, the other for another part of the symptoms of the disease, it is not advisable, after the employment of the more suitable of the two medicines, to administer the other without fresh examination, and much less to give both together (272, note) for the medicine that seemed to be the next best would not, under the change of circumstances that has in the meantime taken place, be suitable for the rest of the symptoms that then remain; in which case, consequently, a more appropriate homoeopathic remedy must be selected in place of the second medicine for the set of symptoms as they appear on a new inspection.

170

Hence in this as in every case where a change of the morbid state has occurred, the remaining set of symptoms now present must be inquired into, and (without paying any attention to the medicine which at first appeared to be the next in point of suitableness) another homoeopathic medicine, as appropriate as possible to the new state now before us, must be selected. If it should so happen, as is not often the case, that the medicine which at first appeared to be the next best seems still to be well adapted for the morbid state that remains, so much the more will it merit our confidence, and deserve to be employed in preference to another.

171

In non-venereal chronic disease, those, therefore, that arise from psora, we often require, in order to effect a cure, to give several antipsoric remedies in succession, every successive one being homoeopathically chosen in consonance with the group of symptoms remaining after completion of the action of the previous remedy.

172

A similar difficulty in the way of the cure occurs from the symptoms of the disease being too few – a circumstances that deserves our careful attention, for by its removal almost all the difficulties that can lie in the way of this most perfect of all possible modes of treatment (except that its apparatus of known homoeopathic medicines is still incomplete) are removed.

173

The only diseases that seem to have but few symptoms, and on that account to be less amenable to cure, are those which may be termed one-sided, because they display only one or two principal symptoms which obscure almost all the others. They belong chiefly to the class of chronic diseases.

174

Their principal symptom may be either an internal complaint (e.g. a headache of many years' duration, a diarrhoea of long standing, an ancient cardialgia, etc.), or it may be an affection more of an external kind. Diseases of the latter character are generally distinguished by the name of local maladies.

175

In one-sided diseases of the first kind it is often to be attributed to the medical observer's want of discernment that he does not fully discover the symptoms actually present which would enable him to complete the sketch of the portrait of the disease.

176

There are, however, still a few diseases, which, after the most careful initial examination (84-98), present but one or two severe, violent symptoms, while all the others are but indistinctly perceptible.

177

In order to meet most successfully such a case as this, which is of very rare occurrence, we are in the first place to select, guided by these few symptoms, the medicine which in our judgment is the most homoeopathically indicated.

178

It will, no doubt, sometimes happen that this medicine, selected in strict observance of the homoeopathic law, furnishes the similar artificial disease suited for the annihilation of the malady present; and this is much more likely to happen when these few morbid symptoms are very striking, decided, uncommon and peculiarly distinctive (characteristic).

179

More frequently, however, the medicine first chosen in such a case will be only partially, that is to say, not exactly suitable, as there was no considerable number of symptoms to guide to an accurate selection.

180

In this case the medicine, which has been chosen as well as was possible, but which, for the reason above stated, is only imperfectly homoeopathic, will, in its action upon the disease that is only partially analogous to it – just as in the case mentioned above (162, et seq.) where the limited number of homoeopathic remedies renders the selection imperfect – produce accessory symptoms, and several phenomena from its own array of symptoms are mixed up with the patient's state of health, which are, however, at the same time, symptoms of the disease itself, although they may have been hitherto never or very rarely perceived; some symptoms which the patient had never previously experienced appear, or others he had only felt indistinctly become more pronounced.

181

Let is not be objected that the accessory phenomena and new symptoms of this disease that now appear should be laid to the account of the medicament just employed. They owe their origin to it[116] certainly, but they are always only symptoms of such a nature as this disease was itself capable of producing in this organism, and which were summoned forth and induced to make their appearance by the medicine given, owing to its power to cause similar symptoms. In a word, we have to regard the whole collection of symptoms now perceptible as belonging to the disease itself, as the actual existing condition, and to direct our further treatment accordingly.

182

Thus the imperfect selection of the medicament, which was in this case almost inevitable owing to the too limited number of the symptoms present, serves to complete the display of the symptoms of the disease, and in this way facilitates the discovery of a second, more accurately suitable, homoeopathic medicine.

183

Whenever, therefore, the dose of the first medicine ceases to have a beneficial effect (if the newly developed symptoms do not, by reason of their gravity, demand more speedy aid – which, however, from the minuteness of the dose of homoeopathic medicine, and in very chronic diseases, is excessively rare), a new examination of the disease must be instituted, the status morbi as it now is must be noted down, and a second homoeopathic remedy selected in accordance with it, which shall exactly suit the present state, and one which shall be all the more appropriate can then be found, as the group of symptoms has become larger and more complete.[117]

184

In like manner, after each new dose of medicine has exhausted its action, when it is no longer suitable and helpful, the state of the disease that still remains is to be noted anew with respect to its remaining symptoms, and another homoeopathic remedy sought for, as suitable as possible for the group of symptoms now observed, and so on until the recovery is complete.

185

Among the one-sided disease an important place is occupied by the so-called local maladies, by which term is signified those changes and ailments that appear on the external parts of the body. Till now the idea prevalent in the schools was that these parts were alone morbidly affected, and that the rest of the body did not participate in the disease – a theoretical, absurd doctrine, which has led to the most disastrous medical treatment.

186

Those so-called local maladies which have been produced a short time previously, solely by an external lesion, still appear at first sight to deserve the name of local disease. But then the lesion must be very trivial, and in that case it would be of no great moment. For in the case of injuries accruing to the body from without, if they be at all severe, the whole living organism sympathizes; there occur fever, etc. The treatment of such diseases is relegated to surgery; but this is right only in so far as the affected parts require mechanical aid, whereby the external obstacles to the cure, which can only be expected to take place by the agency of the vital force, may be removed by mechanical means, e.g., by the reduction of dislocations, by needles and bandages to bring together the lips of wounds, by mechanical pressure to still the flow of blood from open arteries, by the extraction of foreign bodies that have penetrated into the living parts, by making an opening into a cavity of the body in order to remove an irritating substance or to procure the evacuation of effusions or collections of fluids, by bringing into apposition the broken extremities of a fractured bone and retaining them in exact contact by an appropriate bandage, etc. But when in such injuries the whole living organism requires, as it always does, active dynamic aid to put it in a position to accomplish the work of healing, e.g. when the violent fever resulting from extensive contusions, lacerated muscles, tendons and blood-vessels requires to be removed by medicine given internally, or when the external pain of scalded or burnt parts needs to be homoeopathically subdued, then the services of the dynamic physician and his helpful homoeopathy come into requisition.

187

But those affections, alterations and ailments appearing on the external parts, that do not arise from any external injury or that have only some slight external wound for their immediate exciting cause, are produced in quite another manner; their source lies in some internal malady. To consider them as mere local affections, and at the same time to treat them only, or almost only, as it were surgically, with topical applications – as the old school have done from the remotest ages – is as absurd as it is pernicious in its results.

188

These affections were considered to be merely topical, and were therefore called local diseases, as if they were maladies exclusively limited to those parts wherein the organism took little or no part, or affections of these particular visible parts of which the rest of the living organism, so to speak, knew nothing.[118]

189

And yet very little reflection will suffice to convince us that no external malady (not occasioned by some important injury from without) can arise, persist or even grow worse without some internal cause, without the co-operation of the whole organism, which must consequently be in a diseased state. It could not make its appearance at all without the consent of the whole of the rest of the health, and without the participation of the rest of the living whole (of the vital force that pervades all the other sensitive and irritable parts of the organism); indeed, it is impossible to conceive its production without the instrumentality of the whole (deranged) life; so intimately are all parts of the organism connected together to form an indivisible whole in sensation and functions. No eruption on the lips, no whitlow can occur without previous and simultaneous internal ill-health.

190

All true medical treatment of a disease on the external parts of the body that has occurred from little or no injury from without must, therefore, be directed against the whole, must effect the annihilation and cure of the general malady by means of internal remedies, if it is wished that the treatment should be judicious, sure, efficacious and radical.

191

This is confirmed in the most unambiguous manner by experience, which shows in all cases that every powerful internal medicine immediately after its ingestion causes important changes in the general health of such a patient, and particularly in the affected external parts (which the ordinary medical school regards as quite isolated), even in a so-called local disease of the most external parts of the body, and the change it produces is most salutary, being the restoration to health of the entire body, along with the disappearance of the external affection (without the aid of any external remedy), provided the internal remedy directed towards the whole state was suitable chosen in a homoeopathic sense.

192

This is best effected when, in the investigation of the case of disease, along with the exact character of the local affection, all the changes, sufferings and symptoms observable in the patient's health, and which may have been previously noticed when no medicines had been used, are taken in conjunction to form a complete picture of the disease before searching among the medicines, whose peculiar pathogenetic effects are known, for a remedy corresponding to the totality of the symptoms, so that the selection may be truly homoeopathic.

193

By means of this medicine, employed only internally (and, if the disease be but of recent origin, often by the very first dose of it), the general morbid state of the body is removed along with the local affection, and the latter is cured at the same time as the former, proving that the local affection depended solely on a disease of the rest of the body, and should only be regarded as an inseparable part of the whole, as one of the most considerable and striking symptoms of the whole disease.

194

It is not useful, either in acute local diseases of recent origin or in local affections that have already existed a long time, to rub in or apply externally to the spot an external remedy, even though it be the specific and, when used internally, salutary by reason of its homoeopathicity, even although it should be at the same time administered internally; for the acute topical affections (e.g., inflammations of the individual parts, erysipelas, etc.), which have not been caused by external injury of proportionate violence, but by dynamic or internal causes, yield most surely to internal remedies homoeopathically adapted to the perceptible state of the health present in the exterior and interior, selected from the general store of proved medicines,[119] and generally without any other aid; but if these diseases do not yield to them completely, and if there still remain in the affected spot and in the whole state, notwithstanding good regimen, a relic of disease which the vital force is not competent to restore to the normal state, then the acute disease was (as not infrequently happens) a product of psora which had hitherto remained latent in the interior, but has now burst forth and is on the point of developing into a palpable chronic disease.

195

In order to effect a radical cure in such cases, which are by no means rare, after the acute state has pretty well subsided, an appropriate antipsoric treatment (as is taught in my work on Chronic Diseases) must then be directed against the symptoms that still remain and the morbid state of health to which the patient was previously subject. In chronic local maladies that are not obviously venereal, the antipsoric internal treatment is, moreover, alone requisite.

196

It might, indeed, seen as though the cure of such diseases would be hastened by employing the medicinal substance which is known to be truly homoeopathic to the totality of the symptoms, not only internally, but also externally, because the action of a medicine applied to the seat of the local affection might effect a more rapid change in it.

197

This treatment, however, is quite inadmissible, not only for the local symptoms arising from the miasm of psora, but also and especially for those originating in the miasm of syphilis or sycosis, for the simultaneous local application, along with the internal employment, of the remedy in diseases whose chief symptom is a constant local affection, has this great disadvantage, that, by such a topical application, this chief symptom (local affection)[120] will usually be annihilated sooner than the internal disease, and we shall now be deceived by the semblance of a perfect cure; or at least it will be difficult, and in some cases impossible, to determine, from the premature disappearance of the local symptom, if the general disease is destroyed by the simultaneous employment of the internal medicine.

198

The mere topical employment of medicines, that are powerful for cure when given internally, to the local symptoms of chronic miasmatic diseases is for the same reason quite inadmissible; for if the local affection of the chronic disease be only removed locally and in a one-sided manner, the internal treatment indispensable for the complete restoration of the health remains in dubious obscurity; the chief symptom (the local affection) is gone, and there remain only the other, less distinguishable symptoms, which are less constant and less persistent than the local affection, and frequently not sufficiently peculiar and too slightly characteristic to display after that, a picture of the disease in clear and peculiar outlines.

199

If the remedy perfectly homoeopathic to the disease had not yet been discovered[121] at the time when the local symptoms were destroyed by a corrosive or desiccative external remedy or by the knife, then the case becomes much more difficult on account of the too indefinite (uncharacteristic) and inconstant appearance of the remaining symptoms; for what might have contributed most to determine the selection of the most suitable remedy, and its internal employment until the disease should have been completely annihilated, namely, the external principal symptom, has been removed from our observation.

200

Had it still been present to guide the internal treatment, the homoeopathic remedy for the whole disease might have been discovered, and had that been found, the persistence of the local affection during its internal employment would have shown that the cure was not yet completed; but were it cured on its seat, this would be a convincing proof that the disease was completely eradicated, and the desired recovery from the entire disease was fully accomplished – an inestimable, indispensable advantage to reach a perfect cure.

201

It is evident that man's vital force, when encumbered with a chronic disease which it is unable to overcome by its own powers instinctively, adopts the plan of developing a local malady on some external part, solely for this object, that by making and keeping in a diseased state this part which is not indispensable to human life, it may thereby silence the internal disease, which otherwise threatens to destroy the vital organs (and to deprive the patient of life), and that it may thereby, so to speak, transfer the internal disease to the vicarious local affection and, as it were, draw it thither. The presence of the local affection thus silences, for a time, the internal disease, though without being able either to cure it or to diminish it materially.[122] The local affection, however, is never anything else than a part of the general disease, but a part of it increased all in one direction by the organic vital force, and transferred to a less dangerous (external) part of the body, in order to allay the internal ailment. But (as has been said) by this local symptom that silences the internal disease, so far from anything being gained by the vital force towards diminishing or curing the whole malady, the internal disease, on the contrary, continues, in spite of it, gradually to increase and Nature is constrained to enlarge and aggravate the local symptom always more and more, in order that it may still suffice as a substitute for the increased internal disease and may still keep it under. Old ulcers on the legs get worse as long as the internal psora is uncured, the chancre enlarges as long as the internal syphilis remains uncured, the fig warts increased and grow while the sycosis is not cured whereby the latter is rendered more and more difficult to cure, just as the general internal disease continues to increase as time goes on.

202

If the old-school physician should now destroy the local symptom by the topical application of external remedies, under the belief that he thereby cures the whole disease, Nature makes up for its loss by rousing the internal malady and the other symptoms that previously existed in a latent state side by side with the local affection; that is to say, she increases the internal disease. When this occurs it is usual to say, though incorrectly that the local affection has been driven back into the system or upon the nerves by the external remedies.

203

Every external treatment of such local symptoms, the object of which is to remove them from the surface of the body, while the internal miasmatic disease is left uncured, as, for instance, driving off the skin the psoric eruption by all sorts of ointments, burning away the chancre by caustics and destroying the condylomata on their seat by the knife, the ligature or the actual cautery; this pernicious external mode of treatment, hitherto so universally practised, has been the most prolific source of all the innumerable named or unnamed chronic maladies under which mankind groans; it is one of the most criminal procedures the medical world can be guilty of, and yet it has hitherto been the one generally adopted, and taught from the professional chairs as the only one.[123]

204

If we deduct all chronic affections, ailments and diseases that depend on a persistent unhealthy mode of living, (77) as also those innumerable medicinal maladies (v. 74) caused by the irrational, persistent, harassing and pernicious treatment of diseases often only of trivial character by physicians of the old school, most the remainder of chronic diseases result from the development of these three chronic miasms, internal syphilis, internal sycosis, but chiefly and in infinitely greater proportion, internal psora, each of which was already in possession of the whole organism, and had penetrated it in all directions before the appearance of the primary, vicarious local symptom of each of them (in the case of psora the scabious eruption, in syphilis the chancre or the bubo, and in sycosis the condylomata) that prevented their outburst; and these chronic miasmatic diseases, if deprived of their local symptom, are inevitably destined by mighty Nature sooner or later to become developed and to burst forth, and thereby propagate all the nameless misery, the incredible number of chronic diseases which have plagued mankind for hundreds and thousands of years, none of which would so frequently have come into existence had physicians striven in a rational manner to cure radically and to extinguish in the organism these three miasms by the internal homoeopathic medicines suited for each of them, without employing topical remedies for their external symptoms. (See note to 282).

205

The homoeopathic physician never treats one of these primary symptoms of chronic miasms, nor yet one of their secondary affections that result from their further development, by local remedies (neither by those external agents that act dynamically,[124] nor yet by those that act mechanically), but he cures, in cases where the one or the other appears, only the great miasm on which they depend, whereupon its primary, as also its secondary symptoms disappear spontaneously; but as this was not the mode pursued by the old-school practitioners who preceded him in the treatment of the case, the homoeopathic physician generally, alas!, finds that the primary symptoms[125] have already been destroyed by them by means of external remedies, and that he has now to do more with the secondary ones, i.e., the affections resulting from the breaking forth and development of these inherent miasms, but especially with the chronic disease evolved from internal psora, the internal treatment of which, as far as a single physician can elucidate it by many years of reflection, observation and experience, I have endeavored to point out in my work on Chronic Diseases, to which I must refer the reader.

206

Before commencing the treatment of a chronic disease, it is necessary to make the most careful investigation[126] as to whether the patient has had a venereal infection (or an infection with condylomatous gonorrhoea); for then the treatment must be directed towards this alone, when only the signs of syphilis (or of the rarer condylomatous disease) are present, but this disease is very seldom met with alone nowadays. If such infection have previously occurred, this must also be borne in mind in the treatment of those cases in which psora is present, because in them the latter is complicated with the former, as is always the case when the symptoms are not those of pure syphilis; for when the physician thinks he has a case of old venereal disease before him, he has always, or almost always, to treat a syphilitic affection accompanied mostly by (complicated with) psora, for the internal itch dyscrasia (the psora) is far the most frequent fundamental cause of chronic diseases. At times, both miasms may be complicated also with sycosis in chronically diseased organisms, or, as is much more frequently the case, psora is the sole fundamental cause of all other chronic maladies, whatever names they may bear, which are, moreover, so often bungled, increased and disfigured to a monstrous extent by allopathic unskillfulness.

207

When the above information has been gained, it still remains for the homoeopathic physician to ascertain what kinds of allopathic treatment had up to that date been adopted for the chronic disease, what perturbing medicines had been chiefly and most frequently employed, also what mineral baths had been used and what effects these had produced, in order to understand in some measure the degeneration of the disease from its original state, and, where possible, to correct in part these pernicious artificial operations, or to enable him to avoid the employment of medicines that have already been improperly used.

208

The age of the patient, his mode of living and diet, his occupation, his domestic position, his social relation and so forth, must next be taken into consideration, in order to ascertain whether these things have tended to increase his malady, or in how far they may favor or hinder the treatment. In like manner the state of his disposition and mind must be attended to, to learn whether that presents any obstacles to the treatment, or requires to be directed encouraged or modified.

209

After this is done, the physician should endeavor in repeated conversations with the patient to trace the picture of his disease as completely as possible, according to the directions given above, in order to be able to elucidate the most striking and peculiar (characteristic) symptoms, in accordance with which he selects the first antipsoric or other remedy having the greatest symptomatic resemblance, for the commencement of the treatment, and so forth.

210

Of psoric origin are almost all those diseases that I have above termed one-sided, which appear to be more difficult to cure in consequence of this one-sidedness, all their other morbid symptoms disappearing, as it were, before the single, great, prominent symptom. Of this character are what are termed mental diseases. They do not, however, constitute a class of disease the condition of the disposition and mind is always altered;[127] and in all cases of disease we are called on to cure the state of the patient's disposition is to be particularly noted, along with the totality of the symptoms, if we would trace an accurate picture of the disease, in order to be able therefrom to treat it homoeopathically with success.

211

This holds good to such an extent, that the state of the disposition of the patient often chiefly determines the selection of the homoeopathic remedy, as being a decidedly characteristic symptom which can least of all remain concealed from the accurately observing physician.

212

The Creator of therapeutic agents has also had particular regard to this main feature of all diseases, the altered state of the disposition and mind, for there is no powerful medicinal substance in the world which does not very notably alter the state of the disposition and mind in the healthy individual who tests it, and every medicine does so in a different manner.

213

We shall, therefore, never be able to cure conformably to nature – that is to say, homoeopathically – if we do not, in every case of disease, even in such as are acute, observe, along with the other symptoms, those relating to the changes in the state of the mind and disposition, and if we do not select, for the patient's relief, from among the medicines a disease-force which, in addition to the similarity of its other symptoms to those of the disease, is also capable of producing a similar state of the disposition and mind.[128]

214

The instructions I have to give relative to the cure of mental diseases may be confined to a very few remarks, as they are to be cured in the same way as all other diseases, namely, by a remedy which shows, by the symptoms it causes in the body and mind of a healthy individual, a power of producing a morbid state as similar as possible to the case of disease before us, and in no other way can they be cured.

215

Almost all the so-called mental and emotional diseases are nothing more than corporeal diseases in which the symptom of derangement of the mind and disposition peculiar to each of them is increased, while the corporeal symptoms decline (more or less rapidly), till it a length attains the most striking one-sidedness, almost as though it were a local disease in the invisible subtle organ of the mind or disposition.

216

The cases are not rare in which a so-called corporeal disease that threatens to be fatal – a suppuration of the lungs, or the deterioration of some other important viscus, or some other disease of acute character, e.g., in childbed, etc. – becomes transformed into insanity, into a kind of melancholia or into mania by a rapid increase of the psychical symptoms that were previously present, whereupon the corporeal symptoms lose all their danger; these latter improve almost to perfect health, or rather they decrease to such a degree that their obscured presence can only be detected by the observation of a physician gifted with perseverance and penetration. In this manner they become transformed into a one-sided and, as it were, a local disease, in which the symptom of the mental disturbance, which was at first but slight, increases so as to be the chief symptom, and in a great measure occupies the place of the other (corporeal) symptoms, whose intensity it subdues in a palliative manner, so that, in short, the affections of the grosser corporeal organs become, as it were, transferred and conducted to the almost spiritual, mental and emotional organs, which the anatomist has never yet and never will reach with his scalpel.

217

In these diseases we must be very careful to make ourselves acquainted with the whole of the phenomena, both those belonging to the corporeal symptoms, and also, and indeed particularly, those appertaining to the accurate apprehension of the precise character of the chief symptom, of the peculiar and always predominating state of the mind and disposition, in order to discover, for the purpose of extinguishing the entire disease, among the remedies whose pure effects are known, a homoeopathic medicinal pathogenetic force – that is to say, a remedy which in its list of symptoms displays, with the greatest possible similarity, not only the corporeal morbid symptoms present in the case of disease before us, but also especially this mental and emotional state.

218

To this collection of symptoms belongs in the first place to accurate description of all the phenomena of the previous so-called corporeal disease, before it degenerated into a one-sided increase of the physical symptom, and became a disease of the mind and disposition. This may be learned from the report of the patient's friends.

219

A comparison of these previous symptoms of the corporeal disease with the traces of them that still remain, though they have become less perceptible (but which even now sometimes become prominent, when a lucid interval and a transient alleviation of the psychical disease occurs), will serve to prove them to be still present, though obscured.

220

By adding to this the state of the mind and disposition accurately observed by the patient's friends and by the physician himself, we have thus constructed the complete picture of the disease, for which in order to effect the homoeopathic cure of the disease, a medicine capable of producing strikingly similar symptoms, and especially an analogous disorder of the mind, must be sought for among the antipsoric remedies, if the physical disease have already lasted some time.

221

If, however, insanity or mania (caused by fright, vexation, the abuse of spirituous liquors, etc.) have suddenly broken out as an acute disease in the patient's ordinary calm state, although it almost always arises from internal psora, like a flame bursting forth from it, yet when it occurs in this acute manner it should not be immediately treated with antipsoric, but in the first place with remedies indicated for it out of the order class of proved medicaments (e.g., aconite, belladonna, stramonium, hyoscyamus, mercury, etc.) in highly potentized, minute, homoeopathic doses, in order to subdue it so far that the psora shall for the time revert to its former latent state, wherein the patient appears as if quite well.

222

But such a patient, who has recovered from an acute mental or emotional disease by the use of these non-antipsoric medicines, should never be regarded as cured; on the contrary, no time should be lost in attempting to free him completely,[129] by means of a prolonged antipsoric treatment, from the chronic miasm of the psora, which, it is true, has now become once more latent but is quite ready to break out anew; if this be done, there is no fear of another similar attack, if he attend faithfully to the diet and regimen prescribed for him.

223

But if the antipsoric treatment be omitted, then we may almost assuredly expect, from a much slighter cause than brought on the first attack of the insanity, the speedy occurrence of a new and more lasting the severe fit, during which the psora usually develops itself completely, and passes into either a periodic or continued mental derangement, which is then more difficult to be cured by antipsorics.

224

If the mental disease be not quite developed, and if it be still somewhat doubtful whether it really arose from a corporeal affection, or did not rather result from faults of education, bad practices, corrupt morals, neglect of the mind, superstition or ignorance; the mode of deciding this point will be, that if it proceed from one or other of the latter causes it will diminish and be improved by sensible friendly exhortations, consolatory arguments, serious representations and sensible advice, whereas a real moral or mental malady, depending on bodily disease, would be speedily aggravated by such a course, the melancholic would become still more dejected, querulous, inconsolable and reserved, the spiteful maniac would thereby become still more exasperated, and the chattering fool would become manifestly more foolish.[130]

225

There are, however, as has just been stated, certainly a few emotional diseases which have not merely been developed into that form out of corporeal diseases, but which, in an inverse manner, the body being but slightly indisposed, originate and are kept up by emotional causes, such as continued anxiety, worry, vexation, wrongs and the frequent occurrence of great fear and fright. This kind of emotional diseases in time destroys the corporeal health, often to a great degree.

226

It is only such emotional diseases as these, which were first engendered and subsequently kept up by the mind itself, that, while they are yet recent and before they have made very great inroads on the corporeal state, may, by means of psychical remedies, such as a display of confidence, friendly exhortations, sensible advice, and often by a well-disguised deception, be rapidly changed into a healthy state of the mind (and with appropriate diet and regimen, seemingly into a healthy state of the body also.)

227

But the fundamental cause in these cases also is a psoric miasm, which was only not yet quite near its full development, and for security's sake, the seemingly cured patient should be subjected to a radical, antipsoric treatment, in order that he may not again, as might easily occur, fall into a similar state of mental disease.

228

In mental and emotional diseases resulting from corporeal maladies, which can only be cured by homoeopathic antipsoric medicine conjoined with carefully regulated mode of life, an appropriate psychical behavior towards the patient on the part of those about him and of the physician must be scrupulously observed, by way of an auxiliary mental regimen. To furious mania we must oppose clam intrepidity and cool, firm resolution – to doleful, querulous lamentation, a mute display of commiseration in looks and gestures – to senseless chattering, a silence not wholly inattentive – to disgusting and abominable conduct and to conversation of a similar character, total inattention. We must merely endeavor to prevent the destruction and injury of surrounding objects, without reproaching the patient for his acts, and everything must be arranged in such a way that the necessity for any corporeal punishments and tortures[131] whatever may be avoided. This is so much the more easily effected, because in the administration of the medicine – the only circumstance in which the employment of coercion could be justified – in the homoeopathic system the small doses of the appropriate medicine never offend the taste, and may consequently be given to the patient without his knowledge in his drink, so that all compulsion is unnecessary.

229

On the other hand, contradiction, eager explanations, rude corrections and invectives, as also weak, timorous yielding, are quite out of place with such patients; they are equally pernicious modes of treating mental and emotional maladies. But such patients are most of all exasperated and their complaint aggravated by contumely, fraud, and deceptions that they can detect. The physician and keeper must always pretend to believe them to be possessed of reason.

All kinds of external disturbing influences on their senses and disposition should be if possible removed; there are no amusements for their clouded spirit, no salutary distractions, no means of instruction, no soothing effects from conversation, books or other things for the soul that pines or frets in the chains of the diseased body, no invigoration for it, but the care; it is only when the bodily health is changed for the better that tranquillity and comfort again beam upon their mind.

The treatment of the violent insane manic and melancholic can take place only in an institution specially arranged for their treatment but not within the family circle of the patient.

230

If the antipsoric remedies selected for each particular case of mental or emotional disease (there are incredibly numerous varieties of them) be quite homoeopathically suited for the faithfully traced picture of the morbid state, which, if there be a sufficient number of this kind of medicines known in respect of their pure effects, is ascertained by an indefatigable search for the most appropriate homoeopathic remedy all the more easily, as the emotional and mental state, constituting the principal symptom of such a patient, is so unmistakably perceptible, – then the most striking improvement in no very long time, which could not be brought about by physicking the patient to death with the largest oft – repeated doses of all other unsuitable (allopathic) medicines. Indeed, I can confidently assert, from great experience, that the vast superiority of the homoeopathic system over all other conceivable methods of the treatment is nowhere displayed in a more triumphant light than in mental and emotional diseases of long standing, which originally sprang from corporeal maladies or were developed simultaneously with them.

The intermittent disease deserve a special consideration, as well those that recur at certain periods – like the great number of intermittent fevers, and the apparently non-febrile affections that recur at intervals like intermittent fevers – as also those in which certain morbid states alternate at uncertain intervals with morbid states of a different kind.

These latter, alternating diseases, are also very numerous,[132] but all belong to the class of chronic diseases; they are generally a manifestation of developed psora alone, sometimes, but seldom, complicated with a syphilitic miasm, and therefore in the former case may be cured by antipsoric medicines; in the latter, however, in alternation with antisyphilitics as taught in my work on the Chronic Diseases.

The typical intermittent disease are those where a morbid state of unvarying character returns at a tolerably fixed period, while the patient is apparently in good health, and takes its departure at an equally fixed period; this is observed in those apparently non-febrile morbid states that come and go in a periodical manner (at certain times), as well as in those of a febrile character, to wit, the numerous varieties of intermittent fevers.

Those apparently non-febrile, typical, periodically recurring morbid states just alluded to observed in one single patient at a time (they do not usually appear sporadically or epidemically) always belong to the chronic diseases, mostly to those that are purely psoric, are but seldom complicated with syphilis, and are successfully treated by the same means; yet it is sometimes necessary to employ as an intermediate remedy a small dose of a potentized solution of cinchona bark, in order to extinguish completely their intermittent type.

With regard to the intermittent fevers,[133] that prevail sporadically or epidemically (not those endemically located in marshy districts), we often find every paroxysm likewise composed of two opposite alternating states (cold, heat – heat, cold), more frequently still of three (cold, heat, sweat). Therefore the remedy selected for them from the general class of proved (common, not antipsoric) medicines must either (and remedies of this sort are the surest) be able likewise to produce in the healthy body two (or all three) similar alternating states, or else must correspond by similarity of symptoms, in the most homoeopathic manner possible, to the strongest, best marked, and most peculiar alternating state (either to the cold stage, or to the hot stage, or to the sweating state, each with its accessory symptoms, according as the one or other alternating state is the strongest and most peculiar); but the symptoms of the patient's health during the intervals when he is free from fever must be the chief guide to the most appropriate homoeopathic remedy.[134]

The most appropriate and efficacious time for administering the medicine in these cases is immediately or very soon after the termination of the paroxysm, as soon as the patient has in some degree recovered from its effects; it has then time to effect all the changes in the organism requisite for the restoration of health, without any great disturbance or violent commotion; whereas the action of a medicine, be it ever so specifically appropriate, if given immediately before the paroxysm, coincides with the natural recurrence of the disease and causes such a reaction in the organism, such a violent contention, that an attack of that nature produces at the very least a great loss of strength, if it do not endanger life.[135] But if the medicine be given immediately after the termination of the fit, that is to say, at the period when the apyretic interval has commenced and a long time before there are any preparations for the next paroxysm, then the vital force of the organism is in the best possible condition to allow itself to be quietly altered by the remedy, and thus restored to the healthy state.

237

But if the stage of apyrexia be very short, as happens in some very bad fevers, or if it be disturbed by some of the after sufferings of the previous paroxysm, the dose of the homoeopathic medicine should be administered when the perspiration begins to abate, or the other subsequent phenomena of the expiring paroxysm begin to diminish.

238

Not infrequently, the suitable medicine has with a single dose destroyed several attacks and brought about the return of health, but in the majority of cases, another dose must be administered after such attack. Better still, however, when the character of the symptoms has not changed, doses of the same medicine given according to the newer discovery of repetition of doses (see note to 270), may be given without difficulty in dynamizing each successive dose with 10-12 succussions of the vial containing the medicinal substance. Nevertheless, there are at times cases, though seldom, where the intermittent fever returns after several days' well being. This return of the same fever after a healthy interval is only possible when the noxious principle that first caused the fever, is still acting upon the convalescent, as is the case in marshy regions. Here a permanent restoration can often take place only by getting away from this causative factor, as is possible by seeking a mountainous retreat, if the cause was a marshy fever.

239

As almost every medicine causes in its pure action a special, peculiar fever and even a kind of intermittent fever with its alternating states, differing from all other fevers that are caused by other medicines, homoeopathic remedies may be found in the extensive domain of medicines for all the numerous varieties of natural intermittent fevers and, for a great many of such fevers, even in the moderate collection of medicines already proved on the healthy individual.

240

But if the remedy found to be the homoeopathic specific for a prevalent epidemic of intermittent fever do not effect a perfect cure in some one or other patient, if it be not the influence of a marshy district that prevents the cure, it must always be the psoric miasm in the background, in which case antipsoric medicines must be employed until complete relief is obtained.

241

Epidemics of intermittent fever, in situations where none are endemic, are of the nature of chronic diseases, composed of single acute paroxysms; each single epidemic is of a peculiar, uniform character common to all the individuals attacked, and when this character is found in the totality of the symptoms common to all, it guides us to the discovery of the homoeopathic (specific) remedy suitable for all the cases, which is almost universally serviceable in those patients who enjoyed tolerable health before the occurrence of the epidemic, that is to say, who were not chronic sufferers from developed psora.

242

If, however, in such an epidemic intermittent fever the first paroxysms have been left uncured, or if the patients have been weakened by improper allopathic treatment; then the inherent psora that exists, alas! in so many persons, although in a latent state, becomes developed, takes on the type of the intermittent fever, and to all appearance continues to play the part of the epidemic intermittent fever, so that the medicine, which would have been useful in the first paroxysms (rarely an antipsoric), is now no longer suitable and cannot be of any service. We have now to do with a psoric intermittent fever only, and this will generally be subdued by minute and rarely repeated doses of sulphur or hepar sulphuris in a high potency.

243

In those often very pernicious intermittent fevers which attack a single person, not residing in a marshy district, we must also at first, as in the case of acute diseases generally, which they resemble in respect to their psoric origin, employ for some days, to render what service it may, a homoeopathic remedy selected for the special case from the other class of proved (not antipsoric) medicines; but if, notwithstanding this procedure, the recovery is deferred, we know that we have psora on the point of its development, and that in this case antipsoric medicines alone can effect a radical cure.

244

The intermittent fevers endemic in marshy districts and tracts of country frequently exposed to inundations, give a great deal of work to physicians of the old school, and yet a healthy man may in his youth become habituated even to marshy districts and remain in good health, provided he preserves a faultless regimen and his system is not lowered by want, fatigue or pernicious passions. The intermittent fevers endemic there would at the most only attack him on his first arrival; but one or two very small doses of a highly potentized solution of cinchona bark would, conjointly with the well-regulated mode of living just alluded to, speedily free him from the disease. But persons who, while taking sufficient corporeal exercise and pursuing a healthy system of intellectual occupations and bodily regimen, cannot be cured of marsh intermittent fever by one or a few of such small doses of cinchona – in such persons psora, striving to develop itself, always lies at the root of their malady, and their intermittent fever cannot be cured in the marshy district without antipsoric treatment.[136] It sometimes happens that when these patients exchange, without delay, the marshy district for one that is dry and mountainous, recovery apparently ensues (the fever leaves them) if they be not yet deeply sunk in disease, that is to say, if the psora was not completely developed in them and can consequently return to its latent state; but they will never regain perfect health without antipsoric treatment.

245

Having thus seen what attention should, in the homoeopathic treatment, be paid to the chief varieties of diseases and to the peculiar circumstances connected with them, we now pass on to what we have to say respecting the remedies and the mode of employing them, together with the diet and regimen to be observed during their use.

Every perceptibly progressive and strikingly increasing amelioration in a transient (acute) or persistent (chronic) disease, is a condition which, as long as it lasts, completely precludes every repetition of the administration of any medicine whatsoever, because all the good the medicine taken continues to effect is new hastening towards its completion. Every new dose of any medicine whatsoever, even of the one last administered, that has hitherto shown itself to be salutary, would in this case disturb the work of amelioration.

246

Every perceptibly progressive and strikingly increasing amelioration during treatment is a condition which, as long as it lasts, completely precludes every repetition of the administration of any medicine whatsoever, because all the good the medicine taken continues to effect is now hastening towards its completion. This is not infrequently the cause in acute diseases, but in more chronic diseases, on the other hand, a single dose of an appropriately selected homoeopathic remedy will at times complete even with but slowly progressive improvement and give the help which such a remedy in such a case can accomplish naturally within 40, 50, 60, 100 days. This is, however, but rarely the case; and besides, it must be a matter of great importance to the physician as well as to the patient that were it possible, this period should be diminished to one-half, one-quarter, and even still less, so that a much more rapid cure might be obtained. And this may be very happily affected, as recent and oft-repeated observations have taught me under the following conditions: firstly, if the medicine selected with the utmost care was perfectly homoeopathic; secondly, if it is highly potentized, dissolved in water and given in proper small dose that experience has taught as the most suitable in definite intervals for the quickest accomplishment of the cure but with the precaution, that the degree of every dose deviate somewhat from the preceding and following in order that the vital principle which is to be altered to a similar medicinal disease be not aroused to untoward reactions and revolt as is always the case[137] with unmodified and especially rapidly repeated doses.

247

It is impractical to repeat the same unchanged dose of a remedy once, not to mention its frequent repetition (and at short intervals in order not to delay the cure). The vital principle does not accept such unchanged doses without resistance, that is, without other symptoms of the medicine to manifest themselves than those similar to the disease to be cured, because the former dose has already accomplished the expected change in the vital principle and a second dynamically wholly similar, unchanged dose of the same medicine no longer finds, therefore, the same conditions of the vital force. The patient may indeed be made sick in another way by receiving other such unchanged doses, even sicker than he was, for now only those symptoms of the given remedy remain active which were not homoeopathic to the original disease, hence no step towards cure can follow, only a true aggravation of the condition of the patient. But if the succeeding dose is changed slightly every time, namely potentized somewhat higher (269-270) then the vital principle may be altered without difficulty by the same medicine (the sensation of natural disease diminishing) and thus the cure brought nearer.[138]

248

For this purpose, we potentize anew the medicinal solution[139] (with perhaps 8, 10, 12 succussions) from which we give the patient one or (increasingly) several teaspoonful doses, in long lasting diseases daily or every second day, in acute diseases every two to six hours and in very urgent cases every hour or oftener. Thus in chronic diseases, every correctly chosen homoeopathic medicine, even those whose action is of long duration, may be repeated daily for months with ever increasing success. If the solution is used up (in seven to fifteen days) it is necessary to add to the next solution of the same medicine if still indicated one or (though rarely) several pellets of a higher potency with which we continue so long as the patient experiences continued improvement without encountering one or another complaint that he never had before in his life. For if this happens, if the balance of the disease appears in a group of altered symptoms then another, one more homoeopathically related medicine must be chosen in place of the last and administered in the same repeated doses, mindful, however, of modifying the solution of every dose with thorough vigorous succussions, thus changing its degree of potency and increasing it somewhat. On the other hand, should there appear during almost daily repetition of the well indicated homoeopathic remedy, towards the end of the treatment of a chronic disease, so-called (161) homoeopathic aggravations by which the balance of the morbid symptoms seem to again increase somewhat (the medicinal disease, similar to the original, now alone persistently manifests itself). The doses in that case must then be reduced still further and repeated in longer intervals and possibly stopped several days, in order to see if the convalescence need no further medicinal aid. The apparent symptoms (Schein – Symptome) caused by the excess of the homoeopathic medicine will soon disappear and leave undisturbed health in its wake. If only a small vial say a dram of dilute alcohol is used in the treatment, in which is contained and dissolved through succussion one globule of the medicine which is to be used by olfaction every two, three or four days, this also must be thoroughly succussed eight to ten times before each olfaction.

Every medicine prescribed for a case of disease which, in the course of its action, produces new and troublesome symptoms not appertaining to the disease to be cured, is not capable of effecting real improvement,[140] and cannot be considered as homoeopathically selected; it must, therefore, either, if the aggravation be considerable, be first partially neutralized as soon as possible by an antidote before giving the next remedy chosen more accurately according to similarity of action; or if the troublesome symptoms be not very violent, the next remedy must be given immediately, in order to take the place of the improperly selected one.[141]

When, to the observant practitioner who accurately investigates the state of the disease, it is evident, in urgent cases after the lapse of only six, eight or twelve hours, that he has made a bad selection in the medicine last given, in that the patient's state is growing perceptibly, however slightly, worse from hour to hour, by the occurrence of new symptoms and sufferings, it is not only allowable for him, but it is his duty to remedy his mistake, by the selection and administration of a homoeopathic medicine not merely tolerably suitable, but the most appropriate possible for the existing state of the disease (167).

There are some medicines (e.g., ignatia, also bryonia and rhus, and sometimes belladonna) whose power of altering man's health consists chiefly in alternating actions – a kind of primary-action symptoms that are in part opposed to each other. Should the practitioner find, on prescribing one of these, selected on strict homoeopathic principles, that no improvement follows, he will in most cases soon effect his object by giving (in acute diseases, even within a few hours) a fresh and equally small dose of the same medicine.[142]

But should we find, during the employment of the other medicines in chronic (psoric) diseases, that the best selected homoeopathic (antipsoric) medicine in the suitable (minutest) dose does not effect an improvement, this is a sure sign that the cause that keeps up the disease still persists, and that there is some circumstances in the mode of life of the patient or in the situation in which he is placed, that must be removed in order that a permanent cure may ensue.

Among the signs that, in all diseases, especially in such as are of an acute nature, inform us of a slight commencement of amelioration or aggravation that is not perceptible to every one, the state of mind and the whole demeanor of the patient are the most certain and instructive. In the case of ever so slight an improvement we observe a greater degree of comfort, increased calmness and freedom of the mind, higher spirits – a kind of return of the natural state. In the case of ever so small a commencement of aggravation we have, on the contrary, the exact opposite of this: a constrained helpless, pitiable state of the disposition, of the mind, of the whole demeanor, and of all gestures, postures and actions, which may be easily perceived on close observation, but cannot be described in words.[143]

The other new or increased symptoms or, on the contrary, the diminution of the original ones without any addition of new ones, will soon dispel all doubts from the mind of the attentively observing and investigating practitioner with regard to the aggravation or amelioration; though there are among patients persons who are either incapable of giving an account of this amelioration or aggravation, or are unwilling to confess it.

But even with such individuals we may convince ourselves on this point by going with them through all the symptoms enumerated in our notes of the disease one by one, and finding that they complain of no new unusual symptoms in addition to these, and that none of the old symptoms are worse. If this be the case, and if an improvement in the disposition and mind have already been observed, the medicine must have effected positive diminution of the disease, or, if sufficient time have not yet elapsed for this, it will soon effect it. Now, supposing the remedy is perfectly appropriate, if the improvement delay too long in making its appearance, this depends either on some error of conduct on the part of the patient, or on other interfering circumstances.

256

On the other hand, if the patient mention the occurrence of some fresh accidents and symptoms of importance – signs that the medicine chosen has not been strictly homoeopathic – even though he should good-naturedly assure us that he feels better, as is not infrequently the case in phthisical patients with lung abscess, we must not believe this assurance, but regard his state as aggravated as it will soon be perfectly apparent it is.

257

The true physician will take care to avoid making favorite remedies of medicines, the employment of which he has, by chance, perhaps found often useful, and which he has had opportunities of using with good effect. If he do so, some remedies or rarer use, which would have been more homoeopathically suitable, consequently more serviceable, will often be neglected.

258

The true practitioner, moreover, will not in his practice with mistrustful weakness neglect the employment of those remedies that he may now and then have employed with bad effects, owing to an erroneous selection (from his own fault, therefore), or avoid them for other (false) reasons, as that they were unhomoeopathic for the case of disease before him; he must bear in mind the truth, that of medicinal agents that one alone invariably deserves the preference in every case of disease which correspond most accurately by similarity to the totality of the characteristic symptoms, and that no paltry prejudices should interfere with this serious choice.

259

Considering the minuteness of the doses necessary and proper in homoeopathic treatment, we can easily understand that during the treatment everything must be removed from the diet and regimen which can have any medicinal action, in order that the small dose may not be overwhelmed and extinguished or disturbed by any foreign medicinal irritant.[144]

260

Hence the careful investigation into such obstacles to cure is so much the more necessary in the case of patients affected by chronic diseases, as their diseases are usually aggravated by such noxious influences and other disease-causing errors in the diet and regimen, which often pass unnoticed.[145]

261

The most appropriate regimen during the employment of medicine in chronic diseases consists in the removal of such obstacles to recovery, and in supplying where necessary the reverse: innocent moral and intellectual recreation, active exercise in the open air in almost all kinds of weather (daily walks, slight manual labor), suitable, nutritious, unmedicinal food and drink, etc.

262

In acute diseases, on the other hand – except in cases of mental alienation – the subtle, unerring internal sense of the awakened life-preserving faculty determines so clearly and precisely, that the physician only requires to counsel the friends and attendants to put no obstacles in the way of this voice of nature by refusing anything the patient urgently desires in the way of food, or by trying to persuade him to partake of anything injurious.

263

The desire of the patient affected by an acute disease with regard to food and drink is certainly chiefly for things that give palliative relief: they are, however, not strictly speaking of a medicinal character, and merely supply a sort of want. The slight hindrances that the gratification of this desire, within moderate bounds, could oppose to the radical removal of the disease[146] will be amply counteracted and overcome by the power of the homoeopathically suited medicine and the vital force set free by it, as also by the refreshment that follows from taking what has been so ardently longed for. In like manner, in acute diseases the temperature of the room and the heat or coolness of the bed-coverings must also be arranged entirely in conformity with the patients' wish. He must be kept free from all over-exertion of mind and exciting emotions.

264

The true physician must be provided with genuine medicines of unimpaired strength, so that he may be able to rely upon their therapeutic powers; he must be able, himself, to judge of their genuineness.

265

It should be a matter of conscience with him to be thoroughly convinced in every case that the patient always takes the right medicine and therefore he must give the patient the correctly chosen medicine prepared, moreover, by himself.

266

Substances belonging to the animal and vegetable kingdoms possess their medicinal qualities most perfectly in their raw state.[147]

267

We gain possession of the powers of indigenous plants and of such as may be had in a fresh state in the most complete and certain manner by mixing their freshly expressed juice immediately with equal parts of spirits of wine of a strength sufficient to burn in a lamp. After this has stood a day and a night in a close stoppered bottle and deposited the fibrinous and albuminous matters, the clear superincumbent fluid is then to be decanted off for medicinal use.[148] All fermentation of the vegetable juice will be at once checked by the spirits of wine mixed with it and rendered impossible for the future, and the entire medicinal power of the vegetable juice is thus retained (perfect and uninjured) for ever by keeping the preparation in well-corked bottles and excluded from the sun's light.[149]

268

The other exotic plants, barks, seeds and roots that cannot be obtained in the fresh state the sensible practitioner will never take in the pulverized form on trust, but will first convince himself of their genuineness in their crude, entire state before making any employment of them.[150]

269

The homoeopathic system of medicine develops for its special use, to a hitherto unheard-of degree, the inner medicinal powers of the crude substances by means of a process peculiar to it and which has hitherto never been tried, whereby only they all become immeasurably and penetratingly efficacious[151] and remedial, even those that in the crude state give no evidence of the slightest medicinal power on the human body.

This remarkable change in the qualities of natural bodies develops the latent, hitherto unperceived, as if slumbering[152] hidden, dynamic (11) powers which influence the life principle, change the well-being of animal life.[153] This is effected by mechanical action upon their smallest particles by means of rubbing and shaking and through the addition of an indifferent substance, dry of fluid, are separated from each other. This process is called dynamizing, potentizing (development of medicinal power) and the products are dynamizations[154] or potencies in different degrees.

270

In order to best obtain this development of power, a small part of the substance to be dynamized, say one grain, is triturated for three hours with three times one hundred grains sugar of milk according to the method described below[155] up to the one-millionth part in powder form. For reasons given below (b) one grain of this powder is dissolved in 500 drops of a mixture of one part of alcohol and four parts of distilled water, of which one drop is put in a vial. To this are added 100 drops of pure alcohol[156] and given one hundred strong succussions with the hand against a hard but elastic body.[157] This is the medicine in the first degree of dynamization with which small sugar globules[158] may then be moistened[159] and quickly spread on blotting paper to dry and kept in a well-corked vial with the sign of (I) degree of potency. Only one[160] globule of this is taken for further dynamization, put in a second new vial (with a drop a water in order to dissolve it) and then with 100 powerful succussions.

With this alcoholic medicinal fluid globules are again moistened, spread upon blotting paper and dried quickly, put into a well-stoppered vial and protected from heat and sun light and given the sign (II) of the second potency. And in this way the process is continued until the twenty-ninth is reached. Then with 100 drops of alcohol by means of 100 succussions, an alcoholic medicinal fluid is formed with which the thirtieth dynamization degree is given to properly moistened and dried sugar globules.

By means of this manipulation of crude drugs are produced preparations which only in this way reach the full capacity to forcibly influence the suffering parts of the sick organism. In this way, by means of similar artificial morbid affection, the influence of the natural disease on the life principle present within is neutralized. By means of this mechanical procedure, provided it is carried out regularly according to the above teaching, a change is effected in the given drug, which in its crude state shows itself only as material, at times as unmedicinal material but by means of such higher and higher dynamization, it is changed and subtlized at last into spirit-like[161] medicinal power, which, indeed, in itself does not fall within our senses but for which the medicinally prepared globule, dry, but more so when dissolved in water, becomes the carrier, and in this condition, manifests the healing power of this invisible force in the sick body.

271

If the physician prepares his homoeopathic medicines himself, as he should reasonably do in order to save men from sickness,[162] he may use the fresh plant itself, as but little of the crude article is required, if he does not need the expressed juice perhaps for purposes of healing. He takes a few grains in a mortar and with 100 grains sugar of milk three distinct times brings them to the one-millionth trituration (270) before further potentizing of a small portion of this by means of shaking is undertaken, a procedure to be observed also with the rest of crude drugs of either dry or oily nature.

272

Such a globule,[163] placed dry upon the tongue, is one of the smallest doses for a moderate recent case of illness. Here but few nerves are touched by the medicine. A similar globule, crushed with some sugar of milk and dissolved in a good deal of water (247) and stirred well before every administration will produce a far more powerful medicine for the use of several days. Every dose, no matter how minute, touches, on the contrary, many nerves.

273

In no case under treatment is it necessary and therefore not permissible to administer to a patient more than one single, simple medicinal substance at one time. It is inconceivable how the slightest doubt could exist as to whether it was more consistent with nature and more rational to prescribe a single, simple[164] medicine at one time in a disease or a mixture of several differently acting drugs. It is absolutely not allowed in homoeopathy, the one true, simple and natural art of healing, to give the patient at one time two different medicinal substance.

274

As the true physician finds in simple medicines, administered singly and uncombined, all that he can possibly desire (artificial disease-force which are able by homoeopathic power completely to overpower, extinguish, and permanently cure natural diseases), he will, mindful of the wise maxim that "it is wrong to attempt to employ complex means when simple means suffice," never think of giving as a remedy any but a single, simple medicinal substance; for these reasons also, because even though the simple medicines were thoroughly proved with respect to their pure peculiar effects on the unimpaired healthy state of man, it is yet impossible to foresee how two and more medicinal substances might, when compounded, hinder and alter each other's actions on the human body; and because, on the other hand, a simple medicinal substance when used in diseases, the totality of whose symptoms is accurately known, renders efficient aid by itself alone, if it be homoeopathically selected; and supposing the worst case to happen, that it was not chosen in strict conformity to similarity of symptoms, and therefore does no good, it is yet so far useful that it promoted our knowledge of therapeutic agents, because, by the new symptoms excited by it in such a case, those symptoms which this medicinal substance had already shown in experiments on the healthy human body are confirmed, an advantage that is lost by the employment of all compound remedies.[165]

275

The suitableness of a medicine for any given case of disease does not depend on its accurate homoeopathic selection alone, but likewise on the proper size, or rather smallness, of the dose. If we give too strong a dose of a medicine which may have been even quite homoeopathically chosen for the morbid state before us, it must, notwithstanding the inherent beneficial character of its nature, prove injurious by its mere magnitude, and by the unnecessary, too strong impression which, by virtue of its homoeopathic similarity of action, it makes upon the vital force which it attacks and, through the vital force, upon those parts of the organism which are the most sensitive, and are already most affected by the natural disease.

276

For this reason, a medicine, even though it may be homoeopathically suited to the case of disease, does harm in every dose that is too large, the more harm the larger the dose, and by the magnitude of the dose and in strong doses' it does more harm the greater its homoeopathicity and the higher the potency[166] selected, and it does much more injury than any equally large dose of a medicine that is unhomoeopathic, and in no respect adapted to the morbid state (allopathic).

Too large doses of an accurately chosen homoeopathic medicine, and especially when frequently repeated, bring about much trouble as a rule. They put the patient not seldom in danger of life or make this disease almost incurable. They do indeed extinguish the natural disease so far as the sensation of the life principle is concerned and the patient no longer suffers from the original disease from the moment the too strong dose of the homoeopathic medicine acted upon him but he is in consequence more ill with the similar but more violent medicinal disease which is most difficult to destroy.[167]

277

For the same reason, and because a medicine, provided the dose of it was sufficiently small, is all the more salutary and almost marvellously efficacious the more accurately homoeopathic its selection has been, a medicine whose selection has been accurately homoeopathic must be all the more salutary the more its dose is reduced to the degree of minuteness appropriate for a gentle remedial effect.

278

Here the question arises, what is this most suitable degree of minuteness for sure and gentle remedial effect; how small, in other words, must be the dose of each individual medicine, homoeopathically selected for a case of disease, to effect the best cure? To solve this problem, and to determine for every particular medicine, what dose of it will suffice for homoeopathic therapeutic purposes and yet be so minute that the gentlest and most rapid cure may be thereby obtained – to solve this problem is, as may easily be conceived, not the work off theoretical speculation; not by fine-spun reasoning, not by specious sophistry can we expect to obtain the solution of this problem. It is just as impossible as to tabulate in advance all imaginable cases. Pure experiment, careful observation of the sensitiveness of each patient, and accurate experience can alone determine this; and it were absurd to adduce the large doses of unsuitable (allopathic) medicines of the old system, which do not touch the diseased side of the organism homoeopathically, but only attack the parts unaffected by the disease, in opposition to what pure experience pronounces respecting the smallness of the doses required for homoeopathic cures.

279

This pure experience shows UNIVERSALLY, that if the disease do not manifestly depend on a considerable deterioration of an important viscus (even though it belong to the chronic and complicated diseases), and if during the treatment all other alien medicinal influences are kept away from the patients, the dose of the homoeopathically selected and highly potentized remedy for the beginning of treatment of an important, especially chronic disease can never be prepared so small that it shall not be stronger than the natural disease and shall not be able to overpower it, at least in part and extinguish it from the sensation of the principle of life and thus make a beginning of a cure.

280

The dose of the medicine that continues serviceable without producing new troublesome symptoms is to be continued while gradually ascending, so long as the patient with general improvement, begins to feel in a mild degree the return of one or several old original complaints. This indicates an approaching cure through a gradual ascending of the moderate doses modified each time by succussion (247). It indicates that the vital principal no longer needs to be affected by the similar medicinal disease in order to lose the sensation of the natural disease (148). It indicates that the life principle now free from the natural disease begins to suffer only something of the medicinal disease hitherto known as homoeopathic aggravation.

281

In order to be convinced of this, the patient is left without any medicine for eight, ten of fifteen days, meanwhile giving him only some powders of sugar of milk. If the few last complaints are due to the medicine simulating the former original disease symptoms, then these complaints will disappear in a few days or hours. If during these days without medicine, while continuing good hygienic regulations nothing more of the original disease is seen, he is probably

91

cured. But if in the later days traces of the former morbid symptoms should show themselves, they are remnants of the original disease not wholly extinguished, which must be treated with renewed higher potencies of the remedy as directed before. If a cure is to follow, the first small doses must likewise be again gradually raised higher, but less and more slowly in patients where considerable irritability is evident than in those of less susceptibility, where the advance to higher dosage may be more rapid. There are patients whose impressionability compared to that of the insusceptible ones is like the ratio as 1000 to 1.

282

It would be a certain sign that the doses were altogether too large, if during treatment, especially in chronic disease, the first dose should bring forth a so-called homoeopathic aggravation, that is, a marked increase of the original morbid symptoms first discovered and in the same way every repeated dose (247) however modified somewhat by shaking before its administration (i.e., more highly dynamized).[168]

283

In order to work wholly according to nature, the true healing artist will prescribe the accurately chosen homoeopathic medicine most suitable in all respects in so small a dose on account of this alone. For should he be misled by human weakness to employ an unsuitable medicine, the disadvantage of its wrong relation to the disease would be so small that the patient could through his own vital powers and by means of early opposition (249) of the correctly chosen remedy according to symptom similarly (and this also in the smallest dose) rapidly extinguish and repair it.

284

Besides the tongue, mouth and stomach, which are most commonly affected by the administration of medicine, the nose and respiratory organs are receptive of the action of medicines in fluid form by means of olfaction and inhalation through the mouth. But the whole remaining skin of the body clothed with epidermis, is adapted to the action of medicinal solutions, especially if the inunction is connected with simultaneous internal administration.[169]

285

In this way, the cure of very old disease may be furthered by the physician applying externally, rubbing it in the back, arms, extremities, the same medicine he gives internally and which showed itself curatively. In doing so, he must avoid parts subject to pain or spasm or skin eruption.[170]

286

The dynamic force of minerals magnets, electricity and galvanism act no less powerfully upon our life principle and they are not less homoeopathic than the properly so-called medicines which neutralize disease by taking them through the mouth, or by rubbing them on the skin or by olfaction. There may be diseases, especially diseases of sensibility and irritability, abnormal sensations, and involuntary muscular movements which may be cured by those means. But the more certain way of applying the last two as well as that of the so-called electromagnetic lies still very much in the dark to make homoeopathic use of them. So far both electricity and Galvanism have been used only for palliation to the great damage of the sick. The positive, pure action of both upon the healthy human body have until the present time been but little tested.

287

The powers of the magnet for healing purposes can be employed with more certainty according to the positive effects detailed in the Materia Medica Pura under north and south pole of a powerful magnetic bar. Though both poles are alike powerful, they nevertheless oppose each other in the manner of their respective action. The doses may be modified by the length of time of contact with one or the other pole, according as the symptoms of either north or south pole are indicated. As antidote to a too violent action the application of a plate of polished zinc will suffice.

288

I find it yet necessary to allude here to animal magnetism, as it is termed, or rather Mesmerism (as it should be called in deference to Mesmer, its first founder) which differs so much in its nature from all other therapeutic agents. This curative force, often so stupidly denied and disdained for a century, acts in different ways. It is a marvellous, priceless gift of God to mankind by means of which the strong will of a well intentioned person upon a sick one by contact and even without this and even at some distance, can bring the vital energy of the healthy mesmerizer endowed with this power into another person dynamically (just as one of the poles of a powerful magnetic rod upon a bar of steel).

It acts in part by replacing in the sick whose vital force within the organism is deficient here and there, in part also in other parts where the vital force has accumulated too much and keeps up irritating nervous disorders it turns it aside, diminishes and distributes it equally and in general extinguishes the morbid condition of the life principle of the patient and substitutes in its place the normal of the mesmerist acting powerfully upon him, for instance, old ulcers, amaurosis, paralysis of single organs and so forth. Many rapid apparent cures performed in all ages, by mesmerizers endowed with great natural power, belong to this class. The effect of communicated human power upon the whole human organism was most brilliantly shown, in the resuscitation of persons who had lain some time apparently dead, by the most powerful sympathetic will of a man in full vigor of vital energy,[171] and of this kind of resurrection history records many undeniable examples.

If the mesmerizing person of either sex capable at the same time of a good-natured enthusiasm (even its degeneration into bigotry, fanaticism, mysticism or philanthropic dreaming) will be empowered all the more with this philanthropic self-sacrificing performance to direct exclusively the power of his commanding good will to the recipient requiring his help and at the same time to concentrate these, he may at times perform apparent miracles.

289

All the above-mentioned methods of practicing mesmerism depend upon influx of more or less vital force into the patient, and hence are termed positive mesmerism.[172] An opposite mode of employing mesmerism, however, as it produces just the contrary effect, deserves to be termed negative mesmerism. To this belong the passes which are used to rouse from the somnambulic sleep, as also all the manual processes known by the names of soothing and ventilating. This discharge by means of negative mesmerism of the vital force accumulated to excess in individual parts of the system of undebilitated persons is most surely and simply performed by making a very rapid motion or the flat extended hand, held parallel to, and about an inch distant from the body, from the top of the head to the tips of the toes.[173] The more rapidly this pass is made, so much the more effectually will the discharge be effected. Thus, for instance, in the case where a previously healthy woman,[174] from the sudden suppression of her catamenia by a violent mental shock, lies to all appearance dead, the vital force which is probably accumulated in the precordial region, will, by such a rapid negative pass, be discharged and its equilibrium throughout the whole organism restored. So that the resuscitation generally follows, immediately.[175] In like manner, a gentle, less rapid, negative pass diminishes the excessive restlessness and sleeplessness accompanied with anxiety sometimes produced in very irritable persons by a too powerful positive pass, etc.

290

Here belongs also the so-called massage of vigorous good-natured person given to a chronic invalid, who, though cured, still suffers from loss of flesh, weakness of digestion and lack of sleep due to slow convalescence. The muscles of the limbs, breast and back, separately grasped and moderately pressed and kneaded arouse the life principle to reach and restore the tone of the muscles and blood and lymph vessels. The mesmeric influences of this procedure is the chief feature and it must not be used to excess in patients still hypersensitive.

291

Baths of pure water prove themselves partly palliative, partly as homoeopathic serviceable aids in restoring health in acute diseases as well as in convalescence of cured chronic patients with proper consideration of the conditions of the convalescent and the temperature of the bath, its duration and repetition. But even if well applied, they may bring only physically beneficial changes in the sick body, in themselves they are no true medicine. The lukewarm baths at 25 to 27? serve to arouse the slumbering sensibility of fibre in the apparent dead (frozen, drowned, suffocated) which benumbed the sensation of the nerves. Though only palliative, still they often prove themselves sufficiently active, especially when given in conjunction with coffee and rubbing with the hands. They may give homoeopathic aid in cases where the irritability is very unevenly distributed and accumulated too unevenly in some organs as is the case in certain hysteric spasms and infantile convulsions. In the same way, cold baths 10 to 6? in persons cured medically of chronic diseases and with deficiency of vital heat, act as an homoeopathic aid. By instantaneous and later with repeated immersions they act as a palliative restorative of the tone of the exhausted fibre. For this purpose, such baths are to be used for more than momentary duration, rather for minutes and of gradually lowered temperature, they are a palliative, which, since it acts only physically has no connection with the disadvantage of a reverse action to be feared afterwards, as takes place with dynamic medicinal palliatives.

292

Even the external surface of the body, covered as it is with skin and epidermis, is not insusceptible of the powers of medicines, especially those in a liquid form, but the most sensitive parts are also the most susceptible.[176]

293

I find it necessary to allude here to animal magnetism, as it is termed, or rather mesmerism (as it should be called, out of gratitude to Mesmer, its first founder), which differs so much in its nature from all other therapeutic agents. This curative power, often so stupidly denied, which streams upon a patient by the contact of a well-intentioned person powerfully exerting his will, either acts homoeopathically, by the production of symptoms similar to those of the diseased state to be cured; and for this purpose a single pass made, without much exertion of the will, with the palms of the hands not too slowly from the top of the head downwards over the body to the tips of the toes,[177] is serviceable in, for instance, uterine haemorrhages, even in the last stage when death seems approaching; or it is useful by distributing the vital force uniformly throughout the organism, when it is in abnormal excess in one part and deficient in other parts, for example, in rush of blood to the head and sleepless, anxious restlessness of weakly persons, etc., by means of a similar, single, but somewhat stronger pass; or for the immediate communication and restoration of the vital force to some one weakened part or to the whole organism, – an object that cannot be attained so certainly and with so little interference with the other medicinal treatment by any other agent besides mesmerism. If it is wished to supply a particular part with the vital force, this is effected by concentrating a very powerful and well-intentioned will for the purpose, and placing the hands or tips of the fingers on the chronically weakened parts, whither an internal chronic dyscrasia has transferred its important local symptom, as, for example, in the case of old ulcers, amaurosis, paralysis of certain limbs, etc.[178] Many rapid apparent cures performed in all ages, by mesmerizers endowed with great natural power, belong to this class. The effect of communicated human power upon the whole human organism was most brilliantly shown, in the resuscitation of persons who had lain some time apparently dead, by the most powerful sympathetic will of a man in full vigor of vital force,[179] and of this kind of resurrection history records many undeniable examples.

294

All the above-mentioned methods of practicing mesmerism depend upon an influx of more or less vital force into the patient, and hence are termed positive mesmerism.[180] An opposite mode of employing mesmerism, however, as it produces just the contrary effect, deserves to be termed negative mesmerism. To this belong the passes which are used to rouse from the somnambulic sleep, as also all the manual processes known by the names of soothing and venti-lating. This discharge by means of negative mesmerism of the vital force accumulated to excess in individual parts of the system of undebiliated persons is most surely and simply performed by making a very rapid motion of the flat extended hand, held parallel to, and about an inch distant from the body, from the top of the head to the tips of the toes.[181] The more rapidly this pass is made, so much the more effectually will the discharge be effected. Thus, for instance, in the case where a previously healthy woman,[182] from the sudden suppression of her catamenia by a violent mental shock, lies to all appearance dead, the vital force which is probably accumulated in the precordial region, will by such a rapid negative pass, be discharged and its equilibrium throughout the whole organism restored, so that the resuscitation generally follows immedi-ately.[183] In like manner, a gentle, less rapid, negative pass diminishes the excessive restlessness and sleeplessness accompanied with anxiety sometimes produced in very irritable persons by a too powerful positive pass, etc.

OF THE HOMOEOPATHIC DOCTRINES
by J. G. Millingen

It is a matter worthy of remark, that, while the doctrines of homœopathy have fixed the attention and become the study of many learned and experienced medical men in various parts of Europe, England is the only country where it has only been noticed to draw forth the most opprobrious invectives. It is certainly true that no one but an ardent proselyte of the visionary Hahnemann could for one moment become the advocate of all his absurd ideas; yet, while we reject his errors, great and important truths beam from the chaotic clouds that shroud his wanderings; and, however wild his theories may be, incontrovertible facts have been elicited from his apparently inefficacious practice.

Before I enter into an examination of the practical views of the homœopathists, I shall give a brief sketch of their doctrines and of their founder.

Samuel Hahnemann was born in Meïssen in Saxony, on the 10th of April, 1755. His father was an humble porcelain manufacturer. The first rudiments of education that young Hahnemann received were gratuitous; and his master, pleased with the progress of his ambitious but needy scholar, strongly urged him to repair to Leipzig, where, at the age of twenty, he arrived, with exactly the same number of crowns in his pocket as he numbered years. At this university he zealously pursued his favourite studies of the natural sciences, supporting himself by translating French works, and giving lessons; and finally he graduated in the university of Eslan-in 1779.

It was during his arduous studies that Hahnemann was struck with the conflicting systems and the deplorable controversies which for centuries divided in turn the medical schools of Europe, and were triumphant or overthrown by scholastic revolutions; each doctrine being doomed to obscurity and oblivion in the ratio of its ephemeral splendour. The result of his reflections and experiments was the system of homœopathy. Its novelty, its apparent absurdity, soon exposed him not only to opposition, but to violent persecution. As is usual in all cases of oppression, whether justly or unjustly resorted to, proselytes as furious and as fanatical as his persecutors joined their chief. Despite the sanatary regulations of Saxony, which prohibited physicians from dispensing their medicines, Hahnemann prepared and supplied his homœopathic remedies; and, being expelled from Leipzig, sought a refuge at Kœthen, where, exasperated by the harsh treatment he had experienced, he fulminated his anathema on all past and present systems of medicine with no small degree of furious resentment, pronouncing his doctrine to be stamped with the seal of infallibility, and denouncing all others as the aberrations of ignorance and error, or the speculations of imposture and fraud.

As might have been expected, few of his opponents thought it worth their while to study his system calmly and dispassionately; nor, indeed, was such an application necessary, for his doctrines needed no deep investigation on the part of his foes, so fraught were they with apparent errors and false deductions, not only from his own pretended experience, but the experience of ages. Finding that he could not enjoy a despotic sway over the schools, he was resolved at any rate to seek the palm of martyrdom, and had recourse to such violence in words and actions, that many of his enemies maintained he was a more fitting subject for a lunatic asylum than the *soi-disant* founder of a rational doctrine; for he and his fanatical disciples set all ratiocination at nought, considering his *dixit* as a fiat of condemnation passed on all who dared to doubt his infallibility, although at different periods their oracle was obliged to retract many erroneous assertions and contradict fallacious statements.

In the short view of his doctrines which I am about to give, these fallacies will become evident.

Hahnemann had observed in his studies and hospital practice that the prevalent systems of medicine were founded on the rational principle of combating effects by striking at morbid causes. Physicians sometimes endeavoured to attain this desirable end by producing in the system an artificial action differing from the nature of the malady, and founded their practice on the scholastic axiom of *contraria contrariis curantur*; at other times they raised or depressed the vital energies according to the prevalence of excitement or debility, or modified the character of the disease by revulsion and derivation, a practice which received the name of antagonistic, or *allopathic*, —a term used by Hahnemann in contradistinction to homœopathy, and derived from αλλος, *different*, and παθος, *affection*.

In his therapeutic pursuits Hahnemann had been forcibly struck with the long-acknowledged fact that medicinal substances supposed to possess a certain specific property in the treatment of diseases, were known in the healthy subject to produce phenomena bearing a close analogy to the symptoms of those identical diseases. Thus, mercurial preparations occasioned symptoms of syphilis, sulphur produced cutaneous irritation, and, in some instances, the exhibition of cinchona had been known to bring on febrile intermissions. In various works he found these observations established. For instance, amongst many others, he found in the publications of Beddoes, Scott, Blair, and various writers, that nitric acid, which was known to produce ptyalism, relieved salivation and ulceration in the mouth. Arsenic, which, according to Henreich, Knape, and Heinze, occasioned cancerous anomalies in healthy subjects, was stated by Fallopius, Bernharde, Roennow, and many other surgeons, to be efficacious in relieving, if not curing, similar disorders; preparations of copper were asserted by Tondi, Ramsay, Lazermi, and numerous practitioners, to have produced epileptic attacks; and Batty, Baumes, Cullen, Duncan, and several experienced medical practitioners, recommended similar remedies in epilepsy. In short, the illustrations of the power inherent in certain substances to produce accidents analogous to the symptoms of the various diseases in the treatment of which they had proved efficacious, induced Hahnemann to consider whether a treatment founded on *similia similibus curantur* might not be found more effectual than the former practice based upon the *contraria contrariis*. He was of opinion that no medicine was possessed of any *curative property*, but solely acted by its *morbific power* of producing a disordered condition in the system; and on this and other principles, which we shall shortly notice, he asserts that nature does not possess any curative power, totally denying the *vis medicatrix* of the schools. He further maintained, that there does not exist any specific malady; but that which we consider to be a disease is nothing but a complexity of symptoms, and that a cure can only be effected when these complex symptoms are made to disappear.

Impressed with these ideas, he and his disciples proceeded to try various medicinal substances upon themselves and others when in health, and, carefully recording the symptoms which these medicines produced, they drew up a statement of their various powers, that they might be afterwards resorted to, to relieve the same symptoms in a morbid state. Grounding this practice on the principle (in many instances correct) that two similar diseases cannot coexist, they conceived that if, to counteract a natural malady, one can produce by any medication an artificial derangement of the same nature, the artificial disorder will overcome the natural disease, and a radical cure be obtained. To explain more distinctly this idea, I shall quote the author's words.

"The curative power of medicines is thus founded on the property they possess to give rise to symptoms similar to those of the disease, but of a more intense power. Hence no disease can be overcome or cured in a certain, radical, rapid, and lasting manner, but through the means of a medicine capable of provoking a group of symptoms similar to those of the disease, and at the same time possessed of a superior energetic power."[184] And further,

"If two dissimilar maladies happen to be coexisting, possessed of an unequal force, or if the oldest disease is more energetic than the recent one, the latter will be expelled by the former. Thus, an individual labouring under a severe chronic disease will not be subject to the invasion of an autumnal dysentery, or any other slight epidemic. Larrey affirms that the districts of Egypt in which scurvy was prevalent were exempt from the plague. Jenner asserts that rachitis prevents the effect of vaccination; and Hildebrand assures us that phthysical patients never experience epidemic fevers unless of the most severe character."[185]

"If a recent affection, dissimilar to a more ancient one be more powerful than the latter, then will the progress of the latter be suspended until the malady is either cured or has been expended in its career, and then the old one will reappear."[186]

"But the result is totally different when two similar diseases meet in the organism; that is to say, when a pre-existing affection is complicated with one of the same nature, but possessed of more energy."[187]

"Two maladies resembling each other in their manifestation and their effects, that is to say, in the symptoms which they determine, mutually destroy each other, the strongest conquering the weakest."[188]

He further contends that the essential nature of every disease is unknown; that their existence is revealed by alterations and changes in the system perceptible to our senses, and constituting what are called *symptoms*, and it is the series of these symptoms which characterize the disease in its course and its development. According to his notions, the physician has only to follow and study the succession and the grouping of these symptoms; in short, the phases and the phenomena of diseases. Attack and destroy these symptoms, and you will have destroyed the malady.

All classification of diseases, and their various denominations, he therefore deemed absurd, as, according to his doctrines, no one disease resembles another; so various were their modifications, that, with few exceptions, it was idle to give them a particular name, since disease was simply a derangement in our organization manifested by peculiar symptoms.

We are also, according to Hahnemann, ignorant of the essential properties of medicines, and can only observe and record their effects by experimental observation. Like diseases, they also produce a derangement in our organism, manifested by peculiar symptoms, their sole action consisting in developing specific diseases.

In conformity with these notions, to cure disease we have only to produce a similar affection; the primitive one would then give way to the secondary affection artificially produced, and in time the artificial one would cease to exist when the means that produced it were no longer brought into action.

Homœopathic medicines, he maintained, have the property of acting in a direct manner upon the affected part of the system; and this is proved when the disease, and the medicine given to relieve it, produce similar morbid manifestations: and he further contended that our vital organism was less susceptible of the action of natural affections than of those which are artificially produced.

On this basis did the homœopathic doctrinarians ground their practice; but a still more singular theory was broached by their leader; he maintained that medicinal substances, to prove efficacious, should be administered in an attenuated and diluted state, carried to such an extent as to become infinite in their division; he further asserts that this infinite division, far from diminishing their medicinal power and properties, imparts greater energy and certainty of action when these particles encounter in our organization an affinity of disposition, or a homogeny in action; that is to say, that these atomic attenuations act with greater power in those affections which manifest symptoms similar to those which these very medicines are known to produce when experimentally tried upon a healthy subject.

Upon this principle the homœopathist condemns all combinations of medicines as likely to neutralize each other's properties by their various affinities; therefore generally speaking, no fresh medicine should be given until the effects of the former have subsided; and to guide this practice, while they endeavoured to ascertain the symptoms produced by medicines, they also sought to ascribe certain limits to the duration of their action: thus, the influence of aconite lasts forty-eight hours, and that of crude antimony fifteen days.

Dreading all substances that could tend to weaken or neutralize the effect of medicine, the homœopathists made it their particular study to discover the peculiar action of all alimentary substances on the organism, and characterized as antidotes all such articles of food as they considered opposed to this supposed action: thus, wine and vegetable acids were deemed antidotes to aconite; coffee, to Angustura bark; vinegar, to asarum, &c.

I have already stated that the homœopathists conceive that the infinite dilution of their atoms of medicinal substances increase their energy; and this fact they so strenuously maintain, that they assert that accidents of a serious nature may arise when this division is carried too far; and these accidents are then to be met with the medicinal antidotes they pretend to have discovered: thus, camphor is an antidote to cocculus; opium, to the crocus sativus; camomile and camphor, to ignatia amara; and so on.

The minuteness with which the specific actions of various medicinal substances on certain organs is detailed is scarcely credible; and the following extract from the homœopathic materia medica will give a slight idea of their industrious labours. Taking as an example phosphorus, which they affirm produces —

Vertigo, determination of blood to the head, headache in the morning, fall of the hair, difficulty in opening the eyelids, burning sensation and ulceration of the internal canthus of the eye, when exposed to the open air, lachrymation and adhesion of the palpebræ; inflammation of the eyes, with the sensation of particles of sand having been introduced; sparks and spangles floating before the eyes, a dark tinge in objects that are looked on, diurnal cecity, the appearance of a gray veil drawn before the eyes, pulsation in the ears, epistaxis, mucous discharge from the nostrils, foulness of breath, tumefaction of the throat, whiteness of the tongue, ulceration of the mouth, expectoration of glairy mucus, dryness of the mouth by night and by day, spasmodic eructation, nausea, sense of hunger after eating, anxiety after meals; in short, twenty-four octavo pages are devoted to the innumerable effects of this substance on the organism.

Of *magnesia artificialis* three hundred and twelve symptoms are noted; six hundred and fifty of the *rhus radicans*; nine hundred and forty of *pulsatilla*; five hundred of *ignatia amara*; four hundred and sixty of *arsenic*: in short, volumes upon volumes are crowded with these observations, not only recording physical effects, but singular results on our moral faculties; such as serenity or moroseness, gaiety or sadness, a disposition to commit suicide or a fond partiality to life, courage or cowardice, a weak intellect or a vigorous conception. For instance, —common sea-salt occasions irascibility, lowness of spirits, taciturnity, melancholy, palpitation of heart, disposition to shed tears, pusillanimity, and despair; while potash gives rise to ill-temper without apparent cause at noon and in the evening, with violent paroxysms of rage in the morning, impetuous desires, furious passion, with gnashing of teeth, if all around does not yield to the patient's desires; while the vision of a bird hovering about the window produces loud shrieks of alarm, exaltation of the intellects, and a horror of the future. So innumerable, indeed, are all these singular effects attributed to various medicines thus experimented, that no memory, however retentive, could possibly bear them in recollection. The following are the directions laid down for conducting this curious inquiry:

The person upon whom medicines are tried must be free from disease; but weak substances should be given to subjects of a delicate and sensitive constitution. The medicine is to be tried in its most pure and simple state, possessing all its energies, taking special care that it is not combined with any heterogeneous substances during the day it is exhibited, and the time while its action is supposed to last. The diet must be moderate; all spices and high-seasoned food to be avoided, as well as green vegetables, roots, salads, &c. which are known to possess medicinal properties. The dose of the medicine to be similar to that which is usually prescribed by practitioners. If, at the expiration of about two hours, no effect is observed, a stronger dose is to be given. Should the first dose operate powerfully at the commencement, but gradually lose its influence, the second will be given the following morning; and a still stronger one, four times the strength of the first, be administered on the third day.

The result of these experiments being recorded, homœopathic agents are selected to oppose morbid symptoms; and when the choice of remedies has been appropriate, an aggravation of the symptoms is observed. This aggravation is usually considered as an increase of the disorder, whereas it is solely the effect of the homœopathic remedy. "For these phenomena," say the homœopathists, "were frequently observed by physicians, who little thought at the time, that they were the result of the medicines they had given." Thus, when the pustules of itch became more rife after the exhibition of sulphur, it was thought that the increase of the eruption was merely the affection *coming out* more freely; whereas, the aggravation was occasioned by sulphur. Leroy informs us that the heart's-ease, *viola tricolor*, increased an eruption in the face. Lyrons says that elm-bark aggravated cutaneous affections, which were cured by this remedy; but neither of them were aware of the nature of this homœopathic development. For further information on this head, the Organon of Hahnemann must be consulted.

Such were his doctrines for a period of about twenty years, —doctrines which he emphatically pronounced infallible, and founded on the immutable laws of homœopathy. In 1828, however, convinced by numerous failures in the treatment of chronic diseases, that other causes than those which he acknowledged, —such as the improper preparation of the medicine, or dietetic neglect on the part of the patient, —contributed to these disappointments, he announced that he had discovered the hidden source of the obstacles he encountered; and that, after many years of experiments and meditation, he had come to the conclusion that almost all chronic diseases originated from constitutional miasmatic affections or predispositions, which he divided into *sycosis, syphilis,* and *psora,* or, in plain English, the itch. To this latter affection he attributes innumerable disorders. In diseases of a syphilitic character, he had found his mode of treatment infallible; and he therefore concluded that all obstinate and rebellious affections were the result of some other constitutional predisposing circumstances. He tells us that he laboured in profound secrecy to discover this great, this sublime desideratum: his very pupils knew it not; the world was to remain in ignorance of his pursuits until he could proclaim the most inestimable gift that Divinity bestowed upon mankind. This immortal discovery was neither more nor less than the itch; to which malady, according to his views, since the days of Moses, seven-eighths of the physical and moral miseries to which flesh is heir, were to be referred. Whether rendered evident by eruptions, or latent from our cradle, it was a curse transmitted to us, by the modification and degeneration of leprosy, through myriads of constitutions, and which only disappears from the surface to fester in malignity until it bursts forth again in the multifarious forms of innumerable diseases, amongst which we find scrofula, rachitis, phthisis, hysteria, hypochondriasis, dropsy, hydrocephalus, hæmorrhage, fistula, diseases of the head and liver, ruptures, cataracts, tic-douloureux, deafness, erysipelas, cancers, aneurisms, rheumatism, gout, apoplexy, epilepsy, palsy, convulsions, stone, St. Vitus's dance, nervous affections of every description, loss of sight, of smell, of taste, stupidity and imbecility.[189] In support of this doctrine, Hahnemann adduces ninety-five cases recorded by medical writers, in which the disappearance of the itch was followed by various acute and chronic maladies.

The next miasmatic generator is *sycosis,* or the disposition to warty excrescences; but this source of disease Hahnemann does not consider so prolific as syphilis, or his favourite psora.

Such are the principal features of the homœopathic system. I have already stated that its followers consider the most minute particles of medicine more powerful than larger doses; they therefore have recourse to infinite trituration or dilution in three vehicles which they consider free from any medicinal property, —distilled water, spirits of wine, and sugar of milk; by these means they procure a decillionth or a quintillionth fraction of a grain. One drop of their solution is considered sufficient to saturate three hundred globules of sugar of milk; and three or four of these globules are deemed a powerful medicine. To give a better idea of Hahnemann's notions on this subject, I shall quote his own words:

"By shaking a drop of medicinal liquid with one hundred drops of alcohol *once,* that is to say, by taking the phial in the hand which contains the whole, and imparting to it a rapid motion by a single stroke of the arm descending, I shall then obtain an exact mixture of them; but two or three, or ten such movements, would develop the medicinal virtues still further, making them more potent, and their action on the nerves much more penetrating. In the extenuation of powders, when it is requisite to mix one grain of a medicinal substance in one hundred grains of sugar of milk, it ought to be rubbed down with force during one hour *only,* in order that the power of the medicine may not be carried to too great an extent; medicinal substances acquiring at each division or dilution a new degree of power, as the rubbing or shaking they undergo develops that inherent virtue in medicines which was unknown until my time, and which is so energetic, that latterly I have been forced by experience to reduce the number of shakes to two."

As a further illustration of this theory, he affirms that gold is without any action in our organism in its natural state; but that when one grain of this metal is triturated according to the above process until each grain of the last triturated preparation contains a quadrillionth part of the original grain of the mineral, it will be so powerful that it will be sufficient to place this single grain in a phial, to be inspired for a moment, to produce the most amazing results, and none more so than the faculty of restoring to a melancholy individual, disposed to commit suicide, his pristine partiality to life.

Unfortunately for Hahnemann, many of these assertions are unsupported by facts or sound reasoning, and appear mere wanderings of an ardent imagination; and thus soaring in regions of fancy, he himself has struck many fatal blows to his own doctrines. For instance, what are the arguments he adduces to prove that in two similar diseases the strongest will overcome the weakest?

"Why," he exclaims, "does the splendid Jupiter disappear during the twilight of morn to the eyes of the contemplator? It is because a similar power, but possessed of greater energies, the breaking day, acts upon our organs."

This is a defective analogy. Hahnemann tells us that a stronger power banishes a weaker one in a permanent manner, whereas the bright planet he here alludes to will return with the night. Then again: —

"With what do we endeavour to relieve the olfactory nerves when offended by disagreeable odours? By snuff, which affects the nostrils in a similar but in a more powerful manner." This is not correct: when the action of snuff has ceased, the disagreeable effluvia become again offensive. In some instances his poetical vagaries are preposterous. "By what means," he adds, "do we endeavour to protect the ears of the compassionate from the lamentations of the poor wretched soldier condemned to be scourged? Is it not by the shrill notes of the fife united to the loud beat of the drum? How do we endeavour to drown the roar of distant artillery that causes terror in the heart of the soldier? By the roll of the double drum; —nor would this feeling of compassion, this sense of terror, have been checked by admonition or by splendid rewards. In the same manner our grief, our regret, subside, upon receiving the intelligence, true or false, that a more lively sorrow has affected another person." It would be idle to dwell upon the absurdity of such visions and erroneous statements.

To support his doctrines, Hahnemann should have proved, 1st, that medicinal powers do produce an artificial malady similar to the natural affection; 2nd, that the organism only remains under the influence of the medicinal disease; 3rd, that this medicinal disease is of short duration; and 4th, that all these effects can only be produced by a medicine selected according to their similarity of symptoms. Our theorist has utterly failed in his endeavours to establish these facts; therefore have his doctrines been impugned by many of his most zealous disciples, amongst whom may be mentioned Griesselich, Rau, Schroen. The aggravation which he asserts takes place after the exhibition of a homœopathic medicine is not only unsupported by proof, but positively denied by many of their practitioners; and Hartman plainly affirms that, after a homœopathic dose, the patient frequently experiences a state of calm, a disposition to slumber, and often falls into a profound sleep more or less prolonged, in waking from which he finds himself much relieved, if not perfectly cured. Thus several physicians who have adopted his practical views reject many of the doctrines on which they are founded; and a homœopathist has justly compared his works to a wild virgin forest, in which we meet with a number of valuable trees and plants in the midst of arid brushwood and parasitic weeds that would check the growth of the most useful productions.

Yet, notwithstanding the many gratuitous assertions, and consequent erroneous inductions, we meet with in the *Organon*, it is probable that this system is destined to operate a gradual but material revolution in the *practice* of medicine. As to theories, we must agree with Voltaire when he said "En fait de système, il faut toujours se reserver le droit de rire le lendemain de ses idées de la veille."

Hippocrates laid down in his Aphorisms the incontrovertible fact, "Duobus doloribus simul obortis, non tandem eâdem in parte, vehementior alterum obscurat. A. 46." To a certain degree, it was upon this assertion, which the experience of ages has confirmed, that Hahnemann founded the principal and most important point of his doctrine; but, going much farther than the father of medicine, he affirms that similar diseases effectually remove each other. For centuries practitioners have been acting homœopathically; the exhibition of specifics, in fact, being nothing else. As we have already shown, specifics are known to produce symptoms similar to the diseases they cure. Hitherto the number of such medicines has been confined to a very few agents; and perhaps with the exception of mercury, sulphur, and bark, with their several preparations, scarcely any article in the materia medica could have claimed this peculiar property. To extend these limits, which confined in so exiguous a compass our therapeutic agents, has been the laborious and singular study of Hahnemann and his disciples. Haller had first given the example, and they arduously applied themselves to discover by experiments on the healthy subject, both upon their own persons and others, what were the peculiar effects or symptoms produced by various medicinal substances. These observations are so numerous and confused, that, on reading them, we feel plunged in a chaotic labyrinth of symptoms, without any clue to extricate ourselves from its perplexing mazes. Still, from this multifarious catalogue much important information can be collected; and it cannot be denied that the homœopathist has not only thrown a new light on the action of many medicines which we daily prescribe, but brought into practical consideration the necessity of attending to dietetic discipline, by an investigation of the several properties of our usual *ingesta*.

It is obvious that any enthusiast who would blindly embrace the foregoing doctrines without serious and deep investigation, and boldly apply the wild theory to practice, would at once throw open the flood-gates of absurdity, and lend his aid in destroying, if possible, with one fell swoop, the result of ages of mature study and experience. Hahnemann, to fertilize the fields of science, had recourse to inundation instead of wise and cautious irrigation; and the fury with which he and his rash disciples maintained their opinions materially tended to retard their progress. Truth needeth not violence; its own lustre will beam through surrounding darkness, without being dragged into light.

The objections to Hahnemann's doctrines are glaring. The art of healing, from the dawn of science until the present day, has been more or less founded on the faculties of reasoning. We are taught, in the first instance, to observe carefully the phenomena of disease, and, by referring effects to probable causes, endeavour, however difficult the task, to trace their catenation. Many of these causes are perhaps sealed for ever in the inscrutable book of our destinies; yet, if we cannot obtain a knowledge of the origin of these disorders, still when we take into mature consideration the complication of all accidental circumstances, and from visible effects seek invisible relations, guided by our experience in anatomy, physiology, and the revelations of pathology, we may find this pursuit less difficult than it may be imagined. But the homœopathist despises and rejects as idle, all those collateral means of diving into nature's arcana. He bids us dwell only upon evident symptoms, or, in other words, look to the effects alone, and cast away all thoughts of discovering their causes. Nothing can be more illogical than this argument; for certainly we can scarcely hope to remove effects without striking, as far as in our power lies, at their cause. To deny the existence of any specific affection because we cannot account for its origin, is absurd. As well might we reject the use of medicines known to possess specific properties, from our utter ignorance of their *modus operandi.* The exclusive consideration of symptoms would lead us into lamentable error, since the same symptoms are observable in various diseases. Similar pains, for instance, may be the symptoms of rheumatism, nephritic affections, and calculus; headaches may arise from inflammation, and from various and well-known sympathies with distant organs: yet, without seeking to ascertain these relations, the mechanical and empirical homœopathist will prescribe such medicines as are known to occasion pains in the loins, or headaches; only bearing in mind perceptible derangements, heedless of the phenomena of organization, the state of the secretions and excretions, the history, the rise and progress of the disorder, or the idiosyncrasy of the patient. The liver is diseased; the discovery is of no importance. We have only to attend to the pain extending up the clavicle and shoulder, or the uneasiness experienced in the right hypochondrium: the pulse, the respiration, the condition of the excretions, the temperature of the skin, the appearance of the tongue, are all regarded as minor considerations. It is not *hepatitis* that we are called upon to cure; it is to relieve a pain in the shoulder and in the hypochondrium, or a difficulty of lying on the left side.

No one will pretend to deny that our safest, perhaps our sole, guide in the study of disease is the group of symptoms, that become more and more perceptible during the course of our investigations. It was principally on the study of symptoms that the most learned practitioners of every age and country grounded their diagnosis and their prognosis; but they never viewed them either singly, or in their complexity, as unconnected with the particular diseases to which they were not only essentially united, but from which they originated, and of the existence of which they were to be considered the diagnostic signs. Therefore did the ancients classify them as principal and accessory, univocal and equivocal, characteristic or common, as they afforded more or less information in our pathological deduction; and in that light they were weighed with greater or less application, as our judgment could only be formed by the attentive consideration of the phenomena of the organism in health and in disease.

But while the homœopathist's attention is chiefly directed to the discovery of means that can enable him to produce symptoms analogous to those of the disorder, he seems to disregard the laws of sympathy, by which our organism appears to be ruled; a mysterious agency which can only be ascertained by observation and experiment, when, to use the words of a distinguished writer,[190] "by the former we may be said to listen to nature, by the latter to interrogate her." Health depends upon the due co-operation of all these associations; and one organ in the wonderful machinery cannot be deranged in its functions without influencing others, however distant and unconnected they may appear. In this co-ordination, these vital relations have been very properly divided into mechanical, functional, and sympathetic. Their study constitutes the groundwork of all rational induction. It is not by individual or complex symptoms that we can decide where the want of equilibrium is to be traced. Various have been the theories on this most important subject, and great have been the erroneous ideas dogmatically laid down. The illustrious Bichat himself erred when he maintained that sympathies were aberrations-morbid developments of our vital properties. Sympathies, on the contrary, may be considered as constant phenomena, essential and inseparable from our organism, whether in health or in sickness; and are, if I may be pardoned the expression, co-ordinated to co-operate with each other in their mechanical, their functional, and their sympathetic associations.

An incarcerated hernia causes hiccup, nausea, vomiting. Will the homœopathist tell us that we must seek in his catalogue of innumerable effects some substance which is known to produce similar symptoms? Surely the rupture must first call our attention. This example is adduced as referring to nearly every case in which it might be rashly attempted to separate causes from effects. The mammary glands are variously affected in uterine diseases; their impressions are reciprocal, yet the uterine affection must be the chief object of our solicitude. A peculiar pruritus is a symptom of calculus. Are we then to administer a homœopathic dose of *cannabis*, or any other medicine which may give rise to a similar sensation? It may be objected to this observation that these are purely surgical cases, in which we need not be guided by symptoms to discover causes; but it has too frequently happened that nausea and vomiting have been attended to, while the hernia was overlooked, until fatal accidents were manifested. Moreover, a diseased liver, a diseased spleen or kidney, would be just as perceptible as hernia or calculus, if these parts could be brought into view or contact.

It may be said that an erroneous notion of Hahnemann's doctrines on this subject has been taken; it is therefore necessary to quote his own words:

"It may be easily conceived that the existence of a malady presupposes some alteration in the interior of the human organism; but our understanding can only lead us to suspect this alteration in a vague and deceitful manner, from the appearance of the morbid symptoms, the sole guide we can depend on except in surgical cases. The essence of the internal and invisible change is undiscoverable, nor have we any means of guarding against deceptive illusions."[191]

"The invisible substance that has undergone a morbid alteration in the interior of the human body, and the perceptible changes, which are externally developed, —in other words, symptoms, —form by their union what is called disease; but the symptoms are the only points of the malady which are accessible to the physician, the sole indication whence he can derive any intuitive notion, and the principal objects with which he ought to become acquainted to effect a cure. From this incontestable truth there is nothing discoverable in disease beyond the totality of its symptoms to guide us in the selection of our curative means."[192]

It is not to be supposed that an experienced physician, although a homœopathist, will rest satisfied with this study of symptomatic medicine, without endeavouring to attach these effects to some cause, however occult it may appear; but such a doctrine becomes pernicious, since it bids us close the only book of truth that can reveal our errors, —*post mortem* investigations. Surely, if a group of certain symptoms attend a disease which, when terminating fatally, shows disorganization in certain viscera, we are not only justifiable in giving to that disorganization a specific name in our scientific classification and categories, but in considering the symptoms of no other importance than as corroborative of those facts that morbid anatomy daily brings to light.

It is generally admitted that most nosologies are imperfect, and may occasionally lead the young practitioner into error. This is easily accounted for when we consider the Protean forms that the same disease assumes in different individuals; yet, without this classification, the science of medicine could not be studied. A certain arrangement is necessary to simplify all our pursuits in natural science, and to seek a variety we must know the order and the genus.

Had Hahnemann given a better system of nosology than those we possess, and with his truly praiseworthy zeal and industry enumerated the various symptoms of disease as minutely and as accurately as he has recorded the effects of medicinal substances, his labours might have proved a most valuable addition to our store of knowledge.

Let us now direct our attention to the absurdities to which these opinions have led. Solely attentive to effects, and heedless of the disorganization of various important parts of the human economy which morbid anatomy detects, Hahnemann endeavours to discover the occult causes-the original source-the germ-of the malady, which most likely are beyond the reach of our researches; and he boldly affirms that all chronic diseases spring from syphilis, a disposition to warts and the itch. Now experience has proved that such an assumption is unfounded. The most healthy subjects, those who attain the finest old age, are more liable to this disgusting affection than the wealthy and cleanly part of the community. The Irish and Scotch peasantry from their infancy, and through life, are most subject to psora; and certainly our soldiers and sailors, amongst whom the disease is common, are not more predisposed to chronic diseases than any other classes of society, of course not taking into consideration the effects of unhealthy climates.

Syphilis, it will be readily granted, has a considerable share in producing anomalous *sequelæ*, more especially when in combination with mercury. Warts, except of a syphilitic character, were never known to germinate diseases; indeed, they affect the most healthy and robust individuals. Yet to these three miasmatic causes does Hahnemann attribute nearly every disease that was ever known to afflict mankind; while he passes over in silence the predisposition to scrofula, gout, rheumatism, to which we can unfortunately trace with too much certainty the source of much human misery.

That the itch is a disease of great antiquity is a matter of doubt. It has been maintained that it is the same eruptive disorder described by Celsus under the appellation of *scabies*; yet this writer does not allude to its contagious nature, and moreover says, that in some cases it disappears completely, whereas in others it is renewed at certain periods of the year.

Celsus, moreover, includes other forms of pustular eruptions among the different species of scabies, not sufficiently distinguishing them from each other. The character of his scabies is more analogous to the lichen agrius of Willan.

Nor did the ancients consider their *psora* as our itch. It appears to have been the scaly tetter, which they sometimes denominated *psoriasis*, at others *lepra*, a synonymous affection; but neither pustular nor vesicular. Leprosy, indeed, is a malady totally distinct from the itch in all its characters. Hahnemann asserts that the species of leprosy that afflicted the Jews, and which is described by their legislator in the 13th chapter of Leviticus, was the itch; but any one who will peruse this description will perceive that it does not bear the slightest resemblance to that disorder. It appears, on the contrary, to have been that kind of leprosy called *leucé* by the ancients. Nor was leprosy constantly attended with itching, one of the chief characteristics of the malady, and from which sensation it derives its very name. Hippocrates mentions a leprosy that usually occasioned a prurience before rain. There are no diseases in the classification of which more obscurity exists than in cutaneous affections; and Hahnemann's ideas would tend to increase this confusion, since he tells us that he considers the *frambœsia* of America, the *sibbens* of Norway, the *pellagra* of Lombardy, the *plica* of Poland, the *pseudo-syphilis* of the English, and the *asthenia Virginiensis* of Virginia, complications of his three miasmatic principles; and he further informs us, no doubt on the faith of some idle tradition, that *psora* lost its external deformity on the return of the Crusaders, who brought from the Holy Land the use of linen shirts, a cleanly and salutary precaution that eradicated the disease at a period when France had no less than two thousand hospitals for the reception of *itch* patients, —a plain proof that he confounds leprosy with itch, since the hospitals he alludes to were distinctly considered leper-houses.

It is certainly true that there does exist in our system a constant predisposition to eruptive affections of some kind or other. We are born heirs to certain exanthematic affections, such as the measles and smallpox; and it would be as difficult to find a being morally immaculate as an individual free from speck or blemish. Many of these eruptions are considered of a critical and salutary nature; and the ancients fancied that nature relieved herself by throwing upon the surface some "peccant humours." Hence their dread of the retrocession of any of these "breakings out;" and there is no doubt but that accidents frequently followed their sudden disappearance, in the same manner as drying up an issue or a blister established for some time, and become habitual, may occasion internal mischief; but to maintain that all chronic diseases arise from three eruptive principles is a most gratuitous and untenable assertion.

Enthusiastically anxious to support his doctrines, Hahnemann is frequently led into erroneous assertions. Thus he tells us that life will suddenly cease if a little water, or the mildest liquid, is injected into a vein; whereas experience has proved, in the treatment of cholera, and various other instances, that the most stimulating solutions may be thus introduced, not only with impunity, but with salutary results.

It is needless to enter more deeply into the ungracious business of pointing out errors, many of which were evident to Hahnemann himself; since, not only in the several editions of his Organon, but in various paragraphs in the same volume, he contradicts himself.

A much more gratifying and important task is now undertaken, to prove, by the evidence of facts, supported by practical reasoning, that the art of healing is more indebted to the homœopathic doctrines than to any system that has hitherto been delivered in our schools.

That the all-bountiful Creator, in permitting, for purposes unknown to us, mankind to be visited by so many scourges, has also scattered around us means to counteract these evils, cannot be a matter of doubt. Instinct leads animals to find out these salutary agents, and various specifics have been discovered by man. The rudest savage is in possession of curative substances unknown to civilized man, and performs cures where learning and experience have proved of no avail.

To extend the limits of specifics, must therefore be considered a most desirable step towards adding to our means of relieving disease; and in this pursuit it is impossible to bestow too much praise on the homœopathic observer. Enthusiasm-predilection to a favourite but persecuted system-may induce an ardent proselyte not only to deceive others, but unwittingly to deceive himself. It is therefore not only possible, but probable, that in the experimental investigations of the effects of medicine, Fancy, in her multifarious colours, may have depicted, with apparent fidelity, a state of body and mind that only existed in an excited imagination; but when we behold various individuals, distant from each other, and totally unconnected, observing similar results from the exhibition of various medicinal substances, we have no right to call their assertions into doubt. These assertions, moreover, are not laid down dogmatically, but are earnestly recommended to be submitted to the test of experiment. For instance, the homœopathist has found out that certain substances, by diminishing the energy of the heart and arteries, subdue inflammatory action as effectually as venesection. This is a fact daily witnessed, and of which any practitioner may convince himself. It is not asserted, that in cases of sudden determination of blood, which require immediate revulsion and abstraction of the vital fluid, homœopathic remedies will be found possessed of sufficient activity to afford prompt relief; but experience has fully proved that in cases which can admit of a few hours' delay, these medicines very frequently supersede the necessity of debilitating the patient by a copious loss of blood.

Dr. Paris, in his admirable work on Materia Medica, has justly observed, "that observation or experiment upon the effects of medicine is liable to a thousand fallacies, unless it be carefully repeated under the various circumstances of *health* and *disease*, in different climates, and on different constitutions." This has been the main object of the homœopathist; and a further quotation from the above distinguished writer will illustrate the importance of their labours. "It is impossible to cast our eyes over such multiplied groups (of medicinal substances) without being forcibly struck with the palpable absurdity of some, the disgusting and loathsome nature of others, the total want of activity in many, and the uncertain and precarious reputation of *all*, without feeling an eager curiosity to inquire, from the combination of what causes it can have happened that substances at one period in the highest esteem, and of generally acknowledged utility, have fallen into total neglect and disrepute. That such fluctuation in opinion and versatility in practice should have produced, even in the most candid and learned observer, an unfavourable impression with regard to the general efficacy of medicines can hardly excite our astonishment, much less our indignation; nor can we be surprised to find that another portion of mankind has at once arraigned physic as a fallacious art, or derided it as a composition of error and fraud. A late foreign writer, impressed with this sentiment, has given the following *flattering* definition of our profession: *Physic is the art of amusing the patient, while Nature cures his disease.*"

With such a lamentable view of the practice of medicine, can we be too thankful to those observers who strenuously endeavour to rescue it from the dark trammels in which prejudice and interested motives have bound it? In no country more than in Great Britain is such an investigation desirable. We have become proverbial from our incessant abuse of a farrago of medicinal substances; and what is usually termed an *elegant prescription* signifies an amalgam of various drugs and preparations, which most probably, by their affinities, neutralize the expected effects of each other; for, however great and flattering may have been the discoveries of modern chemistry, many of these affinities are unknown to us. Surely when our labours cannot detect any difference in the component parts of the purest Alpine atmosphere and the deleterious air of a loathsome dungeon, we cannot expect to form a correct idea of pharmaceutic combinations.

The mere hopes of being able to relieve society from the curse of constant drugging, should lead us to hail with gratitude the homœopathist's investigations. That many physicians, but especially apothecaries, who live by overwhelming their patients with useless and too frequently pernicious medicines, will warmly, nay furiously inveigh against any innovation of the kind, must be expected as the natural result of interested apprehension; and any man who aims at simplicity in practice will be denounced as guilty of medical heresy. Have we not seen inoculation and vaccination branded with the most opprobrious epithets, merely because their introduction tended to diminish professional lucre?

In these remarks upon medicinal combinations, it is not meant to infer, that, because they are chemically incompatible, they are ineffectual,—experience has proved the contrary; but no one will contend that, if we can attain the same beneficial results from a single ingredient, administered in small quantities and at distant periods, as from the exhibition of repeated and nauseous doses of pills, powders, draughts, potions, &c. which hang over the bed of sickness, nay, of slight derangements, like the sword of Damocles, we have not effected a most salutary reform in the practice of physic. It is related of one of these ingenious and industrious practitioners, that, having seen a prescription, that only contained half a dozen medicines, he exclaimed, "What! nothing more?" To which the prescriber replied, "If you choose, sir, we'll step over to the apothecary, and see what else he has in his shop."

Specifics may be divided into two classes; the one producing a peculiar effect upon particular organs, the other producing general results. Thus, the action of cantharides and digitalis on the urinary system, of emetics on the stomach, of certain purgatives on the small intestines, and of others on the large ones, are generally known; whereas the action of mercury and opium is still a matter of controversy. A study of these effects constitutes the chief object of the homœopathist; and, having determined their peculiar action, these medicinal agents are given singly, and, as we have already observed, in the most minute doses.

It is this division into infinite fractions that has drawn upon the homœopathic practice the denunciation of the allopathic physicians, as it is considered utterly impossible that such imponderable particles can produce any beneficial or prejudicial effect; and the Academy of Medicine of Paris, when officially condemning the doctrine, asserts, in support of this argument, that great danger arises from it "in frequent and serious cases of disease, where the physician may do as much injury, and cause no less mischief, by ineffectual means as by those which are prejudicial."

This is perhaps one of the most important points of the homœopathic doctrine. If these fractional doses are inert, and yet the disease is cured, then must the successful treatment be solely ascribed to the dietetic regimen and the efforts of nature. However, experience has afforded abundant proofs that these infinite atoms do produce positive and evident effects. What appears to our feeble organs an atomic fraction may produce phenomena on the organism which we cannot comprehend, but should not therefore be denied. Let one grain of iodine be dissolved in one thousand five hundred and sixty grains of water, the solution will be limpid; let two grains of starch be dissolved in two ounces of water and added to the first solution, and the liquor will forthwith assume a blue tint. In this experiment the grain of iodine has been divided into $1/15360$. Dissolve the four-hundredth part of one grain of arsenic in four hundred thousand parts of water, and the hydric-sulphite will bring it into evidence. Let a five-thousandth part of arseniate of ammonia be dissolved in five hundred thousand parts of water, and the addition of the smallest proportion of nitrate of silver will obtain a yellow precipitate. Numerous experiments of a similar nature may be daily resorted to, to prove that the most minute particles of two substances possessed of chemical affinities may be brought into action, although diluted *ad infinitum*. But the power that the smallest particle possesses in producing natural phenomena cannot be more evidently proved than by Spallanzani's experiments in fecundation. This physiologist having wrapped up a male frog in oil-silk, fecundation could not take place; but having collected on the point of a camel-hair pencil a particle of the fecundising fluid, he succeeded in vivifying thousands of eggs. Surprised at this result, he dissolved three grains of the secretion in a pound of water, and one globule of the solution was endowed with the same faculty. In this case the globule of water only contained $1/2994687500$ part of one grain. This curious experiment has been tried with a similar result by Prevost and Dumas. How imponderable and impalpable must be the effluvium which enables the dog to track his master for miles! the particle of atter of roses that perfumes a whole chest of clothes! and what must the power of the aroma be which is preserved for thousands of years in some Egyptian mummies! Would the vulgar believe in the wonders of the solar and gaseous microscopes unless they were exposed to view? In these we behold in amazement myriads of individuals in one drop of fluid, each of them as perfect in organization as the mighty mammoth of old or the sagacious elephant of our days, endowed with distinct habits, destructive and reproductive propensities and faculties.

It has been advanced by the opponents of homœopathy that the insignificant dose of three or four medicinal globules cannot possess any power, since one might swallow a thousand of them with impunity. To this it is answered, that it is only under certain morbid conditions that these medicines act by their homœopathic affinities. Moreover, it is well known that small doses of medicinal substances will frequently produce more powerful effects than larger quantities. Tartar-emetic, sugar of lead, calomel, afford daily instances of this fact; and it is also admitted that many substances act differently upon the healthy or the sick. An individual in health can take any food without apprehension; but when his functions are deranged, the slightest imprudence in regimen may lead to serious consequences. There are primordial and inscrutable peculiarities in our constitution that cannot be accounted for; and the medicine which relieves one patient will aggravate the sufferings of others. The exhalations of the American *rhus* are deadly to some persons, but innocuous to others; and many poisons which cause instantaneous death to some animals may be given with safety to others. Whence has arisen the controversy regarding damp sheets, which many maintain are not dangerous, simply from the fact that a healthy person with a vigorous circulation may sleep in them with impunity, when a feeble and languid subject will be exposed to some dangerous determination of blood?

A learned writer already quoted thus expresses himself on this matter:[193] "The virtues of medicines cannot be fairly nor beneficially ascertained by trying their effects on sound subjects, because the peculiar morbid condition which they are calculated to remove does not exist." It may be said that this observation militates against the homœopathic experiments, and to a certain extent it evidently does; but it cannot be inferred that because a medicinal substance will occasionally act differently in health and in disease, that it may not frequently operate in a similar manner when the morbid condition does prevail, since it is generally admitted that medicines act in a relative manner according to the state of the system. Hence classifications of medicines are too frequently erroneous and imperfect. The doses of medicines determine their effects. Linnæus says, "Medicines differ from poisons, not in their nature, but in their dose;" and Pliny tells its aphoristically, "*Ubi virus, ibi virtus.*" According to their doses, medicines will produce a general or a local effect; and Dr. Paris, whom I feel much gratification in quoting, lays down as a rule that "substances perfectly inert and useless in one dose may prove in another active and valuable." It would be foreign to my purpose to enter more fully into this most important subject; but the cases which shall be adduced will be deemed sufficient to convince the most incredulous, of the power of homœopathic doses.

Those who have denied this property have boldly attributed homœopathic cures to dietetic means. Admitting this statement by way of argument, surely, if any observer, by ascertaining the peculiar action of our ingesta, can so regulate the regimen as to produce salutary effects without the aid of medicine, mankind would be most essentially benefited. How many persons do we not daily meet with, who have never taken any medicine since their childhood, when maternal care strove to destroy their digestive organs with apothecary's *stuff*, and who regulate their functions by mere attention to their mode of living. I know one gentleman, a physician, who relieves constipation by green chilies; another, with cold milk; a third, with warm milk: in some habits spinach and sorrel will act as a powerful and safe aperient; in others, cheese, or a hard egg, will operate in a contrary way. Fermented and spirituous liquors all possess specific properties. Some gouty persons cannot drink Claret without bringing on a paroxysm, and others dread a glass of Champagne or Burgundy. Nay, different wines have been known to bring on arthritic attacks in particular parts; and I have known Champagne to produce gout in the wrist, and Burgundy in the knee, in subjects who under other circumstances never experienced the disorder in those articulations. Our peculiar aversion, nay, our dread, of various alimentary substances are well known. The odour of cheese, of strawberries, have occasioned fainting and convulsions; and in certain constitutions, several articles of diet bring on indigestion. In short, the study of our ingesta is one of the greatest importance; and here again the homœopathist is entitled to our best thanks.

This investigation will moreover prompt physicians to be more attentive in inquiring into the various effects of alimentary and medicinal substances on their patients. Instead of hastily drawing out routine prescriptions for such and such a disorder, they will accurately ascertain the physical and moral condition of the subject, taking into due consideration previous habits, predispositions, and pursuits in life. Indeed, it would be desirable that practitioners followed the example of army medical men, who keep an exact register of every individual they attend, and in which is diligently recorded every circumstance connected with the disease and its treatment.

Moral influence has also been called into aid in opposition to this practice, and cures have been attributed to the mere power of fancy and credulity. We have certainly known superstition and mental imbecility to be productive both of good and evil, —to have created some maladies, and cured others; but homœopathy has succeeded when the patient was unaware of the treatment to which he was submitted. But, conceding the point, and admitting that inert substances, such as starch, (and this experiment was resorted to in Paris,) may have obtained singular beneficial results, —the results of a weak imagination, this circumstance alone would be illustrative of the power of moral agency; and who would not gladly wish for a mental relief in lieu of a nauseating and injurious course of medicine?

Others will exclaim, although the homœopathist disavows the *vis medicatrix naturæ*, that he solely succeeds by leaving the malady to the salutary efforts of the constitution. Here again we must admit, that, were we to leave many diseases to run their course, we might be more successful in obtaining a cure than by a rash and detrimental interference, founded on the principle that a physician "must order something."

But the facts I am about to record, —facts which induced me, from having been one of the warmest opponents of this system, to investigate carefully and dispassionately its practical points, —will effectually contradict all these assertions regarding the inefficacy of the homœopathic doses, the influence of diet, or the agency of the mind; for in the following cases in no one instance could such influences be brought into action. They were (with scarcely any exception) experiments made without the patient's knowledge, and where no time was allowed for any particular regimen. They may, moreover, be conscientiously relied upon, since they were made with a view to prove the fallacy of the homœopathic practice. Their result, as may be perceived by the foregoing observations, by no means rendered me a convert to the absurdities of the doctrine, but fully convinced me by the most incontestable facts that the introduction of fractional doses will soon banish the farrago of nostrums that are now exhibited to the manifest prejudice both of the health and the purse of the sufferer.

CASE I.

A servant-maid received a blow of a stone upon the head. Severe headache, with dizziness and dimness of sight, followed. Various means were resorted to; but general blood-letting could alone relieve the distressing symptoms, local bleeding not having been found of any avail. The relief, however, was not of long duration, and the distressing accidents recurred periodically, when abstraction of blood became indispensable. Reduced by these frequent evacuations, I was resolved to try the boasted "bleeding globules" of the homœopathist, when, to my great surprise, I obtained the same mitigation of symptoms which the loss of from twelve to sixteen ounces of blood had previously accomplished. Since the first experiment no venesection became necessary, and the returns of the violent headache were invariably relieved by the same means.

CASE II.

An elderly woman was subject to excruciating headache, with an evident determination of blood to the brain. Numerous leeches were constantly applied. The usual remedies indicated in similar affections were resorted to, but only afforded temporary relief. A homœopathic dose of aconite was given, and the relief that followed was beyond all possible expectation.

CASE III.

My much-esteemed friend Dr. Grateloup of Bordeaux was subject to frequent sore-throats, which were only relieved by local blood-letting, cataplasms, &c., but generally lasted several days, during which deglutition became most difficult. I persuaded him to try a dose of the belladonna, neither of us having the slightest confidence in its expected effects. He took the globules at twelve o'clock, and at five P.M. the tumefaction of the tonsils, with their redness and sensibility, had subsided to such an extent that he was able to partake of some food at dinner. The following morning all the symptoms, excepting a slight swelling, had subsided.

Since this period Dr. G. has repeatedly tried the same preparation in similar cases, and with equal success. In my own practice, I can record seven cases of cynanche tonsillaris which were thus relieved in the course of a few hours.

CASE IV.

H —, a young woman on the establishment of the Countess of —, was suffering under hemiplegia, and it was resolved by Dr. Brulatour and myself to try the effects of nux vomica. At this period the wonders of the homœopathic practice had been extolled to the skies by its advocates, and we were resolved to give one of their supposed powerful preparations a fair trial. The girl was told that the powder she was about to take was simply a dose of calomel; and on calling upon her the following morning we did not expect that the slightest effect could have been obtained by this atomic dose, when, to our utter surprise, the patient told us that she had passed a miserable night, and described to us most minutely all the symptoms that usually follow the exhibition of a large dose of strychnine. It is but fair to mention that the homœopathic treatment did not cure the disease; but the manifest operation of this fractional dose, that could not possibly be denied, is a fact of considerable importance.

CASE V.

Mrs. — — of Brompton, Bow, had laboured under hectic fever for several months, and was so reduced by night perspirations, that she was on the very brink of the grave. Called into consultation, I frankly told her husband that every possible means known in the profession had been most judiciously employed, and that I saw no prospect of obtaining relief. At the same time I mentioned to him that the homœopathic practitioners pretended that they had found the means of relieving these distressing symptoms, which he might submit to an experimental trial if he thought proper. He immediately expressed his wish that it should be adopted. I gave her a homœopathic dose of phosphoric acid and stannum; and, to the surprise of all around her, the night sweats did not break out at their usual hour, —three o'clock in the morning. What renders this case still more interesting is the fact of these perspirations recurring so soon as the action of the medicine ceased; a circumstance so evidently ascertained, that the patient knew the very day when another dose became necessary.

CASE VI.

A daughter of the same lady was subject to deafness, which I attributed to a fulness of blood. This cause I clearly ascertained by the relief afforded by the application of a few leeches behind the ear. I was therefore induced, on a recurrence of the complaint, to endeavour to diminish vascular action by a dose of aconite. The effects were evident in the course of four hours, when the deafness and the other symptoms of local congestion had entirely disappeared.

I could record numerous instances of similar results, but they would of course be foreign to the nature of this work. I trust that the few cases I have related will afford a convincing proof of the injustice, if not the unjustifiable obstinacy, of those practitioners who, refusing to submit the homœopathic practice to a fair trial, condemn it without investigation. That this practice will be adopted by quacks and needy adventurers, there is no doubt; but homœopathy is a science on which numerous voluminous works have been written by enlightened practitioners, whose situation in life placed them far above the necessities of speculation. Their publications are not sealed volumes, and any medical man can also obtain the preparations they recommend. It is possible, nay, more than probable, that physicians cannot find time to commence a new course of studies, for such this investigation must prove. If this is the case, let them frankly avow their utter ignorance of the doctrine, and not denounce a practice of which they do not possess the slightest knowledge.

Despite the persecution that *Hahnemannism* (as this doctrine is ironically denominated) is at present enduring, every reflecting and unprejudiced person must feel convinced that, although its wild and untenable theories may not overthrow the established systems (if any one system can be called established), yet its study and application bid fair to operate an important revolution in medicine. The introduction of infinite small doses, when compared, at least, with the quantities formerly prescribed, is gradually creeping in. The history of medicine affords abundant proofs of the acrimony, nay, the fury, with which every new doctrine has been impugned and insulted. The same annals will also show that this spirit of intolerance has always been in the *ratio* of the truths that these doctrines tended to bring into light. From the preceding observations, no one can accuse me of having become a blind bigot of homœopathy; but I can only hope that its present vituperators will follow my example, and examine the matter calmly and dispassionately before they proceed to pass a judgment that their vanity may lead them to consider a final sentence.

HOMOEOPATHY AS A SCIENCE
by Edward Bayard

"Philosophy and science arc so related as to constitute a unity." —"The Relations of Mind and Brain," CALDERWOOD.

Many of the most important discoveries of the psychologists were rejected by the physiologists, because they could not be proved by their law-and conversely with the psychologists. These contending forces have been brought into lasting alliance by Professor Calderwood. It is believed that as close a relation can be established between Nature's laws and those of homœopathy.

Vaccination, as the sole and sure preventive of small-pox, is one of the great, dominant, fixed facts of the old school. Here is the open and avowed application of the law of cure by similars, *similia similibus curantur*. If it be a law of cure in one case, by what logical process can it be demonstrated to fail in all others? Those most conversant with Nature's laws assert, and truly, that she makes no exceptions: the law of gravity; that water seeks its own level; that the pressure of water is equal in all directions; that sound ascends; that heat expands. It was this universality of the law of Nature which enabled the great naturalist, Cuvier, to construct a whole skeleton from two or three bones. So, with equal certainty, if necessary, could the skeleton of the homœopathic law be evolved from this single bone of its structure-vaccination. Starting from different stand-points, the old and new schools have progressed in the same direction, to diminished doses, both in size and repetition. This is concededly due in the old school to the influence of homœopathy, in the new it is the growth of its own experience.

Messrs. Bell and Laird, in their admirable monograph on diarrhœa, say: "There is indeed a somewhat prevalent opinion that the strength of the dose makes up for want of due care or knowledge in selection. This may be stated in mathematical terms, as follows: If the thirtieth potency of arsenic is equal to a complete knowledge of the drug, one fifth of a grain of arsenious acid is equal to complete ignorance of it. Stated in this, its true form, we grant it."

Homœopathy, as a science, is the law of the vital force; the body is but the mechanism upon which it operates. The dissecting-knife has laid bare to the astonished gaze of the student a perfect organism, while the operating-table presents the companion picture of an organism in total ruins dominated by the vital principle. What, then, is disease-typhoid, pneumonia, scarlet fever? No; disease is the impairment of the equalization of the vital force, and it finds expression where the organism is weakest.

What is cure-to take physic for typhoid or scarlet fever? No; to cure is to locate the center of the disturbance, the diseased nerve cell, and restore the equilibrium.

How do you do this? In spite of its many ramifying influences, the nerve-cell preserves, to the close and exact student, its individuality, often veiled under the apparently familiar features of others, but still recognizable by the differentiating mind. It is this similar of state and remedy which the homœopathic physician, who knows and applies the law, seeks in the patient and in the materia medica; when found, the means of restoring the equalization of the vital current is found with it.

As there is but one nerve-center of a disease, so is there but one remedy.

The system has always a tendency to resist, by reaction, the morbific cause which disturbs it. The similar stimulates reaction. When you put your hot hand into hot water, and take it out and wipe it dry, by the law of reaction it becomes cool. So, if to the frost-bitten ear or hand you apply snow or ice, by the law of reaction the frozen part burns under its stimulus. The power of resistance, which is reaction, is the strength of the constitution, or is the constitution itself. It is this law of reaction under which homœopathy works, by its similars stimulating the additional resistance necessary to aid in nature's cure.

If you go out into excessive cold, and the power of resistance is equal to the demand, you turn red; if not, and this power is overwhelmed, you turn white. And the same difference is markedly observable among those who take sea-baths. By the law of reaction they vary in color from that of a boiled lobster to the livid hue of death, graduated and shaded off by the loss of the power of resistance. All cures are sought by homœopathy under this law, and depend for their success upon this power of resistance, and it is of vital importance that this power be not diminished, for without it there can be no cure. Outside of medicine this law of reaction in the system is recognized as an accepted fact. It is the law of cure, and the study of this law is a science, and that science is homœopathy.

The reason why scarlet fever, measles, chicken-pox, and small-pox do not, as a general rule, recur in the system is that, at the first attack, the system has reacted so strongly against these diseases as to be proof against a second attack. The reaction has so strengthened the system to resist the particular form of morbific influence that it will not readily yield to it again.

"Homœopathy is another form of quackery," says a writer in the June number of "The Popular Science Monthly." It might be objected to his method of treating the subject that no *a priori* argument can suffice in the forum of reason where practical tests and material results may be had, by any one so in love with the truth as to seek it, by going frankly to eminent homœopathic physicians and obtaining permission to study their treatment in a given number of cases, and, with a mind disabused of prejudice, carefully examining and noting each case and giving the results of such observations. There would then, at least, be some facts which would give currency to the alloy of mere argument.

There is certainly no more reason, viewed from a logical standpoint, why the inducing of symptoms or sufferings different from those produced by disease should prove more efficacious in cure than a remedy which produces similar symptoms. It may be so; but the mere assertion does not establish it. The question is one of fact; it does not belong to the domain of reason. However absurd the theory of one school may appear to a disciple of the other, the question remains, Which system cures?

It is asserted that infinitesimal doses, a decillionth part of a grain, can not cure. This statement is based upon the assumption that a dozen, or twenty, or more grains, given by the allopathic school in single or quickly repeated doses, are necessary to effect a cure, and that so given they do cure, which is to assert that allopathy is the only true standard and measure of cure, and that any material deviation therefrom is error. But, if the premise be denied, the conclusion fails.

Of the uncertainty of cure by allopathic remedies, let one of the most eminent of that school speak-that man of attainments and ability, Sir John Forbes. In his work entitled "Nature and Art in Disease," a solemn legacy to his younger brethren, he says:

"And yet what is the character of the results obtained under this system" (homœopathic) "of imaginary medication in the cure of diseases? When fairly weighed do not these results exhibit, if not quite as large a proportion of cures as ordinary medicine, still so large a proportion as to demonstrate at once the feebleness of what we regard as the best form of art and the immense strength of Nature in the same office. . . .

"The favorable results obtained by the homœopaths-or, to speak more accurately, the wonderful powers possessed by the natural restorative agencies of the living body-demonstrated under their imaginary treatment, have led to several other practical results of value to the practitioners of ordinary medicine. Besides leading their minds to the most important of all medical studies, that of the natural history of diseases, it has tended directly to improve their practice by augmenting their confidence in Nature's powers, and proportionately diminishing their belief in the universal necessity of art, thus checking that unnecessary interference with the natural processes by the employment of heroic means, always so prevalent and so injurious. It has been the means of lessening in a considerable degree the monstrous poly-pharmacy which has always been the disgrace of our art, by at once diminishing the frequency of administration of drugs and lessening their dose. . . .

"In a word, almost every drug in our overflowing materia medica, whether inert or active, has been on one ground or another copiously prescribed in every variety of disease under the supposed sanction of this pseudo-specific on empirical indication. Nor let it be supposed that this empirical practice is one of the past day only. It is at this very time in as great vogue as ever, although its employment may be often veiled under the technicalities of newer science.

"Nor is it confined to the ignorant or inexperienced among us, but adopted and followed by men of the greatest abilities and greatest eminence in the profession. . . .

"As in religion and politics, and in those departments of knowledge which are not of a positive or demonstrable kind, early and long continued education, comprising not merely direct instruction, properly so called, but the influence of habitual example, deference to seniority and superiority, unconscious imitation, etc., induce conventional belief of the strongest kind-strong as demonstrated truth itself-and create a sort of wizard circle of power, beyond which the mind of the disciple, however bold, scarcely ever dares to wander. So in medicine, the great majority of practitioners retain the same doctrines and pursue the same practice which they learned in the schools, or, if changing both doctrine and practice, as time and fashion dictate, hold fast, at least, the great fundamental doctrine impressed upon the very core of their professional hearts-viz., that the interference of Art is essential in all cases, and therefore never to be foregone. It need not, therefore, surprise us that it is only a very small minority of medical practitioners who, in ordinary circumstances, can see in disease the true workings of Nature through the artificial veil which conventionalism and professional superstition have thrown over them. . . .

"The conviction of the great autocracy of Nature, in the cure of diseases derived from this source, is much more widely spread among the senior members of the profession than is at all believed by the great body of practitioners. . . . The number of cases that recover and would have died had Art not interfered is extremely small."

These trenchant words from Sir John Forbes carry great weight as a commanding critic in his own profession. Had his strictures upon his brethren and their practices come from an alien pen, they would undoubtedly have been attributed by the allopathic school to malevolence and ignorance; and, doubtless, Sir John Forbes will not escape the same fate, because, if his statements are true, those of whom they are spoken are incapable of perceiving or admitting their truth.

But, conceding the allopathic to be a correct or a possible system of cure, it by no means follows that because it requires large doses to create different symptoms or sufferings, it likewise requires doses of equal quantity to create *similar* symptoms to those to which the system is already so greatly predisposed.

The atomic dose will, however, bear a much closer and more severe test than has been applied to it. It is an approved and well-known fact that a person of iron will will battle long and successfully with a disease which baffles the aid of the most skillful physician, and it is said that his will sustains him. By that is not meant that he leans upon his will as upon a staff, nor that the immaterial, the will, comes in actual contact with the material, the disease; but that the will, acting through the brain, rouses up in the system material resistance to the disease, and effects a cure or prolongs the fight. How much brain would one have to eat in order to obtain a decillionth part of a grain of the will-power which operated in the system in effecting a cure or battling with the disease? The will operating through the brain moves one joint of the little finger, then two, then three, and so on until it moves by one operation of the will the whole fourteen joints of the five fingers, which act in unison at one motion. Yet it is clear that each additional joint moved resulted from the impression made upon a larger area of the nerve-centers in the brain. Assuming for the sake of argument that the correct method of cure is to arouse in the system a direct reaction against disease, and that this can only be accomplished through the brain, it follows that the remedy, which in form is best adapted to act upon the brain, is the best so far as mere form is concerned; and if the immaterial, the will, can produce such positive physical results, the quantity of the medicine operating upon the brain is not required by any law of physics (or physiology) to be many times greater than the nerve-cell, which is the body to be operated upon; especially must this be true when the object sought is not to overwhelm the nerve-center, but simply to stimulate it to increased action.

Professor Calderwood, in his "Relations of Mind and Brain," says of the nerve-cells in the brain: "These are so numerous as to baffle calculation. From the number seen within a small section under the microscope, it is reckoned that there must be many thousands of them in the human brain." Of the nerve-fibers he says: "In the brain itself they are sometimes as minute as a twelve-thousandth part of an inch," and that the smallest of the nerve-fibers in the eye are from $\frac{1}{13000}$ to $\frac{1}{150000}$ part of an inch in diameter. As an adaptation of means to end, a decillionth part of a grain, broken up into many still more minute particles, does not appear to be so much out of proportion to the nerve-cell or to the ducts, the nerve-fibers, as the two, four, six, or more grains given by the allopaths.

The stench contained in a few drops distilled by a skunk attains a potential existence in the air for not less than five hundred feet in every direction. Taking one thousand feet cubed as a minimum, we have one billion cubic feet of air saturated with the smell. Not only is this space filled once, but it is kept filled for an hour, radiating out indefinitely into space; from which it is clear, according to our critic, that a passer-by, an hour afterward, deceives himself by a supposititious shock to the sense of smell caused by the decillionth part of the drop of skunk-odor. But the involuntary clapping of the hand to the nose affords conclusive proof that both the sensor and motor nerves have been sensibly affected.

That in a chemical laboratory there is no appliance so sensitive as a diseased nerve, does not argue the inefficacy of the atomic dose, but proves the want of adaptation of the chemical apparatus to deal with the subject.

Hahnemann's method of trituration is urged as an argument against his principles, without showing that it has anything to do with the principles, or that it fails to accomplish the object sought. The work is now done with great exactness by machinery.

It is said that since the discovery of the *Sarcoptis hominis,* or itch insect, the dogma about psora being such a powerful factor in the causation of diseases has fallen to the ground; that is to say, that those who supported this theory have been, by this discovery, forced to abandon it. Why? Evidently because the theory is inconsistent with the itch-insect. But who proves it? Is the disease the cause of the insect, or the insect the cause of the disease? Do maggots breed carrion, or carrion maggots? Was Hamlet trying to shift the responsibility of Polonius's death from himself to the worms?

"Now, Hamlet, where's Polonius?"

"At supper."

"At supper! Where?"

"Not where he eats, but where he is eaten. A certain convocation of politic worms are e'en at him."

That is, the worms killed Polonius.

But it is clear that Hamlet was not so mad as that, for he said, "For if the sun breed maggots in a dead dog, being a god-kissing carrion —"

So will psora breed the *Sarcoptis hominis,* but so will not the insect breed the itch. Being but the effect, it can not produce the cause. It is not its own *causa causans.*

Homœopathy has suffered, and is likely to suffer, more from its friends than from its enemies.

Persons who adopt it as an easy means of gaining a livelihood are apt to fail, and fall back upon the allopathic school, with its nosology and procrustean prescriptions. Few are those in any calling who have either the frankness to confess or ability to perceive the cause of failure to be from within. The convenience of a name for every disease is apparent. It relieves from further investigation. How little Dr. Shepherd knows of the laws of homœopathy may be demonstrated by a single sentence. He says: "Hahnemann paid no attention to pathology or cause of disease, but only sought for symptoms. For instance, in a case of dropsy, the cause, whether it be from the heart, the kidneys, or the liver, is not inquired into, but the *symptom dropsy is treated.*"

It is clear that the writer here uses the term "cause of disease" as synonymous with the part affected, which is to confound cause and effect, and he substitutes his own nosology "dropsy" for the group of symptoms which indicate, not dropsy, but the remedy to be selected. The fact that the heart or kidneys or the liver is affected does not indicate or prove that the one affected is the cause of disease. It proves that the disease has affected that part, and it follows by an inexorable law that the part affected can only be cured by removing the cause. It is this inversion of cause and effect, of disease and its point of attack or expression, this ignorance of Nature's laws, which induces the allopath to attempt to cut out the core of what he calls cancer; thus trimming the branches of this mighty disease, to strengthen it at the roots, seated deep down in the system. It is like cutting down a locust, and producing a forest from the roots. How can a school, which has been a thousand years dissecting dead bodies to discover the vital principle, hope to free itself from its dogmas? As well might it be expected to discover the electric fluid by dissecting a yard of telegraph wire. Professor Calderwood, who is not a homœopathist, demonstrates, as a scientist, from the discoveries of the foremost physiologists and psychologists, that, by tracing up all of the group of symptoms along the nerve-fibers, we will reach a common nerve-center in the brain, differing in area and location with differing groups of symptoms. This nerve-center is operated upon by certain sensor nerves. The whole object of the homœopathic physician, who is true to the law, is to trace these symptoms to a common nerve-center, and then to select a remedy which, acting upon that nerve-center, will, on the line by which Nature cures, stimulate a reaction, and thus restore the equilibrium, which is perfect health.

The law of Nature's cure is, by rousing up reaction against disease, to restore the disturbed forces to their exact counterpoise, where action and reaction are equal. The allopathic method of creating a new disease to cure the old one is a violation of this law, and at the very outset the regular school must begin by an apology or an excuse, either that Nature has denied to men the means of executing her laws, or that man is ignorant of the means she has placed at his disposal.

As an abstract question, preference must be given to that method of cure which creates the least disturbance in the system, and, as a consequence, leaves it less liable to relapse or a second attack; which does not by antagonizing the vital forces reduce or destroy its economies; which does not work by rule of three; as the remedy is to the disease, so is the constitution to the condition of the patient when the disease shall have left it. Convalescence in homœopathy commences when the correct remedy begins to act. In allopathy, when the remedy and disease have left the patient prostrate, then Nature takes the matter in hand. It is a common error with the ignorant traducers of homœopathy that the higher the potencies or its remedies the weaker they become, as one weakens wine by adding water. It is sufficient answer to quote the following high authority, who discloses the true purpose and effect:

"If it be conceded that the vital principle is identical with electricity, the action of dynamized medicaments becomes easy of comprehension; for in these preparations we have material substances subdivided to a degree that enables them to penetrate the most delicate tissues of the body." —(Dr. Currie's preface to Jahr's "Homœopathic Manual.")

The writer's assertion, that "homœopathy, being a system utterly void of any scientific foundation, is now dying a natural death," receives, to say the least, doubtful support from the animated debate which has been progressing so vigorously in the New York County Medical Society of the regular school in reference to consultation with homœopaths, where the exclusionists accused the more liberal brothers of having an itching palm for the fat fees which now find their way, without chance of tax, to the pockets of the homœopathic physicians, while the argument by the liberal members is that as now homœopathy has progressed and its disciples have a thorough medical education, there is no longer any reason why they should be treated as quacks and impostors. So far as noted, the alleged moribund condition of homœopathy had escaped their observation.

What shall be said of the pretensions to be enrolled with the sciences of that school which has progressed from one stage of universal disease or cause and remedy to another-typhoid, malaria, miasm germ, bleeding, calomel, morphine, quinine-by discarding nearly all that its pioneers held most dear; which, before it can build, must tear down; which retreats from the necessary labor of that scientific investigation which by great diligence and skill eliminates every remedy but one as useless or hurtful, to take refuge in a nauseous mixture of several powerful drugs, administered upon the hit or miss blunderbuss principle-those drugs which are neither allopathic nor homœopathic to the disease, doing more potent injury than the one (which by hap-hazard has some relation) can do good, as Sir John Forbes says, "the monstrous poly-pharmacy which has always been the disgrace of our" (the allopathic) "art"?

It may well be doubted whether homœopathy will ever have enrolled under its banners the same number of practitioners as the regular school. The nearer we approach to an exact science, the fewer are its votaries. The conditions admit fewer. In it there are no formulated diseases nor formulas for prescriptions. It is differentiation as opposed to classification or generalization. The effect, expression, or impression of disease, is not mistaken for disease as a cause. Subject one hundred persons of both sexes and various ages to a cold rain and then to a burning sun, and you will have as many different states as persons. The disturbance of the vital force has found expression in a hundred different forms. It is in the province of the homoeopathic physician to locate the center of disturbance, and then to select as the remedy, by a process of elision from the many similars in the materia medica, the one which most nearly coincides with the expression of the disease or symptoms. When this process sometimes involves the most experienced and skillful physician in a profound study of one, two, and three hours and of re-examination as the expression changes, requiring due weight to be given to each symptom, both relatively and positively, and then to assume the grave responsibility of administering a single remedy and awaiting the result, it will be readily seen that those who are faithful to the law, and able to administer it, will be few.

By operation of the will a strong man liberates from a nerve-center of his brain nerve-energy which, acting along the motor nerves, liberates in its turn sufficient muscular energy to fell an ox. Here the immaterial, the will, has produced a most powerful material result. Suppose for a moment that the nerve-energy had been misdirected, as in case of shock from mental causes, and had all been expended within the man, who would answer for the result?

In the heroic struggle which Nature, unaided, makes against disease, the assistance from Art necessary to speed the cure may in a great majority of cases be set down in decimals, as follows:

Nature	·999
Art	·001

and it will be pretty safe to say that, whenever the proportion is against Nature, there will be no cure.

It is the 11000

which Art is called upon to throw into the scales and make them equal. If she adds more, she destroys the balance.

The atomic dose is adjusted to restore the balance. It is the infinitesimal fraction Nature needs to make the unit health.

If you accept the germ-theory of disease, and attribute to the atomic germs, floating impalpable in the air, or carried long distances through the mails on highly calendered writing-paper, from mere contact with the hands of diseased persons, the power of communicating disease and completely overwhelming the vital power, causing death, you can not logically deny to the atomic dose all aid to the vital power in resisting and defeating the attack of the atomic germ of disease simply because the dose is atomic. Nature, unaided, in a vast number of cases, success-fully resists those diseases which are attributable, by those who maintain the germ-theory in disease, to atomic germs. The number of disease-germs does not matter, as is evidenced by the communication of disease by letter where the number must necessarily be limited. The atomic dose is but a stimulus to Nature. Nature cures, aided or unaided. The atomic dose but excites

118

in a greater degree those powers of reaction and resistance of Nature already set in motion by disease-which is a disturbing cause. Nature always seeks to restore the equilibrium of her forces.

PERSONAL EXPERIENCE OF A PHYSICIAN
by John Ellis

CHAPTER I.

We all admit that every one who attempts to act as a physician, should strive to qualify himself, or herself, for the work by obtaining the best education which our medical schools afford; for to physicians are intrusted, not simply the property or money, but the very lives of their fellow-citizens. As the responsibility is great, so the duty of preparing one's self before commencing practice, and of keeping fully abreast of all new and valuable discoveries in the art of healing, is equally great. A physician should not be led blindly by his teachers and prominent medical writers, and so strongly confirm himself in the theories and views which they proclaim that he cannot, without prejudice, examine new views and theories with due care. It has been said that when Harvey discovered the true course of the circulation of the blood, there was not a single professor in the medical colleges of England over fifty years of age, who ever believed "the heresy," as his discovery was called. However this may have been, it is certain that professors and prominent medical writers are not always the first to see and recognize the truth, even when it is clearly presented to their notice.

A native of western Massachusetts, I studied medicine with an intelligent and worthy physician in my native town, and attended two and one-half courses of medical lectures at the Berkshire Medical College, at Pittsfield, Mass., and graduated in 1841; and during the following winter I attended the Medical College at Albany, N. Y., devoting a large portion of my time to dissecting. After finishing at Albany, I visited various places in western and central Massachusetts, and operated on eyes for strabismus or cross-eyes, —an operation which had then been recently introduced for that deformity; after which I settled at Chesterfield (Mass.), and commenced practicing medicine, where I remained about one year.

One day I visited Northampton, and, calling on a physician with whom I was acquainted, I found upon his table a homoeopathic book. "Why," I exclaimed with astonishment, "you are not studying homoeopathy, are you?" "Yes," he replied, "I am studying it, and trying the remedies cautiously;" and he went on to describe cases which he had treated satisfactorily by the use of the remedies, and among them a case of pleurisy and one of intermittent fever, and he wound up by saying: "Now, if you will go down the street to a book-store and purchase 'Hull's Jahr,' in two volumes, I will give you half a dozen homoeopathic remedies, and you can try them for yourself."

Here was a dilemma. Never until that hour had I ever heard homoeopathy spoken of, by either a medical professor or one of my professional brethren, except with contempt and ridicule. "But," I said to myself, "if there is any truth in homoeopathy I ought to know it, and I cannot treat this physician's testimony with contempt; and it is a duty which I owe to my fellow-men, and especially to my patients, to investigate the new system carefully." I immediately went and purchased the books, and he give me six bottles of medicine, and I took them back with me to Chesterfield. I remember making but one Homoeopathic prescription before leaving Chesterfield, and that was for a case of uterine hemorrhage, which I had treated unsuccessfully for some time with allopathic remedies. I looked over my Homoeopathic books carefully and found that China (cinchona) was indicated. As that remedy was not among the bottles of medicated pellets which my medical friend had given me, I directed that one drop of the ordinary tincture of Peruvian bark should be dropped into a glass of water, and that, after stirring it well, one teaspoonful of the solution thus made should be given three or four times a day. The patient commenced improving immediately, and was soon well.

Soon after that I removed to Grand Rapids, Michigan, and commenced anew the practice of medicine. I then had neither the knowledge nor the faith in homoeopathy which I thought would justify me in treating any serious case of disease with homoeopathic remedies; but I did not neglect to study the new books. One day, a friend of my younger days, who was residing at Grand Haven, came into my office and said that he had been suffering from the toothache for several days, and that he did not like to have the tooth extracted, and he wanted to know if I could do anything for it without extracting it. I told him that I had recently obtained some homoeopathic books and remedies, and that I had noticed that remedies were spoken of for toothache. So I looked over my books and selected Belladonna as the remedy suitable in his case, and gave him a dose of it and other doses to take with him if he needed them. We talked in the office for a short time, and then we walked up to the hotel where he was stopping; as we entered, he stood still a moment and remarked: "Well, my tooth does not ache as severely as it did." I saw him weeks afterward, and he told me that he had not had the toothache from the hour he took the medicine.

Away in that new place, then a village of about one thousand inhabitants, with no homoeopathic physician within a hundred miles of me, I commenced cautiously the use of the new remedies; first in mild cases of disease, and in cases where Allopathic treatment failed to produce the desired effect. Among the first of the serious cases where I used the remedies was a case of pneumonia. A young man had been very sick with that disease for many days. I had resorted vigorously to the antiphlogistic treatment then in vogue; a consulting physician was called, and at last we told the family that our patient could not live until the next morning. I then said to the consulting physician: "I have some homoeopathic remedies; suppose we try them?" His reply was: "It does not make any difference what you try; he will not live until morning." Under such circumstances I felt that I was justified in trying the new remedies. I accordingly dissolved a few pellets of Aconite in a glass of water, and of Bryonia alb. in another glass of water, and directed that a teaspoonful of the solution of Aconite should be given once an hour for five hours, and that a similar dose of Bryonia be given instead of Aconite every sixth hour. I sat down by his bedside and watched his case for two hours. At the end of that period I found that his pulse was five beats less frequent in a minute, and that his breathing was a little easier. The next morning all of his dangerous symptoms had disappeared, and in a reasonable period of time he was restored to health. I talked with the consulting physician about his unexpected recovery, and we were, disposed to think that we had made a false prognosis, and that he would have recovered any way. Still, the case made some impression on me; so that in the next case of pneumonia to which I was called, I resolved to try the same remedies in the same way. The patient was a man about forty years of age. Under the action of the Aconite and Bryonia the patient about held his own, neither gaining nor losing very perceptibly for about three days. At the end of that period I became alarmed, and felt that if the patient were to die I should be guilty of the crime of manslaughter. I discontinued the treatment, and resorted to the then regular antiphlogistic treatment; the patient immediately began to get worse, and at the end of three days more he was a very sick man. I then came to the conclusion that my patient had done much better under the homoeopathic treatment than he had under the Allopathic, and I discontinued the latter and returned to the former, giving the Aconite and Bryonia. The patient ceased to grow worse; he held his own for two or three days, then he began to improve, and was soon restored to health. From that day to this I have never bled a patient suffering from either pneumonia or pleurisy, neither have I applied a blister, or given a cathartic, or an Allopathic dose of tartar emetic, or an opiate, or any form of alcoholic or fermented drinks, either during the continuance of the above-named diseases or during convalescence; nor have I ever regretted, in a single instance, not having done so.

During the fall of the year we had many cases of dysentery which were very obstinate, continuing one or two weeks or longer, attended by a fever approaching a typhoid character. I found the Allopathic treatment unsatisfactory, as there were quite a number of deaths. So I consulted my homoeopathic books and concluded to try the remedies; but at that time I had only the six carefully prepared remedies given me by the physician in Northampton, and I found that I needed some other remedies; so for Arsenicum I used a drop of Fowler's solution of arsenic in a glassful of water, giving a teaspoonful of the solution thus prepared for a dose, and I also used the tincture of Colocynth and other remedies in the same manner. Even with the help of such crude remedies I found that I could generally control the disease far more speedily and with greater certainty and safety than by Allopathic treatment.

I was called to attend a young man who, while stooping over to set a trap in the woods, was mistaken for a bear by a comrade who was hunting with him, and shot through the neck. To restrain secondary hemorrhage I was obliged, in order to save the life of my patient, to ligature both carotid arteries at the interval of only four and one-half days, which, at that time, had never been done successfully at an interval of less than twelve months between the operations. My patient did not suffer from head symptoms, as I was fearful he would, but his lungs became seriously congested. I resorted to the Allopathic treatment without affording any relief; and, as he was steadily getting worse, I consulted my homoeopathic works and gave him Aconite, a drop of the tincture in a glass of water; of the solution thus made I directed a teaspoonful to be given every hour; this gave prompt relief to the active symptoms of congestion. For a cough which remained I gave a few doses of belladonna prepared in the same manner, and all of the symptoms soon disappeared. I reported this case to the New York Journal of Medicine, and it was transferred, even to the homoeopathic prescriptions, to the American edition of Velpeau's great work on surgery.

I found when I went to Grand Rapids that the intermittent, remittent, and pernicious fevers, which prevailed in that place and in the surrounding country, were generally treated by the resident physicians with mercurial or other cathartic remedies, followed or accompanied by Quinine and brandy or fermented drinks containing Alcohol, and opiates where they were supposed to be necessary. As I began to look into homoeopathy, I first prescribed Ipecac for the vomiting which sometimes attended these fevers, one drop of the tincture in a glass of water, and giving a teaspoonful from the glass for a dose. For watery diarrhoeas I gave Fowler's solution of Arsenic in the same manner, and in both instances generally with very satisfactory results. As my confidence in the homoeopathic treatment of diseases increased, I sent to New York and obtained an assortment of the remedies and more books, and was then much better prepared to prescribe successfully. I soon found that by their use I could dispense with cathartic remedies and thus avoid the danger of causing a medicinal irritation of the bowels, which it is sometimes difficult to control. I also found that I could do much better without Alcohol in any form, in the treatment of these fevers, than with it; and I soon ceased to use brandy, wine, beer, etc.

As to Quinine, that remedy will unquestionably interrupt the paroxysms of intermittent and remittent fevers promptly if it is given at the proper time and in suitable doses; and, if the attack is the first the patient has ever had, a return of the disease may at least sometimes be prevented by giving once a week in two or three doses, at an interval of twelve hours, about the quantity which would be required to interrupt the disease in the first instance. These doses should be given the day before the disease is expected to return. I found it much better to give about two large doses of quinine than to give the same quantity in 1 or 2 grain doses. I reported the results of my experiments and observations in the use of Quinine at Grand Rapids to the *New York Journal of Medicine* (allopathic). In all instances where life is in danger from a return of a paroxysm of intermittent or remittent fever, the patient can be rescued from immediate danger by giving Quinine in doses sufficient to prevent a return of the paroxysm. In all other cases, and perhaps even in such, we can rely safely on homoeopathic remedies in minute doses. Quinine in Allopathic doses will rarely cure the disease, excepting, it may be, as named above, in a first attack. If the patient has ever had more than one or two attacks, it is almost sure to return again and again for two seasons, complicated with symptoms caused by the remedy, in spite of Allopathic doses of quinine; whereas by treating the patient homoeopathically, except in old cases, you will not suddenly interrupt the paroxysms, for they may continue one or two weeks, or even a few days longer, but when they cease there is generally the end of the disease, and the patient speedily regains his ordinary state of health instead of lingering along with frequent returns of the disease for generally two seasons, as he does when quinine is used. Old cases of intermittent fever are frequently cured promptly by infinitesimal doses of homoeopathic remedies. I have never seen Allopathic doses of Quinine do any good in typhoid fevers. And, as to the use of cathartics, from my observation I soon became satisfied that a vast number of lives have been lost by their use in cases of remittent and typhoid fevers, the tendency to irritation of the mucous membrane, which exists especially in the latter disease, being often fatally aggravated by cathartic remedies.

I found the prejudice so strong against homoeopathy when I commenced my investigations, that I generally said nothing about the kind of remedies I was using, and sometimes disguised the remedies by mixing with sugar or pulverized liquorice root, or by mixing or dissolving them in water.

I have given the above details to show how carefully and patiently, step by step, I commenced my investigations, and watched the action of remedies when given in accordance with the Homoeopathic law of cure, and compared the results with the results which followed the use of Allopathic remedies.

I remained at Grand Rapids two years. During that period I gradually substituted the Homoeopathic treatment of diseases for the Allopathic, as fast as I found I could cure the various diseases which came under my observation with more safety and certainty by the former method of treatment than by the latter.

Now I ask the intelligent, conscientious, and philanthropic reader, Did I do right or did I do wrong in thus investigating homoeopathy and using cautiously the remedies for the cure of the sick, as I found them more efficacious and safe than the remedies which I had been taught to use and had used previously? If it was my duty to thus critically examine the new method of treatment, when my attention was seriously called to it, and to cautiously try the remedies on the sick, is it not clearly the duty of every Allopathic physician in our land to do the same? To thus earnestly call the attention of physicians of every school to the importance of investigating homoeopathy, and carefully using the remedies for the cure of the sick, and to entreat them not to stop and be satisfied with crude doses, such as drop doses of tinctures and the first, second or third dilutions or triturations of remedies, as some have done, is my sole object in writing these pages. The most decided and satisfactory cures which I have ever witnessed have been effected by the thirtieth and two hundredth dilutions. But, according to my experience, it is not well to confine one's self absolutely to either high or low dilutions, as some have done; but if you are satisfied that you have selected the right remedy, instead of changing the remedy when you do not see relief from its use, change the dilution from low to high or high to low, as the case may be. I could detail many cases to show the importance of doing this. No physician should labor specially to sustain either a theory or preconceived ideas, but to cure his patients promptly. The health and lives of our fellow-beings are too important to be trifled with.

During the early years of my practice of homoeopathy I was called to see a young man recently attacked with "epileptic fits." As he was going immediately to New York, with his sister, I advised them to call on the late Dr. John F. Gray, with whom I became acquainted during my first visit to New York. On reaching New York they called on Dr. Gray, and the young man remained under his treatment for several weeks. Of Dr. Gray's treatment of this patient, so far as remedies were concerned, I know only of a single remedy which he gave, which was Nitrate of silver, which I understood was given in a somewhat crude form, and not even in a low centesimal dilution. The young man, finding little or no benefit from the treatment, went to his home in Georgia, after which I received a letter stating that he had not been essentially benefited by Dr. Gray's treatment, and requesting me to prescribe for him. In response I sent him the 30th dilution of Nux vomica, which he took and soon recovered from the disease, and never had any return of the paroxysms. Dr. Gray was a low dilutionist.

On the other hand, during my second or third visit to New York I called on Dr. Edward Bayard, who was a high dilutionist. I found him in poor health. He had been suffering, as he told me, for some time from a subacute irritation of the mucous membrane of the bowels, with loose passages, and some febrile excitement. He asked me to prescribe for him. After a careful inquiry as to existing symptoms I said to him, "Mercurius vivus ought to cure you." He replied that he had taken it repeatedly without the slightest effect. I asked him what dilution of this remedy he had taken. He replied that he had taken the 30th and 200th dilutions. I suggested that he should take the 3d trituration. "Why," he exclaimed, "I have not prescribed the 3d trituration of mercury for many years, and I do not know as I have any in my office." But, on looking around, he found a bottle of the second centesimal trituration; and I said to him: "That will answer. You can take a dose of that now (which he did) and repeat it three or four times between now and to-morrow night, after which take a dose of the 30th or 200th dilution of sulphur." The next time I saw him he told me that my prescription cured him promptly.

That the careful treatment of diseases by the use of low dilutions of Homoeopathic remedies, when compared with the Allopathic treatment, is wonderfully successful I well know; for it was by the success which attended the use of the low dilutions that I was led into the new practice, as thousands of other graduates of allopathic colleges have been. Still, I know very well by experience that the low dilutionists, in a very large number of cases, fail to cure patients promptly, and in many cases fail to cure them at all when they could cure them promptly by the use of the high dilutions, often by the very same remedy which they have been using. I was called to see a patient suffering from puerperal anaemia, with "nursing sore mouth." She was greatly exhausted; her stomach, which was very acid, would retain very little nourishment. She had been under Allopathic treatment for some time without experiencing any relief. I gave her a low dilution of Pulsatilla, which afforded her no relief. Then I selected other remedies, from which she derived no benefit. After that I gave her the 200th dilution of Pulsatilla, the first dose of which produced, as she declared, a change for the better within an hour, and she rapidly recovered under its use. A lady who had for two winters been sent to Florida by her Allopathic physician for a severe cough, attended by the physical signs of induration of the summit of one of her lungs, called on me early in the fall, saying that her physician advised her to go again to Florida, but that she did not like to go, and wanted me to prescribe for her. After examining her symptoms carefully I gave her a single dose of Sulphur, 200th dilution; at the end of a week she was better, at the end of another week much better, and at the end of the third week she had but few symptoms remaining, for which I gave only one dose of Arsenicum, 200th, which completed the cure.

Having practiced medicine for two years at Grand Rapids, I spent a winter East and visited New York, making the Acquaintance of Homoeopathic physicians, and conversing with them about the new system of treating disease, attending medical lectures and clinics at the two Allopathic colleges. I remember very well attending a clinic at the College of Physicians and Surgeons, held by the late Prof. Willard Parker, when a little child was brought in suffering from whooping cough. Prof. Parker, looking around upon the students, said: "Here, gentlemen, is a case of disease which, like the small-pox, measles, and scarlet fever, runs a definite course; if you will let the patients alone they will generally get well, but if you commence dosing them you will often bring on complications and they will die." This statement, coming from a medical man of his prominence, surely was worthy of consideration.

After spending the winter at the East I went to Detroit, Mich., and opened an office in connection with Dr. P. M. Wheaton. I practiced in Detroit for fifteen years, excepting that during the last six years of that time I spent a part of each year at Cleveland, giving a course of lectures on the Theory and Practice of Medicine at the Western Homoeopathic Medical College, of Cleveland, Ohio.

When I went to Detroit the prejudice against homoeopathy was very strong, especially among physicians. An attempt was made to pass a bill through the Legislature of Michigan which would virtually prohibit the practice in the State. The bill passed the Senate, but, owing to the prompt action of the friends of homoeopathy in exposing the design of the advocates of the bill, it was defeated in the House of Representatives. The presence of the Asiatic cholera in 1849 in the city, and the success which attended the homoeopathic treatment of that disease, was instrumental in calling the attention of large numbers of the most intelligent and influential citizens to the new practice and establishing it upon a firm basis. When the disease first appeared in the city, we furnished the families which we were accustomed to attend, and all others who desired them, with Veratrum album and Cuprum metallicum, which had been earnestly recommended by Homoeopathic physicians elsewhere, who had had experience in treating the disease, as preventive remedies, a dose or two of each to be taken daily. As a result, very few among the families which we were accustomed to attend were attacked with the disease, and in such cases as occurred the disease was generally readily controlled. As a rule, the most troublesome cases which we had to treat were those in which Opium or morphine in some form had been administered before we were called. In such cases it was exceedingly difficult to get a satisfactory response from our remedies, however carefully we selected them.

The Asiatic cholera is a violent disease and rapid in its progress, and if severe cases of this disease are to be treated successfully, it must be by remedies which are prompt in their action. It is here that homoeopathic remedies show their superiority over all other remedies or methods of treatment, for they act upon the diseased organs in the direction of the disease, and thus excite a prompt reaction. Homoeopathic remedies, when properly used, do not benumb, nor do they seriously aggravate existing diseased action; and they neither cause diseased action in well organs, nor reduce the quantity of blood, nor lessen the vitality of the organism and the ability to react against the encroachment of diseased action, as does the allopathic treatment; and, consequently, if a patient dies the physician and his friends have the consolation, at least, of knowing that he did not die from the treatment.

I well remember, while practicing in Detroit, attending a prominent citizen, a lawyer, who had a severe attack of pneumonia; and, while recovering from it, he went one night into a cold room to sleep, and this brought on a relapse which involved both lungs, and my patient became very sick. One day on visiting him I found an Allopathic physician sitting by his bedside. I was told that he simply called as a friend. As I entered he arose and walked out into the hall. I followed him, and asked him what he thought of my patient. He replied very promptly: "He will die! he will die, sir!! He ought to have been bled, blistered, and physicked long ago, but it is too late now." I replied: "He will not die, sir, for the very reason that he has not had the treatment you name; he has his blood and vital energies, unimpaired by the treatment, to sustain him." And he did not die, but recovered, and was appointed Governor of one of the Western Territories long after that.

After having practiced medicine for fifteen years, except the months I was absent at Cleveland the last six years of the time, I was invited to fill the chair of Theory and Practice in the New York Homoeopathic Medical College. This invitation I accepted, and removed to New York and took up my residence there, and commenced practice again in a new field. About the year 1868 I invented a new process for refining petroleum by the aid of superheated steam, and spent eighteen months in developing the process at Binghamton, N. Y., and then returned to my practice in New York City. In the year 1873 I gave up the practice of medicine, and in connection with two gentlemen who were interested in selling oils, I commenced the refining of petroleum, manufacturing therefrom machinery and other oils; to which business I have devoted my attention ever since. I have attended chiefly to the manufacturing department and my partners to the selling.

I have been frequently asked: "Why did you quit the practice of medicine? Was not that a useful business?" Yes, it was; but I had come to feel that there were fields for greater usefulness-in fact, that it was vastly more important to teach people the laws of health and life, and to strive to lead them by precept and example to shun the causes of disease, than it was to cure them when they were sick-that prevention was better than cure. Consequently, when I saw before me a reasonably sure prospect of being able to make a good deal more money at the refining business than I could ever expect to make in the practice of medicine, I could but feel that, by the aid of a reasonable portion of the money thus made, I could perform a far greater use than I could by practicing medicine. This, then, was the reason for my giving up a good and useful profession and practice for my present business. What I have attempted to do for the benefit of suffering humanity since I gave up the practice of medicine, I will name in a future chapter.

CHAPTER II.

WHY EVERY PHYSICIAN SHOULD EXAMINE AND TEST HOMOEOPATHY.

I was born in the year 1815, and on the 26th of November, 1891, was 76 years of age. I have not practiced medicine as a business for many years, and I never expect to practice again. As to money, my present business gives me all I need, and money to spare for benevolent purposes. I do not expect, nor do I desire, to receive one cent, directly or indirectly, for the writing of this pamphlet, or for the money which I expect to spend for paper, printing, binding, and sending it, post paid, to every physician and clergyman in the United States and Canada whose name I can get. I do it because I believe and hope it will be a useful work and instrumental in doing good, and that many who are willing and waiting will find useful suggestions contained in its pages, and that through their instrumentality humanity may be benefited.

A few years after I became a convert to Homoeopathy I met in a railroad car a venerable professor from the college where I graduated. We were mutually pleased to see each other, and after our congratulations were over I remarked to him that, so far as the administration of remedies was concerned, I had departed somewhat from the "general principles" which he used to inculcate, and that I had become a Homoeopathist. The Professor looked up with astonishment and exclaimed most earnestly: "I am sorry to hear that! I am sorry to hear that!" He manifested not the slightest desire to know why I had made the change, but was ready to denounce and condemn. It would be useless to talk to such a man. Before one can see a new truth, however plain it may be, he must be willing to either examine the question carefully himself, or to heed the testimony of those who have examined it. Fortunately, all physicians have not been like the above Professor; for there have been thousands who were educated in and graduated from Allopathic schools, some of them gray-haired men, who, like myself, have carefully studied Homoeopathy and cautiously tested the remedies upon the sick, who have become converts to the new practice, and who have ever after relied upon its remedies in the treatment of the sick. No intelligent physician of any other school has ever carefully read the Homoeopathic works, and has to any considerable extent cautiously used the remedies in the treatment of severe cases of various diseases, without being able to see the vast superiority of the Homoeopathic over the Allopathic treatment of disease; and no one, without prejudice, and willing to see the truth, will ever do so without being convinced. Can a man, with eyes open, on a clear day, go out at noon time and declare that the sun does not shine? He may make such a declaration while shut up in a cellar or cavern, or if he never opens his eyes. As one who has patiently and diligently studied and practiced both systems, I say without the slightest hesitation that Homoeopathy, as a system of practice, is as superior to Allopathy as the direct light of the sun is to the reflected light of the moon; in fact, much of the allopathic practice of to-day is but a reflection of the homoeopathic light. What intelligent physician to-day bleeds, blisters, salivates, or vomits his patients, as students were taught to do by preceptors, professors, and books fifty years ago? And why is such treatment so frequently, to say the least, discarded now by Allopathic physicians? Is it not largely because the success which results from the Homoeopathic treatment of diseases, has convinced Allopathic physicians and their patients that such violent disease-creating measures and remedies are unnecessary?

Homoeopathy is strictly a scientific system of medicine. It is based upon a law of nature — "*Similia similibus curantur,*" or the law that remedies will cure symptoms and diseases similar to those which they will cause when taken by healthy persons. It is wonderful with what care, skill, and perseverance the new Materia Medica has been developed, mostly by intelligent physicians, commencing with Hahnemann, taking the different remedies in varying doses, and carefully and patiently watching the symptoms that follow, and writing them down day after day; and then, when similar symptoms occur in case of disease, giving the remedies and carefully watching and writing down the results. Allopathic physicians, as a rule, have not the slightest conception of the vast amount of patient and persevering labor in this direction which has been done by physicians as well educated as they are, and most of whom have graduated in the same schools, who have devoted their lives to this work. Are not these facts worthy of the consideration of every physician in the world who desires the highest good of his fellow men? It is well known to every intelligent physician that there is some truth in the homoeopathic law of cure, and that it has to some extent been recognized from the earliest periods of medical history. A cathartic remedy, even in Allopathic doses, will sometimes cure a diarrhoea, and an emetic will sometimes cure a nauseated stomach; but such remedies when given in large doses do not always cure, or they would generally be used by Allopathists; they sometimes seriously and even dangerously aggravate the disease, so that the vital forces do not react and thus effect a cure. Nitrate of silver and acetate of zinc, which applied to well eyes will cause irritation and inflammation, are often applied to inflamed eyes. The kine pox, which is a similar disease, is well known to either prevent or materially modify smallpox; and so I could go on enumerating cases where Allopathic physicians treat their patients in accordance with the Homoeopathic law of cure. The great discovery of Hahnemann was not so much the Homoeopathic law of cure, for some knowledge of that was possessed before his day, but the practical application of that law to the cure of disease. He found by careful experiments that diseases can be cured by remedies, which when given to the well will produce similar symptoms or diseases, in doses so small as not to seriously aggravate the existing disease or symptoms; and that all diseases may be thus treated with a success hitherto unknown. This discovery was accompanied by the most careful experiments by him and his followers upon themselves, to ascertain with the greatest possible care the effects of various remedies upon the healthy, so as to be able to make accurate prescriptions for the sick. Here you have most careful scientific investigation and experiments as to the action of remedies upon the well and sick, made, not by pretenders or quacks, but by well educated physicians, that should command the admiration and respect of every intelligent man and educated physician.

As to the doses given to the sick, which have been such a stumbling-block to our Allopathic brethren, their size is simply the result of the most careful experiments. Everyone can understand that if we give an Allopathic dose of Ipecac to a patient already sick and vomiting, or of Veratrum album to a patient suffering from Asiatic cholera or cholera morbus, we will almost certainly aggravate the disease, perhaps to a fatal extent; for it is the reaction of the vital forces of the system against the new excitement caused by the remedy, which overcomes this new excitement and the diseased action at the same time. Now, if the action of the remedy is so severe that no reaction follows, then, of course, no cure follows, and even death may result.

The great beauty and excellence of the Homoeopathic system of medicine consists in the ability to treat patients successfully thereby, without making well organs sick, or aggravating existing diseased action, or creating an opposite diseased state, as you do when you give a cathartic remedy in a cathartic dose for constipation; in that case the reaction, if reaction follows, is not in the right direction, consequently the constipation is often aggravated. I have hardly ever seen, excepting in cases of mechanical obstruction, a severe and troublesome case of constipation that had not been caused by the use of cathartic remedies. So if we give an opiate, or an astringent, for a diarrhoea, we can see that it is a direct effort to restrain the disease by force, as it were, and we necessarily have to give large doses; and, if the vital forces react against this medicinal intrusion, the reaction is not in the direction of health. It is true that the vital forces sometimes overcome the diseased action in spite of the medicinal action; but it does not always do this, and subacute and chronic diarrhoeas are the result of the use of such remedies in some cases. To create disease of a well organ for the sake of curing disease in another organ, as is done when blisters are applied to the skin for diseases of internal organs, and when cathartics are given for diseases of the head or lungs, every one can see is a roundabout treatment; and while patients may sometimes be benefited by this calling off, as it were, the attention of the vital forces from the diseased action in other organs, still it is not a very satisfactory treatment as a whole; for you may lessen the vital power of resistance against diseased action, and may even cause serious disease of the organ assailed. I repeat, one of the great beauties of Homoeopathy lies in the fact that when remedies are given in accordance with its law of cure, they do not have to be given in disease-creating doses.

Hahnemann tells us that a single dose of the 30th dilution of Aconite, which contains but the decillionth of a drop of the tincture of the remedy, will cure acute pleurisy in twenty-four hours. I have thus treated patients suffering from pleurisy with a single dose of that remedy (it should be given soon after the commencement of the disease), and at the end of twenty-four hours have found the pain and fever all gone, and the skin moist and cool; and in one instance within two days the patient was on his way to California. I have never seen any such satisfactory cures of that disease from any kind of Allopathic treatment, nor from the low dilutions of Aconite or any other Homoeopathic remedy.

Hereafter I shall call attention of both physicians and the clergy to the causes and different methods of restraining or curing both spiritual and natural diseases; for there is the most beautiful analogy or correspondence between the methods of treating natural and spiritual diseases, and they must be considered in connection if we would clearly see the truth.

CHAPTER III.

THE DANGERS THAT RESULT FROM THE ALLOPATHIC TREATMENT OF DISEASES.

This treatment of diseases, more in the past than at present, consists largely in giving and applying remedies in disease-creating doses. The antiphlogistic treatment consists of blood-letting and the use and application of reducing remedies which directly or indirectly lessen the inflammatory or febrile action; but it is manifest that while it may lessen the activity of the diseased symptoms it also lessens the vitality of the system as a whole, and consequently its power to resist and overcome the existing diseased action; so that it is a serious question whether in many cases more is not lost than gained, and it is certain that, owing to the loss of blood and strength, convalescence will be more tedious. Then the use of remedies which cause active diseased action is not always safe. My own mother, at the age of 51 years, while in delicate health, was taken with a severe pain in her side. A physician was called. She thought an emetic would do her good. The physician gave her one, and she died during its operation, or immediately afterward. Her physician was so affected by this sudden and unexpected result that he had to go and lie down. At that time I was but 10 years old.

In typhoid fever there is a tendency to irritation of the mucous membrane of the small intestines; and, as I have already stated, I am satisfied from observation that when cathartics are given during this disease this irritation is often most seriously aggravated, and death not unfrequently follows as a result.

But the greatest danger and evil which result from the Allopathic treatment of disease lie, not in the direction of the sudden deaths which sometimes result from the use of its remedies, but in the liability of patients to be led into the habitual use of a drug that has afforded them palliative relief during sickness, and the countenance thus given for the use of such drugs by the laity during health. Perhaps as a rule poisonous substances palliate the symptoms which they cause, or which follow their use. A cathartic remedy will palliate the costiveness which frequently follows the use of cathartic remedies. Opium will palliate the sleeplessness and suffering that follow when the patient leaves off the use of opiates which he has been taking for disease; and alcohol and all fluids and remedies which contain an appreciable quantity of alcohol will palliate the coldness of the surface, craving, and distress which follow when a patient who has been taking such remedies attempts to discontinue their use. And thus the patient is led to continue the remedy because it makes him feel better every time he takes it; and, consequently, he is led on as naturally as water runs down hill, until he becomes a slave to his appetite.

Now, cannot every conscientious and intelligent man see what an immense blessing to his fellow men it would be if all physicians were able to treat their patients as successfully by the use of Homoeopathic remedies and doses as by the use of the so-called Alcoholic stimulants and Narcotics, which are enslaving and ruining so many, and thus be able to discard and discountenance the use of all such remedies? How can honest, conscientious physicians disregard and treat with contempt the testimony of physicians who have been educated in the same schools with themselves, but who have used their reason and freedom to investigate the new practice and test the curative action of its remedies, when they assure them that they have treated their patients far more successfully by the use of Homoeopathic remedies than they ever have done by the use of narcotics, alcoholic and fermented drinks, and other Allopathic remedies? How can physicians disregard the testimony of multitudes of patients who have been thus cured?

Why should not every physician study Homoeopathy and test the remedies on the sick? He can do it cautiously; he has all of his old remedies by him; what has he to lose? If they do not relieve his patient's sufferings more safely and promptly, he is not obliged to continue to use them. Is it a sensible and rational course for any one to allow himself to be so strongly confirmed in the views of prominent professors, teachers, and books, that he cannot without prejudice examine new truths and new methods of treating diseases, and even new theories? Should not a man strive to keep abreast of the age in which he is living? Take it, for instance, in regard to the action of alcohol on living structures. No other man has ever experimented so carefully, patiently, and thoroughly as has Dr. Richardson, of England, and the results of his experiments appeal to the common sense and observation of every unbiased man. He shows conclusively by its action that it should never have been given in a vast majority of the cases of disease where it is given by physicians; yet what attention is paid to his testimony and demonstrations, which every disinterested physician can see to be true if he will?

Dr. Richardson has also shown conclusively that alcohol paralyzes the minute capillary vessels, so that while the blood is forced into them through the arteries by the heart, it does not flow out of these minute vessels into the veins as rapidly as it does during their healthy action; consequently these vessels are congested and unnaturally distended with blood; the face and surface of the body become red, owing to the presence of an unnatural quantity of blood in these vessels. Nor is this all. The heat of the body is generated by changes going on in the blood and flows with the blood, and consequently the surface of the body becomes, from the presence of this excess of blood, unnaturally warm; but the heat is rapidly radiated from the surface, consequently the body, as a whole, becomes cooler. Dr. Richardson found by careful experiment that, while the surface was warmer, internally the body was cooler and less able to stand the cold; and he also substantiated the truth of his experiments by experiments on pigeons.

I will allow Canon Wilberforce, of South Hampton, England, to describe his experiment. While attending a reception during his recent visit to New York he was asked the following question: —

Dr. E. P. Thwing: "I would like to ask the Canon, as a physician, if the feeling as to alcoholic medication in England has changed for the better; for instance, the aspect of the British Medical Association toward this subject?"

Canon Wilberforce: "I believe that is one point in which we are going furthest ahead. I think that the whole aspect of the medical question is changing, mainly under the influence of that distinguished man of science, Dr. Richardson. He is one of the leading scientific minds of Great Britain. He has been successful in his experiments and as bold as a lion in his utterances, and he is leading scientific thought in this direction. He has proved over and over again, to use a common phrase, that from the monarch on the throne down to the maggot in the cheese, every healthy being is better without alcohol. The other day he was staying with me. I have the greatest possible objection to experimenting upon living animals, but he described to me an experiment on pigeons. It was not a very painful experiment; indeed, there are some people who, I am afraid, would like to have the experiment made upon them. He tried to induce the pigeons to take peas soaked in alcohol. They refused to do so at first; but after a while they were pleased, and they selected the peas saturated with alcohol. One cold night he turned the pigeons out, and on the following day, when he was examining them, strange to say, all those pigeons that ate the alcoholized peas were frozen to death, and those that remained teetotalers were perfectly safe and sound."

The drinking of alcoholic liquors generates no heat, it simply holds the heat in the congested blood-vessels upon the surface of the body, where it is wasted, and thus the temperature of the body as a whole is lowered.

The greatest mortality which results from the use of intoxicating drinks does not result from what is recognized as drunkenness, but from what is recognized as moderate but steady drinking. The drunkard after his sprees usually has seasons of abstinence, during which he has a chance to recuperate or regain strength and vigor, and consequently drunkards often live to an advanced age; but the steady drinker has no such seasons of rest, but his face, by its almost constantly congested appearance, shows the condition of his internal organs; for the effect of alcohol is to paralyze the minute capillary vessels throughout the body and fill them with blood, which produces redness upon the surface and a sensation of warmth. The separation of waste and worn-out materials and their removal is largely effected through these minute blood-vessels, and it is through them that nourishment reaches all the structures of the body; consequently, the almost constant state of congestion of these minute vessels, which results from regular, moderate drinking, interferes very seriously with this change or purification and renewal of all the structures of the body. As a result, while some drinkers die from drunkenness, many more die from apoplexy, paralysis, laryngitis and bronchitis, heart failure, fatty degeneration of the heart, diseases of the stomach and liver, Bright's disease of the kidneys, etc., and especially from an inability to either resist or withstand epidemic, contagious, or inflammatory diseases, or even mechanical injuries.

There are life insurance companies that give special privileges to total abstainers over moderate drinkers (they never insure drunkards). Such companies find that they can give a bonus of from 17 to 23 per cent. to total abstainers as compared with moderate drinkers.

I remember very well attending the family of a brewer. He was standing by when I advised his wife not to drink beer, for it was not good for her, as it would increase her debility and retard her recovery. With astonishment and great emphasis he exclaimed: "Tell me that beer is not good for her!" Striking his chest with his fist, he said: "Just look at me and see what beer has done for me!" He was born in Scotland, and manifestly inherited a good, strong constitution. I replied to him: "You are a large, strong man, but a little too fleshy; what beer has done for you time will tell better than I can." A few months, perhaps a year or two, after that conversation, I was riding up a street which led toward his residence when I was called in a hurry into a saloon to see a man who was said to have fallen down "in a fit." On reaching his side I found the above brewer dead upon the floor. Without much question he died of heart failure, from fatty degeneration caused by the steady use of beer. I never heard of his being intoxicated.

Dr. W. B. Carpenter, who stands at the very head of the physiologists of our century, says: —

> "That the taking of alcoholic stimulants is in any way useful in keeping up the heat of the body, may now be considered as a myth altogether exploded."

Again he says: —

> "Now, it is the result of many observations that the introduction of alcohol specially deranges the vaso-motor system; this derangement showing itself alike in disturbance of the heart's action, and in relaxation of the capillary vessels, which become filled with blood, especially in the nervous system and in the skin. This causes one to feel that warmth and exhilaration which is the first effect of the introduction of these disturbing agencies, and which are appealed to as evidence that drink does us good. Well, what are the facts? The fresh glow is simply the result of relaxation of the capillary vessels of the skin, allowing a large quantity of blood to come to the surface, so as to give the feeling of superficial warmth. But if a larger amount of blood comes to the surface, it robs the parts within; and the feeling of genial warmth gives way to a general depression, especially when we are exposed to severe cold. The temporary exhilaration of the nervous system, too, is followed by a corresponding depression. Hence a person feels 'sick and sorry' the next morning after taking alcoholic stimulant."

As to alcohol giving strength, it is well known that it supplies no substance to the tissues; therefore it meets no want, and consequently can give no strength. Every one can see that blood-vessels, when paralyzed and congested with blood by alcohol, cannot perform their function in the metamorphosis of the tissues of the body, or of conveying nourishment to them and removing worn-out, effete substances from them, as during health. If you would see the legitimate effects of alcohol, look at the permanently congested face of the steady drinker, or his "rum blossoms," and remember that the capillary vessels of his brain and other internal organs are in a similar state, and then say if you think he has been strengthened by alcoholic drinks.

I remember very well when a young man, when a neighboring farmer was sick and unable to gather his hay, that the young men in the neighborhood set a day when they would meet and gather his hay for him. When, on the day set, we met in the field, and the neighboring young men noticed that my brother and myself had no bottle of cider brandy with us, they exclaimed with delight, "We will lay you out before noon." A spirited contest with our scythes commenced in good earnest. But they did not lay us out; they were glad to seek and lie in the shade of trees to rest, while we were able to continue our work. It is well known that men who are preparing themselves for, or engaging in, feats requiring great strength and endurance are beginning to find that they must let intoxicating drinks alone. It is something marvelous to see with what tenacity so many physicians hold on to the idea that fermented wine, beer, brandy, and whiskey are strengthening. This idea comes, to a great extent, from the custom which prevails of giving such drinks to patients who are recovering from fevers, acute diseases, and from the effects of other debilitating causes. Many physicians have been so accustomed to give these drinks to patients, under such circumstances, that they have not the slightest idea how much better they would do without them.

A few years ago I met a German woman whose husband I knew well, and had reason to fear that beer drinking was doing him great harm. I said to her that, on her husband's account, she should never let another drop of beer enter her house if she could help it. "Why," she exclaimed, "I cannot do without beer. I suffer so much during and after confinement, and am so weak, and have so little milk for my child, that my doctor says that I must have beer to give me strength." She was then expecting to be confined within a few months. I replied to her by saying: "I have attended a great many more patients during confinement than your physician has ever attended, and after the first three years of my practice, I never gave to a single patient beer, fermented wine, whiskey, or brandy, or any other intoxicating drink. Now, if you will follow my advice, you will have a very different time from what you have ever had before; and my advice is that from this time forth you do not taste a single drop of beer, wine, or any other intoxicating drink." She said she would follow my suggestions. I met her again when her child was a few months old, and she looked like another woman. She came up to me and said: "Well, Doctor, I have followed your advice strictly. I have not tasted beer, wine, or any other intoxicating drink, and I never before had such a comfortable time during my confinement. I never was so strong or gained my strength so rapidly. I never had so much nurse for my child, and I never had such a good-natured baby before." She was the mother of several children.

Such are the results of the two methods of treatment.

There is no surer way to retard and often prevent recovery than to give patients drinks or even remedies which contain an appreciable quantity of alcohol. Where the tendency to recovery is strong they will recover sooner or later in spite of the treatment; but in some cases the physician may keep a delicate, nervous patient sick as long as he gives alcohol in any form; and in the most critical stage of typhoid fever, pneumonia, and other diseases where the patient needs nourishment, and that impurities should be removed, there is no more dangerous treatment than to give alcohol in any form, which interferes with these processes by paralyzing and congesting the capillary vessels. Hot water and nourishment, cautiously supplied, are what such patients require, not alcoholic stimulants.

The habit of taking either opium or morphine in our country has very generally resulted from the prescriptions of physicians. The patient may obtain palliative relief from its use, but suffers when he attempts to leave it off; consequently, without fully realizing the danger which he incurs, he continues the remedy until he is enslaved.

With the exception of alcohol, I know of no more dangerous medicine to give during the critical stages of inflammatory, febrile, and other diseases than Allopathic doses of opium in any form. This anodyne, by its retarding, benumbing, and stupefying effects upon the body, often destroys the power of reaction at the critical stage of the disease when the vital forces should be left free to act, and consequently in many cases patients die who would not die if they were not under the influence of this drug. Patients will often go very near to the border line and yet rally if kept free from the so-called "stimulants" and narcotics, and simple, plain nourishment is cautiously given and the body kept warm.

Physicians are sometimes responsible for the habit of using tobacco among their patrons. It is generally in chronic cases of disease where tobacco is prescribed, and, as a rule, when it is once prescribed by a physician the patient never thinks of giving up the use of the remedy; nor, so far as I have known, are physicians who prescribe tobacco often, if ever, careful to direct patients to discontinue using the remedy as soon as the symptoms of the disease from which they are suffering are relieved. Of course, a physician who neglects to do this seriously neglects his duty. It is safe to say that few physicians ever prescribe the smoking or chewing of tobacco as a remedy for diseases who do not use the weed themselves, for they can generally find much better and safer remedies.

If a physician loves intoxicating drinks and has become a slave to them, he actually feels that they do him good every time he drinks, for by relieving the symptoms temporarily which they have caused they actually make him feel better; and what is more natural than that he should prescribe them for his patients? Here, then, it can be clearly seen that there is great danger in employing physicians who love intoxicating drinks, tobacco, or opium in any form; for they believe in the efficacy of these poisons, and they will often prescribe them when a physician not addicted to their use would not think of doing so.

I have alluded to some of the dangers which attend and the evils which often result from the Allopathic treatment of diseases. Every one can see that they are formidable enough and that they merit the serious attention of every lover of his race. The skillful homoeopathic physician is able to avoid these dangers and evils, for he does not use disease-creating or appetite-begetting doses of any remedy.

We notice that those having the management of our railroads are beginning to see that, for the protection of the property of the owners and lives of their patrons, it is not safe to employ men who drink intoxicating drinks at all; for it is well known that large numbers of those who drink are sooner or later sure to become unreliable and careless. Is it not time that physicians should cease to accept as students, and that our medical colleges should cease to graduate and send forth as physicians, men who drink intoxicating drinks? Should not medical professors and teachers have as much regard for the health and lives of men, women, and children as the managers of our railroads?

Again, it is well known that the use of tobacco tends to prevent development, impair health, and to make men moody, if not careless, and it not unfrequently leads them, especially when young, to disregard the rights and feelings of others. We see men and boys smoking wherever it is not strictly prohibited, even lighting their cigars and cigarettes as they leave our elevated railroad stations, and walking down the stairs before ladies and gentlemen, thus compelling those who follow to breathe the atmosphere which they have polluted. As a fair illustration of the spirit so frequently manifested, I will describe a little incident which occurred in my presence. A young man, perhaps twenty years old, stood in a line of men approaching the paying teller's window in one of our banks, vigorously smoking his cigar. An elderly gentleman behind him asked him if he would be so kind as not to smoke. The young man immediately straightened himself up in a most self-important manner and exclaimed: "What do you think I care if it is offensive to you?"

In our railroad cars smokers have to separate themselves from wives, children, and friends and go by themselves into a smoking-car or apartment, and why? simply because tobacco smoke is unpleasant to every man, woman, and child who is not accustomed to it; and the smoker's breath often smells so strong of the smoke when his cigar is gone that it is exceedingly unpleasant to sensitive persons. Why should our medical colleges graduate young men to go forth for the purpose of attempting to heal sick, sensitive, and nervous patients, who smoke or chew tobacco, and thus are unpleasant to many and a bad example to all? Have we not enough cleanly young men, of good habits, to supply all the physicians we need in our country? A smoking physician, by his breath and bad example to the young, may do a vast deal more harm than he can ever do good as a physician in the world.

The use of an intoxicating wine as a communion wine in so many of our churches, and the efforts of so many clergymen to justify its use, together with the prescription of intoxicating drinks by physicians, are the chief supports which to-day sustain our distilleries, breweries, and saloons, and the prevalent drinking habits and consequent drunkenness. Let all of our clergy, churches, and physicians withdraw their patronage and sanction of intoxicating drinks, and it would not be many years before the manufacture and sale of such drinks would be prohibited throughout the length and breadth of our land. That day will surely come, for a new age is opening up before us very different from the past. The Lord is coming at this day in the "clouds of heaven" with power and great glory. Old things are passing away and all things are being made new-new heavens and a new earth.

Sir Astley Cooper says: "I never suffer ardent spirits in my house, thinking them evil spirits. If the poor could witness the white livers, the dropsies, or the shattered nervous systems which I have seen, the consequences of drinking, they would be aware that spirits and poisons are synonymous terms."

Again he says: "We have all been in error in recommending wine as a tonic. Ardent spirits and poisons are convertible terms."

Dr. Benj. Richardson declares it to be his opinion that the administration of alcohol will become, like blood-letting, a thing of the past, that it is passing into the same position as blood-letting. He, as a student, was educated to bleed; he was educated in the employment of alcohol; he saw the effects of the application of these tested by comparison, and he has, in one instance as much as in the other, come to consider them as behind the age, and both as remedies belonging to a departed and deceived generation. —The Dawn (English), Nov. 19, 1891.

I cannot close this chapter without again earnestly calling the attention of all physicians to the great danger to life which results from giving alcohol in any form to patients in very critical cases, or as they are at or approaching the crisis in their disease, in fevers and in inflammatory diseases, such as pneumonia, etc.

Since writing the preceding pages, in fact, since most of them were in type, my attention has been called by notices in our papers to the fact that champagne was given to a starving man, and that a few drops of brandy were mixed with the milk given to a child in a similar condition, or suffering from marasmus; and within a week a physician who has traveled extensively and lectured before medical, theological, and literary organizations, and who has frequently been in consultation in critical cases, described in my hearing several cases of pneumonia which he visited, which were, as he expressed it, drunk. When asked by the attending physician what he would suggest, he always replied, "Stop giving your patients alcoholic liquids;" and with a single exception, out of a large number, and that was a complicated case, recovery followed. While practicing in Detroit I was called to see a prominent citizen who was suffering from typhoid fever. His physicians had told his family that he would die, but that the "stimulants" they were giving him might keep him alive a few hours. I found him delirious, with cold, clammy extremities and almost pulseless. I stopped his "stimulants" at once and gave him Homoeopathic remedies and nourishment, and the next day he was out of danger. No more dangerous treatment has ever been adopted than to give a patient in a critical stage of disease alcohol in any form or quantity. Every intelligent physician ought to be able to see that this is true. I repeat, alcohol paralyzes the minute capillary vessels and veins (look at the face of the drinker) on the surface of the body, in the brain (look at a drinker's words and actions), stomach, lungs, and kidneys, and congests them with blood, through which the structures are nourished with food and drink and purified by the removal of decomposed and effete substances. Cannot every one see that these vessels, when thus paralyzed and congested, cannot perform their duty as well as they can in a natural state? Then, again, the temperature of the body is lowered internally and its heat wasted from the surface. What patients in the critical stages of disease require are warmth applied, if needed, to the surface of the body and limbs, and hot water (not scalding hot, of course), milk, unfermented wine, and other simple, easily digested articles which will nourish and strengthen the body taken internally.

It is possible that in sudden, severe cases of hemorrhage, alcohol may sometimes rescue a patient from fainting and bleeding to death, by storing the blood in the capillary vessels of the brain and surface of the body temporarily while the bleeding vessels contract; but even in such cases other remedies, if at hand, may prove more reliable.

In cases of marasmus in children, if Homoeopathic remedies and nourishing articles fail to give relief, and the child becomes greatly emaciated, give the child cautiously salt fat pork, fried, but not to a crisp; give him a piece in his hand, too large for him to swallow, and see with what avidity he will chew and suck it. The fat in combination with the salt will supply a want in the child's system, and patients will often be restored by this simple treatment after other measures have failed.

Even if alcohol were a stimulant, as some claim, we can certainly see that to give it to a patient in a state of great exhaustion, either from lack of nourishment or from an inability to take nourishment owing to diseased action, is to most seriously endanger the life of the patient and often to destroy life; for alcohol gives no nourishment, and all unnatural excitement is necessarily followed by corresponding depression, which often carries patients in critical cases below the living point, and death follows.

I will close with the following from the *Health Monthly*: —"The theory that whiskey is necessary in the treatment of pneumonia has received a blow from Dr. Bull, of New York, who discovers that in the New York hospitals sixty-five per cent. of the pneumonia patients die with alcoholic treatment, while in London, at the Object Lesson Temperance Hospital, only five per cent. die. —*Ex.*"

CHAPTER IV.

PERSONAL RELIGIOUS EXPERIENCE OF A PHYSICIAN; AND AN APPEAL IN BEHALF OF A NEW DISPENSATION.

We know that in various ages of the world the Lord has revealed a knowledge of Himself to man. In the Ten Commandments we have the laws of spiritual life, in accordance with which we must live if we would enjoy spiritual health, precisely as we must live in accordance with the laws of natural life and health, if we would enjoy natural health.

We are dependent upon revelation for a knowledge of the laws of spiritual health, and of the causes and methods for the cure of spiritual diseases; but the Lord gives us, if we will keep His sayings, the ability, by careful scientific study and investigation, to obtain a knowledge of the physical laws of health, and the causes and methods of curing physical diseases. And it is wonderful how the natural in all respects symbolizes or corresponds to the spiritual.

To the Jewish Church the Lord revealed so much knowledge of Himself, and how they should live if they would be prosperous and happy here and hereafter, as that Church was prepared to receive; and He also promised to manifest Himself in person. All Christians believe that He fulfilled His promise when Jesus Christ appeared on earth; but He did not come in the manner which the Jews at the time of His advent expected. He came, not as a temporal ruler or prince; consequently they took Him for an impostor and crucified Him. To His followers and disciples He promised to come again in the clouds of heaven; but the clouds of heaven may not be the clouds of the material earth, any more than the spiritual kingdom which He came to establish was a natural kingdom; and it is possible that His second coming may not be in the manner anticipated by the Christian Church at the time of His second coming. He intimated as much when He inquired if He should find faith on earth. Should Christians, then, not watch and pray, and heed the signs of the times, lest they follow the example of the Jews, and reject Him at His second coming? Should not clergymen, as well as physicians, be led in freedom according to reason, and not blindly by prominent religious professors, clergymen and writers, and creeds formulated in an age of comparative darkness? Should the traditions and creeds of men be allowed to make of none effect the Word of God? Do we not see all around us signs of a most wonderful change going on in the world? Are these changes which we behold from the Lord, or from man?

I was reared in the Baptist Church. My father was a deacon, and labored faithfully to bring his children into the Church. I was taught that I must be converted, or get religion, before being baptized or joining the Church. What was meant by being converted I never fully comprehended, but I inferred from the instruction I received that it meant a radical change in one's feelings, the result of faith in the Lord's "atoning blood;" and that when this change was effected, I should be able to tell an experience similar to what I had heard others tell before joining the Church, which sometimes seemed quite marvelous. I attended "protracted meetings" and "revival meetings." And, one evening, I remember hoping and almost feeling that I felt a little change, and I even thought of announcing my feelings in the meeting; but caution prevailed, and I concluded to wait until the next day and see if there really was any change in my feelings. When the next day came, I could see no change, and consequently I made no announcement. Thus, I grew up and continued, until I was over thirty years of age, outside of the organized Church. I always respected religion, the Bible, and religious teachers, but I never got converted.

I had many things during childhood and early youth to be thankful for. My father and grandfather before him were accustomed to gather the family, night and morning, and read, or have some member of the family read, a chapter in the Bible, and then prayer was offered. Now, when this is done regularly, and especially if the Bible is read, in course, with here and there a few kindly remarks by the father or mother, no one can tell the good impression which is made on the children; they learn to reverence the Bible, and, what is of exceeding great moment, they hear it read through and through several times before they reach manhood, and they become comparatively familiar with the good and living precepts therein contained. The Sabbath-school, once a week for an hour or two, is all very well; but, in my estimation, it is very little, compared with daily family worship and acknowledging the Lord, and asking a blessing. O, that all Christian men and women could be aroused to the importance of such religious observances?

Some years ago, I went with my wife and a friend for a summer outing to the Catskill Mountains, and spent a few days at the Mountain House. There were a large number of guests there, of the various religious denominations. Those religiously inclined had established the custom of meeting every morning around a table, in a large room, when a chapter from the Bible was read, followed by singing and prayer. There have been few, if any, incidents of my whole life that I have more frequently thought of, or with greater pleasure and delight, than of those large, non-sectarian, and, as it were, family gatherings and simple services.

My mother died, as stated in the first part of this work, when I was ten years old. After remaining a widower for three years, during which period my grandparents, who lived with us, died and my only sister was married, my father married a widow, the mother of several children, a good Christian woman and a member of the Baptist Church.

I have always been thankful that I had a step-mother. No own mother could have been more kind, or have exercised a stronger influence for good over a son than she strove to exercise over me. She entered our home when I was thirteen years of age, when I needed a mother's influence and care perhaps as much as at any period of my life after I had ceased to draw my nourishment from my mother's breasts. Tears come into my eyes as I recall the pleasant, useful, and happy evenings and Sunday afternoons which I spent with her, when we happened to be alone in the house, reading and conversing about the interesting stories in the Bible and other religious books and papers that she thought would interest me. She may have had faults, yet I was about to say I do not remember one; but, unfortunately, she had one-she was a smoker of tobacco. Years before she had been troubled with "water brash," and a physician who, without much question, was himself a smoker, advised her to smoke; so she commenced smoking. He did not tell her to stop smoking as soon as she felt relief, as any intelligent physician should have done, if he was so unwise as to make such a prescription; but it is a question whether she ever experienced any permanent relief; for she was a bright, intelligent woman, and would have been likely to stop smoking of her own accord if she had been cured. In my estimation the physician who made the prescription was much more to be blamed than she was for the habit which followed. But seventy years ago very little was known as to the fearful slavery and diseases and mortality which result from the use of tobacco, compared with what is known to-day. The sin of ignorance cannot be pleaded in extenuation of such habits to-day, as it could then.

As to intoxicating drinks, I remember hearing my grandfather, when he was over eighty years old, after taking a drink of cider-brandy, exclaim: "A good gift of God, if taken with faith and prayer."

Fortunately, or providentially, I would say, the temperance reformation commenced soon after, and my father and other prominent members and the clergymen of the Baptist and Congregational churches in our town took an active part in the new movement. My father signed the pledge not to drink intoxicating drinks, and I followed his example; and I thank the Lord that I did so, for it gave me the strength and courage to say, "No, I thank you, I never drink," when invited and tempted to drink intoxicating drinks. No intoxicating drinks have been publicly sold in that town (Ashfield, Mass.) for many years. During a recent visit there I found that, within the past three years, there have been 61 deaths in the town, of whom 15 only were under 50 years of age, whereas 20 were over 80 years, of whom 4 were over 90 years of age. What do you think of that, Christian brother?

I remember very well the first ideas I had of God when a boy, which I derived from the preaching and praying of ministers. It was that God and our Lord Jesus Christ were two distinct

Beings. We had for a time a venerable gray-headed old man who preached one Sabbath, and a young man who preached the next. I thought the old man represented God the Father and the young man represented Jesus Christ.

When I arrived at manhood and came in contact with men of different religious views, and read some of their writings, the doctrine of the Trinity became more and more a mystery to me. At one time I was slightly inclined to Unitarianism, but I could not reconcile their doctrines with the Bible. Yet the Trinitarians seemed to teach distinctly that there are either two Gods, possessing different attributes, or that Jesus Christ was not God. It does not make any difference what we say with our lips; the question is, What do we "think in our hearts"? When I heard a bishop of one of the prevailing denominations stand up in his pulpit, as I have, and represent Jesus Christ as standing with one hand upon the throne of Jehovah, and the other hand resting upon the sinner's head, pleading with the Father to forgive him for his (Christ's) sake, was there not in the mind of that bishop a distinct idea of two Beings, possessing different feelings and passions? Now, were both of them Gods, or was one of them not God? And when I heard prayers so frequently terminated by the phrase, "Forgive us for Christ's sake," the question naturally arose, to whom were such prayers addressed? If there are any intelligent rational ideas connected with the phrase in the mind of the one using it, has not his prayer unquestionably been addressed to some God outside of the Lord Jesus Christ? Who is that God? Can Christian men safely reject the express teaching of our Lord Himself when on earth, when He declared: "I and my Father are One;" "Whose hath seen me, hath seen the Father"? and the apostle's teaching, that "God was in Christ, reconciling the world unto Himself"? Is there any other way to the Father at this day except through the person of the Lord Jesus Christ-God manifest in the flesh? Is He not the "Alpha and Omega, the beginning and the end, the first and the last"? Why, then, pray to an unknown God? In the Old Testament, we are told that "I, Jehovah, am your Savior, and beside me there is no Savior," and in the New Testament we are told that in Jesus Christ dwelt all the fullness of the Godhead bodily. He is "Immanuel-God with us." Let us, then, worship Him-One God in One Divine Person.

The doctrine of election and predestination early troubled me. I could not reconcile it with the loving kindness which the Sacred Scriptures proclaim as characteristic of our Heavenly Father.

The doctrine of justification by faith alone, "without the deeds of the law," as the old hymn read, was not a doctrine which appealed to my reason, but it was a very consoling doctrine. Every young man who has been carefully reared by religious parents, and under the influences of a church, expects to be converted and get religion some time before he dies, and to join a church. But if he enjoys good health and the prospect of living for many years, especially if he is taught that, by merely believing or having faith at any time in the "atoning blood of Christ," he can escape the consequences of his evil deeds, there is great danger of procrastination.

A clergyman once said to me: "If a man repents and gets converted one hour before his death, the worse he has been or lived, the happier he will be." It seems to me better to be guided by the Word of the Lord, and to believe that the evil doer shall not go unpunished. The Lord came into the world to save men from sin and from the penalty only so far as they co-operate with Him. Sin is the cause, the penalty is the effect; and effect follows cause as a normal and necessary consequence.

The young, as well as the old, should be taught the great truth, that every thought we harbor, and every word we speak, and every act we do, aid in building up our spiritual organism, and will tell on our eternal destiny, just as the natural food and drink we use, and the exercise we take, will tell on the future health of our material bodies, for good or evil; and there is no avoiding it. If a man or woman, young or old, would be right in the future, he must do right in the present. No one should forget that, even if we reach heaven, the mansion which we will occupy there will depend on our lives here-every one will unite with those like Himself. No one can tell the immense harm which has been done to our race, by teaching that either by faith alone, or through the influence or efforts of the clergy, men can be saved from the penalties or consequences which are sure to follow an evil life. The "willing and obedient" shall eat the good of the land. Our blessed Lord tells us: "If ye keep my commandments, ye shall abide in my love" (John xv: 10). Thus beautiful, symmetrical, spiritual organisms are built up, not by "sowing wild oats" during youth, and disobeying the divine commandments during the subsequent period of life. It is well for all, young or old, to remember the Word: "Be not deceived; God is not mocked: for whatsoever a man soweth, that shall he also reap." (Gal. vi: 7.) At this day we need practical doctrines, which shall unite religion and life, or faith and charity, and such alone will command the respect of non-churchgoers.

While a young man my attention was early called to the doctrines of the Universalists, but their doctrines did not seem to me to accord with the Sacred Scriptures; nor did I think that all men could be equally happy hereafter, when there is such a vast difference in their conduct and lives here. Genuine happiness is the result of right willing and doing; in other words, of keeping the commandments. I have no doubt but the Lord desires that all men should thus live and be happy; but we know that all men are not willing. Having created them free agents, God does not compel them here to love the Lord and their neighbor, which loves manifestly constitute heaven; what reason, then, have we to think He will compel them to do it hereafter? If a man deliberately leads an evil life here, growing ever stronger and more confirmed in that life, until he has made evil his good and rejoices in it, what reason have we to suppose or assume that he will change when he enters the next life? I am willing to leave him in the hands of the Lord-he has passed from my sight. I well remember the remarks of my grandmother when she was eighty-six years of age, a few days after the death of her husband, my grandfather. She said: "I do not fear to die, for I feel that God will do me no injustice." Within a few days she departed in peace.

The Millerite excitement commenced when I was a young man. When I was about twenty years old I was traveling in central Massachusetts. One night there was a meeting of Millerites in the neighborhood where I was stopping, and I attended the meeting. The speaker was very zealous and earnest in his remarks. There was a comet with quite a long tail then visible, and he seemed to think that that comet, with its tail, might sweep across the track of our earth and work its destruction, which he anticipated. I remember very well my reflections on leaving that meeting. A few days before I had stood upon the side of a hill near the track, and had seen for the first time a railroad train on its way from Boston to Worcester. I said to myself: "Now we have railroads, steamboats, friction matches, temperance societies, Sunday-schools, the Bible translated into various languages, which but a few years ago were unknown. This great continent, from being a wilderness, inhabited by a comparatively few wild Indians, has been discovered and is being developed and cultivated by civilized and Christian people, and gradually being made capable of containing and sustaining hundreds of millions of inhabitants." With all these facts before me, I said to myself, "It looks a great deal more as though the world is just beginning to live; in fact, that a new era is dawning, than it does that the world is going to be destroyed." From that night the Millerite doctrine never troubled me any more, for I felt that I beheld, in all the wonderful inventions being made and changes going on in the world, the dawning light of a better day for the inhabitants of our earth.

CHAPTER V.

THE DAWN OF A NEW DISPENSATION.

We behold the dawn of a new day before we see the sun, from whence the light proceeds.

The young in the Baptist Church, not having been baptized in infancy, are brought up to feel that they are out of the Church, and that they have to be converted, or "to get religion," before they join the Church, instead of being brought up to feel that, having been baptized, they belong to the Church and must believe its doctrines, and live the life which they teach. Thus I remained out of the Church until I was over thirty years of age. After I was twenty-three years old I attended different churches, as was most convenient. For a time I attended the Episcopal Church, while studying medicine; and after I graduated I attended the Congregational Church for several years more frequently than any other; but I had no thought of joining that Church, for during those days I always thought that immersion was the only true mode of baptism.

While practicing medicine in Detroit, a gentleman whose family I was attending asked me if I would not like to read a work on "Heaven and Hell," written by Emanuel Swedenborg, who claimed, he said, to have had open intercourse with the spiritual world, and to have written of what he had seen and heard in that world. He said that he had read it, and believed that the views therein contained were rational and true. If I had ever heard of them at all, at that time, I had never heard the writings of Swendenborg spoken of favorably before. Out of respect to the gentleman, I took the book home with me, but did not feel sufficient interest in it to attempt to read it through in course, but read here and there a few pages; and, after keeping it a few weeks, I returned it to the owner, feeling from what I had read no interest in its contents. Not long after this a lady whom I was attending asked me if I would not like to read Professor George Bush's reasons for accepting as true the revelations contained in the writings of Emanuel Swedenborg. Well, I thought to myself, if the gentleman who lent me "Heaven and Hell," if my patient here, who is a very intelligent woman, and Professor Bush, whom I had understood was a very learned man, believe that Swedenborg's writings contain truths good and useful, it may be well for me to read the pamphlet then before me. So I took the book home with me and commenced reading it. About that time Rev. George Field commenced the delivery of a course of lectures on Creation and the first chapters of Genesis, treating the subject from the standpoint of Swedenborg's writings. I attended his lectures, which added very much to my interest, and I read Bush's reasons with care. Then I obtained "Heaven and Hell," and read it carefully through with the greatest interest. When a small boy I remember very well listening with fear and trembling to a discourse delivered by a clergyman, on "God is angry with the wicked every day," in which the speaker dwelt upon the fearful sufferings which the Lord had in reserve for the wicked in a hell of fire and brimstone, where they were to be tortured forever and ever.

When I came to read Swedenborg's "Heaven and Hell," I found a very different and more rational doctrine taught-that heaven consists in loving the Lord and the neighbor, or in religious obedience to the divine commandments; and that hell consists in loving one's self and the world supremely, or sensual and selfish gratification, without regard to use; that either heaven or hell is within us, according to the character of our ruling love; that the Lord casts no one into hell, but does all He can, without interfering with man's freedom, to prevent men from going to hell; if they go there, they go of their own free choice, among their like, where selfishness in some form rules the hearts of the inhabitants; they would not and could not be happy among those who are ruled by love to the Lord and the neighbor; or by obedience to the divine commandments. The spiritual world is a more real world than this; therefore, in that world the motives, thoughts, and intentions of men cannot be hidden as readily as in this world; consequently, there is a great gulf between heaven and hell. One is opposite to the other. When love to the Lord and to the neighbor rules in the hearts of all the inhabitants, there is no need of penal laws or punishments, for each one is a law unto himself, and all are striving to do good to each other and to all; consequently, unity, peace, and harmony prevail.

How different from this is hell, where selfishness prevails; where the love of dominion over others, or the love of vain show, the love of acquiring unfairly that which belongs to others, the love of riches for the sake of being rich, and of selfish and sensual gratification without regard to use, rules in the hearts of all the inhabitants. We know that such perverted passions make a hell hot enough here; and, as death does not change the character of a man's ruling love, they will make a hell hot enough hereafter. But the Lord, in His mercy which endureth forever, by His angels governs the hells as well as the heavens, and does not permit vindictive punishments. All punishments are for the benefit of evil doers, to restrain and prevent them from doing evil to others and themselves, and from sinking to greater depths of wickedness; we may, therefore, safely leave the inhabitants of that world in His care.

No man or woman can read "Heaven and Hell" attentively, carefully, and prayerfully without great benefit. It is clearly shown that, to escape hell, an evil man has but to repent, to look to the Lord and shun evils as sins against Him, and that the Lord is no respecter of persons, but that He gives to every man the ability to do this, if he is willing. When we examine ourselves carefully in the light of the Sacred Scriptures, and discover an evil, if we shun that evil as a sin against the Lord, He keeps us in the effort to shun all evils, and enables us more clearly to see other evils to which we are inclined. Here is an open door for approaching the Lord, free to all; there is no mystery about it. If an evil man is to be reformed, he must repent or face about and commence a life of shunning evils as sins against God; otherwise, there will be no radical change, but a miserable shuffling from one evil habit to another. Even if a man shuns one evil habit, like the smoking or chewing of tobacco, because it injures his health and is likely to destroy his life, and not because it is a sin, and without the acknowledgment that it is a sin, he is almost sure to seek as a substitute some form of intoxicating drinks-opium, strong coffee, or tea. We make a great mistake, as Christians, if we try to substitute coffee- or tea-houses for saloons; not that the effects of coffee and tea are as pernicious as intoxicants, but they are unnecessary, and often diseases and great suffering result from their use. We should strive to show men and women, in the light of this day, what substances are unmistakably injurious to health and endanger life, and strive to lead them, by precept and example, to shun their use as sins against God.

After reading "Heaven and Hell" I read the "True Christian Religion," which is the last work that Swedenborg published, containing the essential doctrines of the New Christian Church, or the New Jerusalem now descending from God out of Heaven, "making all things new." In this work it is clearly shown that God is one in essence and in person, and that in the Lord Jesus Christ that one God is manifested to men. God is love. "In the beginning was the Word and the Word was, with God and the Word was God." Here we have the Father or Divine Love, the Son or Divine Wisdom, and the Holy Spirit or Divine Proceeding, flowing from the Father because He is a being of infinite love, wisdom, and power, through the Son, a trinity in unity. The Divine Being is no more three persons than a man is three persons, because he is created in the image of God and has affection or love, an understanding, or thoughts, words, and acts that flow from his love through his understanding out toward his fellow men. All the doctrines of the New Christianity are based upon the Sacred Scriptures and appeal to our highest reason; and we are to receive them because we see them to be true and in strict harmony with the Word when the latter is correctly understood.

But I have neither time nor space to discuss these doctrines here. I will simply say, that when we come to see clearly that there is but one God whose name is one, who was manifested in the person of the Lord Jesus Christ, and that whoso seeth Him seeth the Father, then a number of false doctrines which proceed from and cohere with the doctrine of a tri-personal Deity will disappear like mists before the rising sun; and we shall be prepared to see and understand the rest of the beautiful and rational doctrines taught in "The True Christian Religion," and the mystery of Babylon and all man-made creeds will disappear before this new revelation from our Lord Jesus Christ.

After reading the "True Christian Religion" I read the work on Divine Providence, which gives such a clear view of the Lord's providential care over men that it strengthens and encourages the earnest seeker after truth wonderfully. It is a book which should be read by every Christian man and woman.

Next, "The Angelic Wisdom Concerning the Divine Love and Wisdom" throws a flood of light on the origin of the material universe and all created things. In this work we are clearly shown that the Lord is Love itself, because He is Life itself: and "that angels and men are recipients of life;" and "that all created things in a certain image represent man," and "that Love is the life of man."

But Swedenborg's "Apocalypse Revealed" was one of the most satisfactory works I ever read. It opened up to me a new world of thought, of expectation, hope and joy. The reading of this work and the first volume of his "Arcana Celestia" satisfied me that the Sacred Scriptures are divine or a special revelation from God to man, and differ from all merely human writings as much as a living man differs from a statue; for they are filled with a Divine spirit. The Lord says: "My words are spirit and life."

The Sacred Scriptures are written in accordance with the law of correspondence between spiritual and natural things. The spiritual is the cause, the natural is the effect; and effects must correspond to their causes in every particular. The Lord is the sun of the spiritual world and the creator of all things: consequently our natural sun corresponds to the spiritual sun, or the Lord. From the Lord, or the spiritual sun, love and wisdom proceed, and give life to man's spiritual body; from the natural sun flow natural heat and light which enable the natural body to live; natural heat and light therefore correspond to spiritual heat and light, or to love and truth, which are heat and light to the spirit of man. Through the natural clouds and atmosphere which surround the earth we receive natural heat and light from the natural sun, as we receive spiritual heat and light or love and truth from the Lord through the literal sense of the Sacred Scriptures; Consequently the clouds of heaven in which the Lord was to come are the literal sense of his holy Word, unfolding its spirit and life and manifesting the Father clearly to His children. The sun which was to be darkened was not the natural but the spiritual sun, or the Lord obscured to man's spiritual perception. When men in their creeds separated the Lord into three persons, and framed doctrines in accordance therewith, which, in their estimation, would enable them to reach heaven by believing certain dogmas, instead of by a life according to the Divine Commandments, then was the sun indeed darkened in the minds of men. Then a true faith or knowledge of the Lord was destroyed and the moon became as blood. A true faith reflects the light or wisdom of the Lord upon man, as the natural moon reflects the light of the natural sun. Water corresponds to truth upon the natural plane of the mind, for it cleanses the natural body as truth cleanses his spirit; it also circulates throughout the natural body, conveying nourishment to all the structures of the body as truth circulates through the spiritual body, conveying that which is good and true to strengthen and develop the spiritual body. It is owing to this correspondence that water is used in the ordinance of baptism, for it performs the same office for the natural body that truth does for the spiritual body; it cleanses and conveys nourishment; and therefore baptism by water signifies that man is to be regenerated by receiving and living according to the truth. It is also the Christian sign —a sign that one baptized is of the Christian Church, or professes the Christian religion.

The "Fruit of the Vine," or pure unfermented or unleavened wine, has been organized by the Lord in the vegetable kingdom; it therefore not only contains water, but also organized nourishment for the structures of the body, which supply in a most remarkable degree the wants of the body, like a mother's milk to her infant child; it therefore most beautifully symbolizes blood, and corresponds to spiritual truth, united with good from the Lord, which nourishes and builds up the spirit of man, when he drinks or appropriates it, or when he lives as divine truth teaches, shunning evils as sins against God. It is consequently used appropriately in the Most Holy Supper.

It has been my aim above to simply give the reader a glimpse of this most wonderful and beautiful of all sciences, and really the foundation of all sciences-the science of correspondence between natural and spiritual things. He who reads carefully and without prejudice the "Apocalypse Revealed" and the "Arcana Celestia," with a desire to know and live according to the truth, cannot fail to see that the Sacred Scriptures are plenarily inspired, and are a special revelation from God to man; and that, different from all merely human writings, they contain within the letter a connected spiritual sense. That the science of correspondences was once understood by the inhabitants of our earth, is to be seen in the relics which remain in a more or less perverted form in the hieroglyphics of Egypt, the idolatry among many nations, and sun-worship, where the spiritual signification has often been lost and men have come to worship the natural objects instead of the spiritual, which they represent. The mythological writings of many nations, and even Masonry, contain remains of this once well known science. The first chapters of Genesis and the entire Word are written in strict accordance with this science. The first chapters of Genesis, like the Parables of our Lord, were not intended to be understood literally; the very names therein show this clearly. A tree of life, a tree of knowledge of good and evil, a talking serpent, how can any man for a moment suppose these to be natural trees and a natural snake? Do serpents ever talk? the garden eastward in Eden, and an Ark which would not hold the hides and teeth of all the animals on earth-were these to be understood literally?

CHAPTER VI.

A NEW DAY TO OUR EARTH.

> "'Behold He cometh with clouds,' signifies that the Lord will reveal Himself in the literal sense of the Word, and will open its spiritual sense at the end of the church." —*A. R. 23.*

A church, we are taught, comes to its end when the true doctrines of the Word are falsified by its members, to justify evils of life; or when the members of a church who are in the love of ruling over others in civil and ecclesiastical affairs, for their own aggrandizement, or for vain show, or who love money or sensual gratification without regard to use, strive to justify the gratification of their perverted loves and appetites by an appeal to the Sacred Scriptures, and thus frame creeds and doctrines which exalt faith and ceremonials above a life of charity, and when men come to live in accordance with such false doctrines the church comes to its end. At the same time, there remain some who are still in the good of life, or striving to live good lives in obedience to the Divine commandments. Such comprise the common people who receive the Lord with joy at His coming, and follow Him, among whom a New Dispensation of Divine Truth commences. Such may be found both among the clergy and laity. The end of the world is the end of the Dispensation or Age, and not of the material earth —"The earth endureth forever."

We are told by Swedenborg that the angels rejoiced greatly that it had pleased the Lord to reveal a knowledge of correspondences so deeply concealed during some thousands of years; "and they said it was done in order that the Christian Church which is founded on the Word, and is now at its end, may again revive and draw breath through heaven from the Lord." —*Conjugial Love,* 532.

So we are not to look for the destruction of the prevailing religious organizations, but for the rejection of their false and irrational doctrines, and the receiving of new light and life from the Lord. And how is such a result to be brought about?

It was apparently the opinion of Swedenborg that his writings would be read by the clergy, who would teach the doctrines therein contained to their congregations; and thus the glorious truths for this new Era or crowning Church would be spread among the people; for, in speaking of the descent of the New Church, or New Jerusalem, from God out of Heaven, he says it can only take place "in proportion as the falses of the former Church are removed; for what is new cannot gain admission where falses have before been implanted, unless those falses are first rooted out; and this must first take place among the clergy, and by their means among the laity."

That Swedenborg's anticipations are surely and somewhat rapidly being realized at this time seems beyond question; for over 30,000 clergymen of the various religious denominations of our country have already sent for and obtained Swedenborg's "True Christian Religion" and "Heaven and Hell," and over 25,000 have received his "Apocalypse Revealed." It is known that large numbers are reading the above works with great interest, and that hundreds if not thousands are full receivers of the doctrines therein contained, and that they are teaching them to their people as fast as they find they can receive them. In fact, many of Swedenborg's writings were translated into English by the late Rev. John Clowes, Rector of St. John's Church, Manchester, England, who, for many years, without ever being required to sever his connection with the Church of England, openly and boldly taught the doctrines revealed through Swedenborg. Mr. Clowes says: —

> "Nothing, therefore, can be plainer than that the New Jerusalem Dispensation is to be universal, and to extend unto all people, nations, and languages on the face of the earth, to be a blessing unto such as are meet to receive a blessing. Sects and sectarians, as such, can find no place in this General Assembly of the ransomed

of the Lord. All the little distinctions of modes, forms, and particular expressions of devotion and worship will be swallowed up and lost in the unlimited effusions of heavenly love, charity, and benevolence with which the hearts of every member of this glorious New Church and Body of Jesus Christ will overflow one toward another. Men will no longer judge one another as to the mere externals of church communion, be they perfect or imperfect; for they will be taught that whosoever acknowledges the incarnate Jehovah in heart and life, departing from evil, and doing what is right and good according to the commandments, he is a member of the New Jerusalem, a living stone in the Lord's new Temple, and a part of that great family in heaven and earth whose common Father and Head is Jesus Christ. Every one, therefore, will call his neighbor *Brother*, in whom he observes this spirit of pure charity; and he will ask no questions concerning the form of words which compose his creed, but will be satisfied with observing in him the purity and power of a heavenly life."

"The Gentiles," says Swedenborg, "cannot profane the holy things of the Church like Christians, because they are not acquainted with them." "They are afraid of Christians on account of their lives." "Those who have lived well, according to their religious principles, are instructed by the angels, and easily receive the truths of faith, and acknowledge the Lord," "for they have not formed for themselves any principles of falsity opposed to the truths of faith, which would need to be first removed."

"Although Gentiles are not in genuine truths during their life in the world, they receive them in the other life from a principle of love."

"The Church of the Lord exists with all in the universe who live in good according to their religious principles, and acknowledge the Divine Being; and they are accepted of the Lord and go to heaven."

The above is in strict accordance with all that Swedenborg has written; for he says: —

"In the spiritual world to which every man goes after death, it is not the character of your faith into which inquiry is made, nor of your *doctrine*, but of your *life*, whether it has been of this character or that; for it is known that such as a man's *life* is, such is his faith-nay, more, such is his doctrine; for life forms its doctrine and faith for itself." (*D. P.* 101.) "For the good of life according to one's religion contains within it the affection of knowing truths, which such persons also learn and receive when they come into the other life." (*A. C.* 455.)

"Evils which belong to the will, are what condemn a man and sink him down to hell; and falsities only so far as they become conjoined with evils; then one follows the other. This is proved by numerous instances of persons who are in falsities, and yet are saved." (*Ibid.* 845.)

"It has been provided that every one, in whatever heresy he may be as to the understanding, can still be reformed and saved, provided he shuns evils as sins, and does not confirm heretical falsities in himself; for by shunning evils as sins the will is reformed, and through the will the understanding, which then first comes out of darkness into light. There are three essentials of the Church: the acknowledgment of the Divine of the Lord, the acknowledgment of the holiness of the Word, and the life which is called charity. According to the life, which is charity, every one has faith; from the Word is the knowledge of what the life must be; and from the Lord are reformation and salvation. If the Church had held these three as essentials, intellectual dissensions would not have divided but only varied it, as light varies its colors in beautiful objects, and as various diadems give beauty in the crown of a king." (*D. P.* 259.)

Here, then, we have a broad spirit of charity which acknowledges every man as a brother who believes in a Supreme Being, shuns evils as sins, and strives to live conscientiously and honestly according to the light he possesses.

As many who will be likely to receive this pamphlet may know little, if anything, in regard to the claims which Swedenborg makes, that he was the human instrument chosen by The Lord through whom to reveal to the world the truths of a New Dispensation, even of the Second Coming of the Son of Man, it may be well to allow this chosen servant to speak for himself as to his mission. He says: —

> "I have been called to a holy office by the Lord Himself. I can sacredly and solemnly declare that the Lord Himself has been seen of me, and that He has sent me to do what I do, and for such purpose has opened and enlightened the interior part of my soul, which is my spirit, so that I can see what is in the spiritual world and those that are therein; and this privilege has now been continued to me for twenty-two years. But in the present state of infidelity, can the most solemn oath make such a thing credible or to be believed? Yet such as have received true Christian light and understanding will be convinced of the truths contained in my writings, which are particularly evident in the book of 'Revelations Revealed.' Who, indeed, has hitherto known anything of importance of the spiritual sense of the Word of God, of the spiritual world, or of heaven and hell; the nature of the life of man, and the state of souls after the decease of the body? Is it to be supposed that these, and other things of like consequence, are to be eternally hidden from Christians?"

Again, in the "True Christian Religion," at a later date, toward the close of his life in this world, he says: —

> "I foresee that many who read the relations after the chapters, will believe that they are inventions of the imagination; but I assert in truth that they are not inventions, but were truly seen and heard; not seen and heard in any state of mind buried in sleep, but in a state of full wakefulness. For it has pleased the Lord to manifest Himself to me, and to send me to teach those things which will be of His New Church, which is meant by the New Jerusalem in the Revelation; for which end He has opened the interiors of my mind or spirit, by which it has been given me to be in the spiritual world with angels, and at the same time in the natural world with men, and this now for twenty-seven years."

In a letter to the King of Sweden, with characteristic simplicity and boldness, he says: —

> "When my writings are read with attention and cool reflection (in which many things are to be met with hitherto unknown) it is easy enough to conclude that I could not come to such knowledge but by a real vision and converse with those who are in the spiritual world. I am ready to testify with the most solemn oath that can be offered in this matter, that I have said nothing but essential and real truth, without any admixture of deception. This knowledge is given to me by our Saviour, not for any particular merit of mine, but for the great concern of all Christians' salvation."

When asked why a philosopher was chosen to this office he replied: —

> "To the end that the spiritual knowledge which is revealed at this day might be reasonably learned and naturally understood; because spiritual truths answer unto natural ones, inasmuch as these originate and flow from them, and serve as a foundation for the former."

To the Swedish clergymen who visited him a short time before his death, and who urged him to recant what he had written if it was not true, he replied, with great zeal and emphasis: —

> "As true as you see me before you, so true is everything that I have written, and I could have said more had I been permitted. When you come into eternity you will see all things as I have stated and described them, and we shall have much to discourse about with each other."

Here, then, we have in this illustrious seer the unparalleled instance of a man, not in the enthusiasm of youth, but at the mature age of fifty-six years, standing among the first in the philosophical world, with reputation unsullied, high in office in his native country, with proffered promotion, giving up all, and proclaiming to the world that he was called by the Lord to the important office of revealing new truths of vast moment to his fellow-men —even the truths of a new dispensation, or of the second coming of our Lord and Saviour Jesus Christ.

Now, I appeal to you, one and all, Clergymen of the Christian Church, of every name, to obtain and read his writings. In the good Providence of the Lord, three among his most important works can be obtained without money and without price by the clergy and theological students of our country, by simply ordering them and sending the postage-as will be seen on the second page of the cover of this pamphlet.

Swedenborg does not require or desire you to believe anything contained in his writings on his simple declaration, but you are to believe the statements made, and doctrines proclaimed, in his writings, only as you perceive them to be true, and in strict accordance with the Sacred Scriptures. What have you to lose by reading his writings? Thousands of laymen and clergyman testify to you that they have found the greatest help and strength from reading them, even where they may not have read enough to fully recognize his claims.

Canon Wilberforce, of Southampton, England, one of the most distinguished clergymen of the English Church, visited this country a few years ago; and while he was here, being a prominent temperance man, the National Temperance Society gave him a reception, during which some one introduced me to him as a believer in the writings of Emanuel Swedenborg. Stopping a moment, and looking steadily at me and those in the immediate vicinity, he exclaimed, most emphatically: "Emanuel Swedenborg has done the Christian Church an immense service! an immense service!! especially in his explanation and illustration of the doctrine of the Lord." These words were spoken manfully and boldly in the presence of members and clergymen of his own and other Churches. The doctrine of the Lord is the chief corner-stone of the New Jerusalem now descending from God out of Heaven. Let that doctrine be accepted by our Churches, and their creeds, so far as they are based on a tri-personal God, will need no revision; they will disappear.

"All things," says a great authority, "are of God, who hath reconciled us to Himself by Jesus Christ, and hath committed unto us the ministry of reconciliation; to wit, that God was in Christ reconciling the world unto Himself, not imputing their trespasses unto them." (2 Cor. v: 18, 19)

The late Professor George Bush and a large number of distinguished scholars and clergymen, after a most thorough and careful examination of Swedenborg's writings, assure us that in them they find the truths of a New Dispensation, even of the Second Coming of the Son of Man in the clouds of heaven. The light of a New Day is shining. Christian brethren, will you close your eyes against it?

Was there ever any greater need of a new revelation from God to teach men anew that, if they would reach heaven and happiness, they must repent and shun evils as sins against God, and strive to live a life according to the commandments? Look at the fearful evils which prevail in our beloved country; the love of rule, civil and ecclesiastical; the miserly love of money, selfishness, vanity and sensualism, in their worst and most degrading forms! Customs and habits prevail which threaten the extinction of at least the Protestant portion of the community in large sections of our country. A Catholic bishop stated, a few years ago, that one quarter of the inhabitants of New England are Catholics, and that one-fourth of the population give birth to 70 per cent. of the children born in New England. More recent inquiries, it is stated, show that the average number of children in a family among the Canadian French settled in New England, averages 5; whereas among the native New Englanders the average number of children in a family is 1-1/2. It is not difficult to see by whom the land of the Puritans will be ruled within the next quarter of a century. Seventy years ago, the average number of children to a family among New Englanders was fully equal to the number among the French to-day. Why this change? Fashionable habits of dress-tight lacing, which is worse to-day than ever before-has, to a large extent, destroyed the ability of the New England and other native American women to bear healthy and well-developed children, and to properly nurse them after they are born. Among our present deformed women, child-bearing is attended with much more danger and suffering than among well-developed, symmetrical, and beautifully formed women. No man who desires peace, health, and happiness in his home, and desires to leave children behind him, and to thus perform the most important use which can be performed in this life, should ever think of marrying a small-waisted woman.

Then again, to have a good family of children is thought not to be fashionable, among those who are led by fashion, as it interferes too much with one's selfish pleasures, they think; most dearly do they pay in after life, if they live many years, for their folly. Children are a blessing; and yet the most unnatural and injurious measures are adopted to prevent bearing children, even to the destroying of the unborn. The Catholic Church, through the confessional, holds some restraint over Catholics; but what restraint do our Protestant Churches hold over their members in regard to such evils? Look at the miserable caricatures of the female form printed in our fashionable magazines, and even in our daily papers, and sent forth and freely spread before our young girls, for them to pattern after, and thus deform themselves.

Look at the drunkenness, the leaden and congested faces of our steady drinkers of intoxicating drinks, and the innumerable deaths and the wretchedness and sorrow which follow such drinking; and remember that the chief support of such drinking at this day is the use of the drunkard's cup instead of "the fruit of the vine" as a communion wine in so many of our churches, and the example of so many of our clergy, backed up by the prescribing of such drinks by so many of our doctors. Do away with these two chief supports, and prohibition would be enacted and enforced throughout our land within five years.

Look at the use of tobacco, which is to-day recognized as one of the most deadly poisons, which when used by the young prevents the development of the human body, and at all ages causes innumerable diseases and deaths and an inability to withstand the encroachment of other causes of disease; and the smoke and saliva from the nostrils and mouths of those who use it, which are so unpleasant and disagreeable to those who are not accustomed to them, but who yet are so frequently compelled to breathe a polluted atmosphere. Please read the following and tell us whether to thus prevent the development of the body and lessen one's ability to withstand the causes of diseases should be shunned as a sin against God or not: —

SMOKING AND PHYSICAL DEVELOPMENT.

From the records of the senior class of Yale College during the Past eight years, the non-smokers have proved to have decidedly gained over the smokers in height, weight, and lung capacity. All candidates for the crews and other athletic sports were non-smokers. The non-smokers were 20 per cent. taller than the smokers, 25 per cent. heavier, and had 62 per cent. more lung capacity. In the graduating class of Amherst College of the present year, those not using tobacco have in weight gained 24 per cent. over those using tobacco, in height 37 per cent., in chest girth 42 per cent., while they have a greater average lung capacity by 8.36 cubic inches. —*Medical News.*

Just see the countenance which is given to this habit by too many of our clergymen-the example which they set! Yes, in many of our denominations, young men who are known to be smokers, or chewers of tobacco, with their breaths smelling of this filthy, poisonous weed, are deliberately licensed and ordained by Clergymen, when it is known that they will go in and out before young and old, setting them an example which will unquestionably do untold injury to the rising generation, and confirm old smokers and chewers in their injurious and destructive habits, and thus be instrumental in destroying many lives. What are the fathers and mothers in our churches thinking about when they consent to such an example being set before their children? Is it not time that they awake to the importance of choosing and introducing into office their own ministers, instead of entrusting this duty to the clergy? Swedenborg has given us the true signification of ordination by the laity. In speaking of the ordination of the Levites by the laity he says: "By the sons of Israel laying their hands upon the Levites was signified the transference of the power of ministering for them, and the reception of it by the Levites, thus separation." —A. C. 10,023. It will be seen that it was not Aaron the priest who laid his hands upon the Levites when they were introduced into the office of the priesthood, but the laity, or the children of Israel; and we can all see how appropriate and significative the ceremony was; and it was strictly in accordance with republican usages of this day. It does not exalt the officer above the office which he fills.

Is there a race of men on earth to-day who stand in greater need of light on spiritual subjects, and of the services of good, earnest, clean, pure-minded Christian Missionaries, who shall call men and women to repentance, and by precept and example lead them to shun the fearful evils named above, and many others, as sins against God, more than the people of the United States? Look at our children, many of whom, if they live at all, grow up with crooked legs and spines, delicate muscles and irritable brains, imperfectly developed jaws and consequently crowded teeth, which commence decaying and torturing the young before they are twenty years old, instead of lasting during life as they should; all of which results principally from feeding children with starvation bread, or superfine flour bread, cakes, and puddings, instead of the "full corn in the ear," or unbolted flour or meal, as the Lord has organized it in the kernel of grain. Many years ago scientific investigation demonstrated the fact that the portions of the grain which nourish the brain, muscles, and bones is principally confined to the dark, hard portion of the kernel immediately beneath the hull; this is not easily pulverized or rolled into superfine flour, and if it were the flour would not be white; but it goes principally into, the second and third runnings or as canal, shorts, and bran, and is fed to the horses, cattle, and hogs, causing them to be well developed, strong, and healthy, while our children, for the want of it, are half starved. Even a dog, it has been found by experiment, will starve to death on superfine flour bread, but will live well enough on Graham or unbolted flour bread. I have seen a child come near starving to death on such bread, and only rescued her from impending death by mixing mashed potatoes with the flour from which the bread was made. The little girl thought she could eat no other food but such bread, and if she ate anything else she threw it up. And yet, strange to say, I have known in one or more institutions under the care of physicians, which were devoted to the treatment of deformed and crippled children, superfine flour bread to be given them to eat.

It is fashionable and customary to use superfine flour bread; and as a physician, and an employer of men, I know how difficult it is to induce or persuade fathers and mothers, even for the sake of their children, to use Graham or unbolted flour bread, cakes, and puddings, which will give nourishment to the brain, muscles, teeth and bones, and all the fat and heat-producing material they need, instead of superfine white flour bread, cakes, and puddings, which give comparatively little more than fat and heat-producing material.

I remember very well when my wife and myself were traveling in Egypt up the Nile, and were at ancient Thebes, mounted on donkeys, going to the tombs of the kings, the young Arab girl, with a vessel of water upon her head, balanced by the ends of the fingers of one hand, who ran beside us over the sand, stones, and hills; for she was one of the most beautiful and symmetrical female forms I have ever seen. There was no contracted waist or humped shoulders, but a beautiful female figure, full of life, with splendid teeth and sparkling eyes. And on a visit to the house of our Arab dragoman, or guide, we saw how the flour or meal was made upon which that young girl was fed. In the court-yard two women were grinding at a mill as they ground thousands of years ago. There were two circular mill stones, perhaps 20 inches in diameter, standing in a basin; through the centre of the upper stone there was an opening through which the wheat was poured, and upon two sides were erect wooden handles, by which the women turned the stone round and round, and back and forth, and the meal escaped into the pan at the circumference. I said to our dragoman: "We have not had a bit of good bread in Egypt. We have been stopping at hotels where they think they must give the Americans and Englishmen white bread. Now, I wish you would bring me some bread made from that flour to-morrow morning;" and he brought us some bread, and it was by far the best bread that we had in Egypt.

The fearful evils which I have hastily named in the preceding pages, and many others which cause the prevailing deformities, diseases, insanity, and premature deaths, are not to be dragged along into the Church of the New Jerusalem now descending from God out of heaven; but our race is to be purified, renovated, and developed into a healthy, noble, symmetrical, graceful manhood by the new inflowing of truths from the Lord, pointing out the evils and falses which are causing the present suffering and wretchedness, and calling on men and women to shun such evils and falses as sins against God. A reformation from worldly motives is but "skin deep," and generally only results in the changing of one bad habit for another. Men and women must be earnestly called to repentance, and to the absolute necessity of shunning the evils which prevent the development of the body, impair health and reason, and so fearfully shorten the average duration of human life, as sins against God, which will tell on their eternal destiny. The fact that individuals who drink intoxicating drinks, smoke or chew tobacco, or deform their bodies by tight dressing, sometimes live to old age under otherwise favorable circumstances, amounts to nothing. The simple question is, do such habits shorten the average duration of human life? If they do, they are a violation of the laws of God as manifested in the organization of the human body and in His Word.

CHAPTER VII

THE WANTS OF THE CHRISTIAN CHURCH.

The Christian Church at this day, first of all, needs true doctrines which are in harmony with the Sacred Scriptures, and which all men who are willing to see and obey, using the reason with which God has endowed them, can accept and see to be true.

Second, such a law or principle of interpretation of the Sacred Scriptures, that when they are interpreted in accordance with it, every man and woman who is willing to see and obey the truth will find there is actually no conflict between the Word of the Lord and His works, and no real contradictions to be found in the Sacred Scriptures.

In the writings of Swedenborg the Lord has shown us that "all religion has relation to life, and that the life of religion is to do good;" and that, if we would enter into the heavenly life, or have heaven within us, we must strive faithfully and honestly to keep the commandments, not simply in external acts, but also in our motives, thoughts, and words, as well as in act. In the writings of Swedenborg the Lord has clearly revealed Himself and has come down to the comprehension of man-God in Christ and in His Word.

The Science of Correspondences enables us to see that the first eleven chapters of Genesis are purely allegorical, and in their spiritual and true sense treat of the regeneration of man, and his fall through the seduction of his lowest or sensual nature and appetites, as men are seduced to-day; and of a flood of evils and falses, similar to the flood which threatens to overwhelm the Christian world, at least in our land, at this day; and a New Church as an ark of safety. While the Science of Correspondences shows that there are no more contradictions in the Word of the Lord than in His works, there are apparent truths and real truths in both. It is an apparent truth that God is angry with the wicked every day; but the real truth is that God is never angry, but when man disobeys His laws and brings upon himself consequent suffering, it appears to him that God is angry. So it appears to us that night and darkness are caused by the going down of the sun, but the real truth is that the sun always shines and that night and darkness are caused by the earth's diurnal revolution on its axis. It will therefore be seen that if the Sacred Scriptures are the Word of God and in accordance with His works, they must contain both apparent and real truths.

No man who has ever diligently and faithfully, without prejudice, read the Sacred Scriptures in the light of the Science of Correspondences, as revealed by the Lord through Emanuel Swedenborg, has ever failed to be satisfied that the Sacred Scriptures are Divine and plenarily inspired, and that they differ as much from the writings of men as do the works of God from the works of men. At this day, when so many of our clergy and intelligent laymen are beginning to doubt the special inspiration of the Sacred Scriptures, a knowledge of the Science of Correspondences, in accordance with which they were written, is wanted above every thing else, that the Christian Church "may revive again and draw breath through heaven from the Lord."

The Lord speaks to man in parables, and "without a parable," we read, "spake He not unto them." The Lord intimates in many passages that the Sacred Scriptures, or His words, contain a spiritual sense, as in the following: "It is the spirit that quickeneth; the flesh profiteth nothing; the words that I speak unto you, they are spirit and they are life." "The letter killeth, but the spirit giveth life."

"The early Christian Fathers, Clement of Alexandria, and Origen, understood that the Sacred Scriptures have a spiritual sense; and Origen-when that shrewd enemy of Christianity, Celsus, ridiculed the stories of the rib, the serpent, etc., as childish fables-reproaches him for want of candor in purposely keeping out of sight, what was so evident upon the face of the narrative, that the whole is a *pure allegory.*" —*Noble's Plenary Inspiration.*

"The idea of a spiritual sense in every part of the Scripture was the generally received doctrine of the Primitive Church-believed and taught by Origen, Ignatius, Justin Martyr, Jerome,

Augustine, Pantaenus, Tatian, Theophilus, Pamphilius, Clement and Cyril of Alexandria, and nearly all the early Christian Fathers. And the same belief has been held by many eminent theologians ever since. Dr. Mosheim, speaking of the illustrious writers of the second century, says: 'They *all* attributed a double sense to the words of Scripture; the one *obvious* and *literal*, the other *hidden* and *mysterious*, which lay concealed, as it were, under the veil of the outward letter.' But the Fathers had no recognized rule for eliciting the spiritual sense. Each one's own spiritual perception was his only guide. A hundred different expositors, therefore, might give as many different expositions of the same text." —*Rev. B. F. Barrett.*

Every natural object is the form and embodiment of some spiritual idea or principle; and therefore it is the most perfect expression or type or picture of that idea.

"Inasmuch as the end of the creation is an angelic heaven out of the human race, and thus the human race itself, therefore all other things that are created are mediate ends, which being referable to man, look to these three things of man, his body, his rational part, and his spiritual part, for sake of conjunction with the Lord. For a man cannot be conjoined to the Lord unless he be spiritual; nor can he be spiritual unless he be rational; nor can he be rational unless his body is in a sound state. These things are like a house, of which the body is the foundation, and the rational is the house built upon it; the spiritual comprises those things which are in the house, and conjunction with the Lord is being at home in it."

Here are outlined clearly and distinctly three fields for much needed labor.

We see above, clearly taught by Swedenborg, that "a man cannot be spiritual unless he be rational, nor can he be rational unless his body be in a sound state." The reason is plain: for the natural corresponds to the spiritual; natural diseases and natural causes of disease correspond to spiritual diseases and spiritual causes of spiritual disease.

Swedenborg says that: "Diseases correspond to the lusts and passions of the mind; these, therefore, are the origins of diseases; for the origins of diseases in general are intemperance, luxuries of various kinds, pleasures merely corporal; also envyings, hatreds, revenges, lasciviousness, and the like; which destroy the interiors of man, and when these are destroyed the exteriors suffer and draw man into diseases, and thereby into death." — *Arcana Coelestia*, 5712.

For this reason, if a man is to be reformed and regenerated, his reformation must commence by his shunning natural falses and bad habits of life, which correspond to his spiritual evils.

Swedenborg's writings give us a wonderful insight into the causes and cure of both spiritual and natural diseases, as we shall hereafter see, and many suggestions which it would be well for us to heed. He says: —

> "The man who is willing to be enlightened by the Lord, must take especial heed lest he appropriate to himself any doctrinal which patronizes evil; for man in such case appropriates it to himself, when he confirms it with himself, for thereby he makes it a principle of his faith, and still more so if he lives according to it. When this is the case, then evil remains inscribed on his soul and his heart; and when this effect has place, he cannot afterwards in any wise be enlightened by the Word from the Lord; for his whole mind is in the faith and in the love of his principle, and whatsoever is contrary to it, this he either does not see, or rejects, or falsifies." (A. C. 10,640.)

Every one can see how true this is in regard to evil habits which destroy health, reason, and life, such as the prevailing use of tobacco and the drinking of intoxicating drinks. If a man drinks thoughtlessly, without knowing any better, he can be taught and shown that it is wrong and a sin to drink poisonous fluids which are entirely unnecessary, and which endanger health, reason, life, and the welfare and happiness of all associated with him, and actually destroy vast multitudes of those who drink them moderately. All children and young persons who are free from bad examples and false teachings can be taught and can readily see that it is wrong and a sin to use such drinks; but let a man strive to justify such habits by the Sacred Scriptures, and to make them accord with his religious principles, and we all know how difficult it is for him ever to see the truth upon this and kindred subjects.

MUCH-NEEDED INSTRUCTION.

Inquiry should be made into the natural causes of disease, into which spiritual causes flow and cause the suffering, wretchedness, and premature deaths which prevail, and men and women should be led by precept and example to see them as evils and to shun them as sins against God. Swedenborg says: —

> "Thus, by washing the feet, is meant to purify the natural principle of man; for unless this principle appertaining to man, when he lives in the world, is purified and cleansed, it cannot afterwards be purified to eternity; for such as the natural principle of man is when he dies such it remains; for it is not afterwards amended, inasmuch as it is that plane into which interior things, which are spiritual, flow in-it being their receptacle; wherefore when it is perverted, interior things, when they flow in, are perverted like it." (A. C. 10,243.)

There are two great hindrances to the reformation of the world at this day; the first is false teaching in regard to evils, by which unlawful indulgences are justified, and in moderation held to be good; for by this the individual is strongly confirmed in their favor and prevented from seeing the truth. The second is the love of the evil which the truth condemns, which closes the mind against the truth, and, as it were, binds and imprisons the individual (see A. C. 5096). It must be self-evident to every intelligent Christian that if it is wrong to deliberately appropriate falses and evils "temperately" or moderately to the building up of our spiritual organizations, it is equally wrong to appropriate temperately those natural substances which correspond to falses and evils in a vain attempt to build up healthy natural bodies. Total abstinence in both cases is the only law of life. The lover of intoxicating drinks can never be radically reformed or regenerated until he resolves, with the help of the Lord, to stop drinking intoxicating drinks and sets himself honestly about it; so the thief must stop stealing, the vain woman must stop her tight dressing and habits of idleness; and so of all other evils affecting physical and spiritual health and life.

But to-day the great difficulty is, that multitudes of the young and of all ages become "bond-servants" to evil habits, which impair health and reason and shorten life, through ignorance, hereditary inclination, and the bad example of others. And how are they to regain their freedom, and the innocent to be protected from contamination and from a like slavery? The truth can alone make them free; and even when received by the willing and obedient, line upon line and precept upon precept may be required. And they will often have to endure many a hard struggle; and those who are free should have sympathy and charity, and judge them not. Men, women, and children must be taught that they have no right to follow habits which will endanger health and reason, and which observation and carefully collected statistics show will shorten the average duration of life; for to thus act is to violate the command, "Thou shall not kill." The causes of ill health, deformity, and the prevailing insanity and premature deaths must be sought out and exposed, and a call to repentance must be made.

In the good providence of the Lord, we have men who, by education, diligent investigation, and careful observation, are most admirably adapted to give the needed instruction-physicians. Let physicians arm themselves with true doctrines, with the spiritual sense of the Word, with the Science of Correspondences and a knowledge of natural sciences, and they will be able to combat the prevailing evils as no other men can; and they should lead in all the great necessary reforms of this age that have regard to physical health, life, and morals. In almost every society of our Churches of any size will be found one or more medical men who have devoted their lives to the study of anatomy, physiology, the causes of disease, diseases and their cure, and the effects of poisons and the bad habits of dress, and other habits injurious to health; and they are able to speak with authority in regard to the prevailing evils of life, which are so destructive to our race. These men, thus providentially prepared, should be called into the field as lecturers. There is not a religious society which does not actually need the services of such teachers; and we can send no other missionaries to those outside of our church organizations who will, to the same extent, command their attention and respect. In order that the body with its environment may be a fit dwelling place for the Spirit, there are provided —

"*Uses for sustaining the body*, comprising its nourishment, clothing, habitation, recreation and enjoyment, protection and conservation of state. The uses created for the nourishment of the body comprise all things of the vegetable kingdom which are good for food and drink; fruits, berries, seeds, pulse, and herbs; all things of the animal kingdom which serve for meat, oxen, cows, calves, deer, sheep, kids, goats, lambs; not to mention milk; also fowls and fish of many kinds." (D. L. W. 331.)

"Good uses," says Swedenborg, "are from the Lord, and evil uses are from hell. Evil uses were not created by the Lord, but they originated together with hell." (D. L. W. 336.) Among the evil uses he enumerates all kinds of poisons-in a word, "all things that do hurt and kill men." (*Ibid.* 339.) Here, then, is a criterion by which we must judge of the suitability of any article for nourishing and supplying the wants of our natural bodies. It should be evident to every one that substances which have their origin from hell, which, when used as we use legitimate articles of food and drink, seriously endanger, hurt, and kill men, should never be used for such purpose.

Who are better qualified to judge as to what are evil uses than the physician, who has made them the study of his life? The men and women who are violating the laws of life cannot see that such violations injure them; for such violations palliate the sufferings which they cause, and make the transgressors feel better every time they indulge. The true physician, by precept and example, is qualified to lead all who are willing to be led to a higher life and to protect the innocent and the young.

That such teachers are most important at this day is manifest "from the signification of physicians as denoting preservation from evils-the evils which obstruct conjunction. In the Word, physicians, the art of physic and medicine, signify preservation from evils and falses.... That in the Word, physicians, the art of physic and medicine, signify preservation from evils and falses, is manifest from the passages where they are named.... Hence it is evident what *medicine* signifies, viz., that which preserves from falses and evils; for when the truth of faith leads to the good of love, it preserves, because it withdraws from evils." (A. C. 6502.)

Here, then, we have the men suitable for this use. Shall we call them into the fields which are ripe and ready for the harvest?

A clergyman who has a knowledge of the medical profession and of medicine, in speaking of the importance of such teachers, says: "Moreover, from their relation to the sick and suffering, from their habit of analyzing the mental and moral states of their patients, and from the deep, tender sympathy which sincere, God-fearing physicians have for suffering human beings, they are placed in a much closer relation to the people than any other vocation could give them. How many persons have been comforted, strengthened, instructed, and turned to uprightness of life through the kindly ministrations of their physicians!"

And church organizations are languishing for the want of such teachers, and can never thrive in true doctrine and good lives, as they should, without them.

Surely every one can but see of what immense benefit such lecturers would be, especially to the young in our churches. One physician might be employed by and serve several societies, giving to the different societies once or twice a week a lecture in each society, fully illustrated by drawings, plates, stereoscopic and microscopic views, which would attract young and old, and fill our churches to overflowing with those who now attend no church; and the latter, when they found a physician, with the consent of the church, thus clearly pointing out the great evils of life which cause so much suffering, wretchedness, sorrow, and so many premature deaths, and calling young and old, from a religious standpoint, to shun them as sins against God, could but feel that our churches are striving to elevate humanity, and are a great blessing, and that it would be desirable to belong to them, and especially to have their children brought up under the influence of the Church.

Nearly the same could be said in regard to the important services which a second class of teachers of which I am about to speak could render. By the lectures of the two new life would be infused into our churches, and they would stand upon a sure foundation by manifesting love to God and man in our external natural lives, by teaching and leading men to act from spiritual motives, and to be willing to see their evils, and to commence by shunning well-known evils as sins against God. What a glorious day would this open up to our churches and for the elevation of our race through them!

THE SECOND CLASS OF TEACHERS REQUIRED.

Physicians as teachers in our churches should have for a special work the teaching of truth as to the physical life of man in connection with his spiritual life-the laws of health, the causes of prevailing diseases, deformities, insanities, and premature deaths, together with the methods and the duty of shunning them as sins against God. But there are other evils and questions which require careful consideration in our churches, such as the true relation, according to the laws of justice, mercy, and right, which should exist between men as neighbors, citizens, and Christians; and the clear light of this New Day should be brought down to guide men into a life of peace and harmony and good-will in this wilderness state of the world. Important questions are pressing for a solution, and for a careful consideration, by the religious teachers of our churches, such as the ecclesiastical and civil government best adapted for men of different countries and races, especially for our own country and churches; the relation of capital and labor; the right of single individuals to hold an unlimited amount of real estate, and transmit it to their children; the rights of corporations and of women; and our duties to others in all the relations of life. Fortunately, we have in our churches legal men or lawyers, who, while familiar with the doctrines of the Church, have devoted their lives to the consideration of such questions. It would not be difficult to point out several members of the legal fraternity belonging to our church organizations who would be able to perform a great use to the Church as lecturers and acting as missionaries among those who do not attend church as opportunity may offer. They would enter into a field of usefulness almost altogether beyond the reach and influence of our present ministers. Their advice, their counsel, their discourse, in their legal practice, are channels for the introduction of Christian thought and doctrine otherwise closed. There is one passage in the Writings which indicates this use: —

> ”*And strengthen the things which remain that are ready to die* —that hereby is signified; that the things which pertain to the moral life should be vivified, appears from the signification of strengthening, as denoting to vivify the moral life by truths; *for truths from the Word vivify that life*, which, when it is vivified, is also strengthened, for it then acts as one with the spiritual life.” (A. E. 188.)

To meet and vivify the moral life of man with truths from the Word is a use eminently adapted to the position and mind of the legal profession. We need the services of such ministers, especially at this day, when we inherit from the fallen churches of the past an inclination to the love of spiritual and temporal dominion or rule, and the love of money and of vain show without regard to use. The evils that result from the gratification of such perverted affections must be fearlessly exposed, and a call to repentance made, before the injustice, oppression, and wrong which exist all over the world can be materially lessened. Lawyers, by making a special study of the Word in connection with their professional-studies, could not fail to impart much valuable instruction both to the Church and the world.

Christian physicians and lawyers would take hold of men in their present low state, showing them what acts are evil and wrong, and why they are so; and would call on them to repent and stop doing the evil acts which the truth condemns, fully realizing that a man must cease doing evil before he can cease thinking and willing evil; or, in other words, that reformation must commence on the natural plane, and from the highest motives of which the individual at present is susceptible.

It is the duty of our clergy to teach spiritual truths and the spiritual sense of the Word, and to lead men and women to live good lives, in obedience to the Divine commandments, from spiritual and celestial motives. But it is difficult for them to fill the entire field where religious instruction is needed, for we are living in the midst of the most direful evils of life, which must be put away before the New Jerusalem can descend and have an abiding place with men. Evils so terrible as to destroy vast multitudes of men and women of all ages, and even innocent children, all around us, too frequently go unheeded by our clergy and the periodicals under their charge. I know that in this respect there are some noble exceptions among our clergy and editors; but however willing and anxious they may be, it is impossible for one man to possess the knowledge and to impart all the necessary instruction as perfectly as three men thoroughly educated and trained for the different fields for labor could do it.

To recapitulate: The physicians are required to teach and to lead men to obey, from a principle of obedience, the spiritual and natural laws of health and life; the lawyers are required to teach and lead men by spiritual truths to act from a principle of justice, truth, and neighborly love in all their relations with others; our ministers are required to teach and lead men to act from love to the Lord and thence the neighbor, and to do right because it is right, and to administer the ordinances of the Church.

While some church organizations are laboring earnestly for the reform of men and women addicted to evils, and are striving to guard the innocent and young; and while in many of the churches in England they are organizing their temperance societies and "Bands of Hope," many of our organizations are as silent as the grave in regard to these evils. Can our churches prosper without teachers who are able to point out the evils of life which are so destructive to our race, and who are sufficiently free themselves to be able earnestly and consistently to call men to repentance, and to lead them to live orderly lives?

Various denominations of Christians, in sending forth missionaries to distant lands, have, of late years, been sending, among others, some well-educated physicians as missionaries, and have found them very efficient in reaching and influencing the people among whom they labor. May not all take a hint when some of the religious organizations around us are beginning to see the advantages of sending out medical missionaries? If we would reach the Gentiles, or non-church goers, in our midst, should we not follow their example? A vast number of children and young people are growing up in our country, who are more ignorant of the spiritual and natural laws of health and life than many in Gentile lands; many of them rarely read or hear the Sacred Scriptures read, and do not even know the Ten Commandments.

CHAPTER VIII

METHODS FOR RESTRAINING AND CURING SPIRITUAL AND NATURAL DISEASES.

As there is a correspondence between the natural and spiritual causes of disease, so there must be a correspondence between the methods of restraining and curing natural and spiritual diseases.

First: Spiritual diseases or evils are restrained by punishments which, by force, as it were, counteract the inclination to do evil; corresponding to this method we have the Antipathic method of restraining natural diseases, which is one of the prevailing methods; for instance, for constipation cathartics are given, for a diarrhoea astringents, and opiates are given to forcibly relieve or restrain the symptoms of disease. Every one can but see that such remedies for the cure of natural diseases, like punishments for the cure of spiritual diseases or evils, are but palliative; for the reaction, if reaction ensue, is not in the right direction. It is true that a cure sometimes results in spite of the treatment, especially in transient cases, the vital forces restoring health during the temporary restraint of the diseased action; but in many cases the constipation is only aggravated by cathartics, and diarrhoeas are not benefited by astringents; and the evil man often becomes more vicious after punishment.

Second: Spiritual evils are often restrained by exciting one passion to restrain evil acts in another direction; for instance, acquisitiveness and vanity are often excited to restrain evil men from evil acts, which might result from hatred and a desire for revenge, thus calling off the attention from the prevailing evil inclination. Corresponding to this method of restraining spiritual diseases we have the Allopathic method of restraining diseased action in one organ by exciting diseased action in another organ or part, as is done when a cathartic is given for disease of the head or lungs, or when a blister is applied to the skin in case of internal diseased action; thus, as it were, calling off the attention of the vital forces from the diseased structures, and thus palliative relief is often obtained in natural as in spiritual diseases.

Third: Either from afflictions, suffering, disappointments, or from voluntarily hearkening to the truth, a man begins to feel a desire to change his life, and looking to the Lord he repents and resolves to obey the Divine Commandments by shunning evils as sins against God. But when he commences to do this, evil spirits flow into his mind and tempt him to again do evil acts; if the temptations are too strong he falls, but he may fall to rise again; he will either do this by renewing his resolution to overcome the evil inclination, or he will fall to rise no more, and keep on in his old course of life, perhaps worse than before. Thoughts come before actions; if a man, when tempted to do evil, resists the thoughts of doing the evil acts, every one can see that he is striking a blow at the perverted affection through which he has been tempted to do evil; consequently the step toward a cure is far more radical and permanent than it would have been if he had done the evil act.

Children and the young should be taught that to violate the Divine Commandments is a sin against God, and that they should resist their hereditary or acquired inclination to speak wrong words or do evil acts the moment such inclinations are manifested in their thoughts, which is far better than to allow them to move them to do evil acts. The cure of spiritual diseases by the resisting of temptation is a genuine method of cure. Corresponding with this for the treatment of natural diseases, we have their treatment by the use of Homoeopathic remedies. Only spirits of a similar inclination can tempt a man to do an evil act and thus manifest his unsubdued inclination to him, which enables him to see and overcome the inclination by resisting it. So, on the natural plane, it is only a poisonous substance or remedy, which is capable of causing a similar disease to the one existing, which can manifest the disease to the vital forces and thus enable them to react against the disease. But if the dose of the remedy given is too large it will aggravate the disease, as a cathartic dose of a cathartic remedy will aggravate a diarrhoea; but the vital forces may react and overcome the disease, or they may not, and the disease continue even worse than before. It is the reaction of the vital forces that overcomes the diseased action and effects the cure, and not the remedy, any more than it is the evil spirit that tempts man that overcomes his spiritual evils during regeneration. As it is not necessary that the temptation should be so strong as to make a man take the first step toward performing an evil act, to enable him to resist it if he will the moment the inclination is seen in his thoughts, so it is not necessary that a dose of a Homoeopathic remedy should be so strong as to aggravate the natural diseased action in the slightest degree before it can be seen by the vital forces, and a reaction follow. The size of the dose must be determined by experience; but we know that its effects need only to equal the effects of temptations which proceed no further than the thought of doing evil before reaction may follow, therefore we can form no conception of the minuteness of the dose which may be sufficient for a cure to follow.

But if a man would be restored to spiritual health by getting rid of his hereditary and acquired inclinations to do evil, he must acknowledge the Lord, diligently search His Word, and be willing to see and obey His commandments, which are the laws of spiritual health and life, and must be obeyed conscientiously, in intention, thought, word, and deed, if health is to be restored; otherwise, punishment, hope of reward, and temptations can only afford palliative relief at best. So in regard to natural diseases. If a man would be restored to physical health by getting rid of his hereditary and acquired inclinations to diseases, he must recognize that the laws of nature are the laws established for his good by the Lord, and he must diligently study the laws pertaining to health and life, and be willing to see and obey those laws as to sunlight, air, exercise, clothing, and in eating and drinking, etc., if he would be restored to health; otherwise, antipathic, allopathic, and even homoeopathic remedies will prove only palliative at best. If we expect to be well, spiritually or naturally, we must strive to know and obey the laws of health and life.

Temptations by evil spirits permitted and controlled by the Lord for the sake of removing many spiritual evils, and a corresponding action of homoeopathic remedies administered by a skillful hand, for the sake of removing natural diseases, are curative methods which belong to the New Jerusalem Dispensation, now descending from God out of heaven, making all things new-the Church of the future.

CHAPTER IX.

PERSONAL EXPERIENCE CONTINUED-AND EFFORTS.

Soon after I commenced reading the writings of Emanuel Swedenborg, while residing in Detroit, I was invited to attend a social gathering at the residence of one of the members of the congregation of believers in his writings in that city. During the evening, to my astonishment, fermented wine was passed around to the guests, of which quite a number partook. As already stated in the preceding pages, while a young man, through the efficient teachings of Baptist and Congregational clergymen and prominent members of the churches, and the results of drinking which I witnessed, I was providentially enabled to see that to use drinks which endangered health, reason, and life was wrong, and consequently a sin; and with many others I signed a pledge never to drink intoxicating drinks during health. The reader can imagine how I was shocked to see intoxicating wine presented and partaken of among gentlemen and ladies who professed to be receivers and believers in a new revelation of Divine truth from God to man. I immediately saw the clergyman of the society, and asked him if Swedenborg teaches that it is right and proper to drink an intoxicating wine. He replied that he did.

He and members of his society were holding Sunday afternoon meetings for the purpose of reading the writings and discussing such questions as might arise, which meetings I attended. I said to the reverend gentleman that I would like to have this wine question discussed at our next meeting, to which he assented. At that meeting, I brought up the medical and scientific aspects of the question, and endeavored to show that fermented wine was a dangerous poison, it having destroyed vast multitudes of the human race, and that it performed no use when taken into the stomach of healthy men and women; and, consequently, that it is wrong to drink a wine which does so much harm. The clergyman tried to justify its use by quoting certain comparisons which Swedenborg had made between the apparent combat which takes place during fermentation and the combat which ensues during the regeneration of man, and the clearness of resulting wine after fermentation and that of truth in the mind after regeneration, and also of the purity of alcohol after it has been through certain processes, which he named, compared with pure truth.

But we know that pure alcohol cannot be used as a beverage, and therefore it is certain that these comparisons were simply as to the clearness of fermented wine after fermentation, and the purity of alcohol after being purified; and that they have nothing to do with the inherent quality of these fluids, or their ability to affect man when he drinks them. We had an earnest discussion of the question from our different standpoints, but neither of us was satisfied with the result; and, consequently, we adjourned the discussion of the subject until the next Sabbath afternoon. In the meantime, the clergyman prepared a discourse, which he delivered on Sunday morning, in which he endeavored to show that fermentation was caused by an influx of angels from the highest heaven into the juice of the grape, stirring it up and cleansing it from "inherent impurities." Providentially, during the week, I had obtained a copy of Swedenborg's work on the "Angelic Wisdom Concerning the Divine Love and Wisdom," in which he teaches that all poisonous substances which do harm and kill man derive their life from or through hell. When we came together in the afternoon to discuss the question, we were about as far apart as it was possible to be, as the reader can readily see. He took the ground that fermentation was caused by influx from the highest heaven, and I took the ground that it was caused by influx from the lowest hell, and we had an earnest discussion; but he certainly did not satisfy me nor many of his audience, if any, that his position was true. How could he? for there is no doubt but that fermented wine has harmed and killed more of the human race in ages past than any other poison. As a result of that discussion, within my knowledge, fermented wine was never again used at the sociables of that society during my residence in Detroit.

Within perhaps a year after that discussion, I was baptized and united with the Detroit Society of the New Church. When I came to understand, from the writings of Swedenborg, the true signification of water and the ordinance of baptism-that water signified natural truth and that baptism introduced one into the Church, and signified that man is to be regenerated or purified by living a life according to the truth, and that the head represented the man —I did not regard immersion as so important as I had previously, consequently I was baptized by the application of water to the head. There is, I think, no serious objection to any one being baptized by immersion who prefers it. Children should, I think, be baptized into the Church, and be brought up to feel that they belong to the Church, and are expected to live the life of the Church. More and more have I seen the importance of bringing children up under the influence of the Church, where they should be instructed and entertained and thus kept away from bad company.

WHY A SEPARATE NEW-CHURCH ORGANIZATION.

Swedenborg made no attempt to organize the believers in the revelations made by the Lord through his instrumentality into a separate church organization, and nowhere in his writings does he express the opinion that such a separate organization would ever be needed or desirable. And he apparently expected that the prevailing false doctrines of the churches would, in the increasing light of the New Jerusalem, be seen to be false by the clergy of existing church organizations; and that through them the laity would be enabled to see that they are false, and thus they would be put away, as is manifest in passages which I have quoted elsewhere; also see T. C. R. 784.

When individual men or churches put away false doctrines, they are prepared, if in the good of life, to see and receive the truth; consequently Swedenborg says that although the First Christian Church has come to its end through false doctrines and evils of life, yet it is to revive again through the instrumentality of the newly revealed science of correspondences; consequently it is not to utterly perish, for there is a remnant within its borders.

Then the reader will inquire, "Why was an external New-Church organization ever formed?" We have not to look far to find the reason. First, there was a vast multitude of intelligent men and women who did not belong to any church organization, and when some of them came to see and believe the new doctrines, they naturally desired to be baptized and to join a church organization; but seeing clearly in the light of the new revelations that, according to the Sacred Scriptures, God is one in essence and in person, and that that one God was manifested to man in the person of the Lord Jesus Christ, and that He made that human form Divine and is henceforth to be worshiped as one God in His Divine Humanity, and that a life according to His sayings and the commandments is essential to salvation, they could not join the prevailing churches, for they could not assent to their creeds.

Second. When, as soon occurred, both clergymen and laymen, belonging to various church organizations, began to read the writings, and to see that the Lord is in very deed now coming in the clouds of heaven, and desired to let the new light shine among their brethren, they found that they were often not free to do so without giving offense; and in not a few instances clergymen found that they were silenced as preachers, and sometimes both clergymen and laymen were expelled, for believing the Heavenly Doctrines instead of the creeds; consequently the receivers of the doctrines of the New Dispensation had no choice but to form a new church organization. But at this day there is a vast change, and I trust that from but a very few if any church organizations would a lay member be expelled for believing in the Supreme Divinity of the Lord Jesus Christ, and that the Sacred Scriptures are Divine and plenarily inspired, and that a life according to the Lord's sayings and His Commandments is essential to salvation. Consequently there are thousands of earnest receivers of the Heavenly Doctrines of the New Jerusalem scattered throughout the various churches, gradually leavening, as I trust, the whole lump; and there are clergymen not a few who are gradually beholding, with more or less fullness, the light of this New Day; and as they receive it, large numbers of them are not slow to let the light shine among their fellow-men, as they are prepared to receive it.

The Lord has given to men freedom and reason, and they are responsible for their acts. To whom do a clergyman and members of a church organization owe fealty, to the Lord and His Word and the members of the congregations where they worship, or to a creed and church or a church organization formulated and organized during darker ages of the world and Church? Should men or should they not, when they behold the glorious light of the Lord's Second Coming in the clouds of heaven, stand in their place and proclaim the glad tidings to all who are willing to hear?

Swedenborg, in giving the spiritual sense of the second chapter of the Apocalypse, in No. 69 of the *Apocalypse Revealed*, says: —

"This and the following chapter treat of the seven churches, by which are described all those in the Christian Church who have any religion, and out of whom the New Church, which is the New Jerusalem, can be formed; and this is formed by those who APPROACH THE LORD ONLY, AND AT THE SAME TIME PERFORM REPENTANCE FROM EVIL WORKS. The rest, who do not approach the Lord alone, from the confirmed negation of the divinity of His humanity, and who do not perform repentance from evil works, are indeed in the Church, but have nothing of the Church in them."

If all clergymen and members of our churches, the moment they begin to see that portions of their creeds are false and injurious in their tendency, instead of trying, by proclaiming the truth among their brethren, to have the false doctrines removed and true doctrines substituted, were to immediately forsake the church organization in which, in the good providence of the Lord, they stand, what hope would there be for the perpetuation of existing churches as Christian organizations at all? The great danger at this day is that false doctrines will be seen faster than true doctrines will be seen to take their place, and thus our churches and members will be left desolate and return to a Gentile state. For instance, if our clergy and intelligent laymen begin to see, as many of them seem to be doing already, that the doctrine of a tri-personal God, instead of a trinity in unity, and the doctrine of the vicarious atonement are contrary to the teachings of the Sacred Scriptures, and unreasonable and inconsistent, and do not at the same time see clearly the scriptural doctrine that God is one in essence and in person, and that in the person of our Lord Jesus Christ that one God was manifested for the purpose of reconciling the world unto Himself, such individuals are almost sure sooner or later to deny the Divinity of the Lord Jesus Christ, and that the Sacred Scriptures are divine and special revelations from God to man, and consequently plenarily inspired.

The doctrines which are false in the prevailing church organizations must go-they are going-from the minds of their members if not from their creeds. Then are these organizations to become Gentile and stand like the remnants of the Ancient Church, which we behold in southern and eastern Asia? I think not; for we are told, as has been already stated in the revelations made by the Lord through Emanuel Swedenborg, that the science of correspondences was revealed that the Christian Church "may revive and again draw breath from the Lord through heaven." Gentiles received the Lord at His first coming with joy; and so I believe the Gentiles in and out of our church organizations will receive Him now as He comes in the clouds of heaven. In the light manifested in the Sacred Scriptures by the aid of the science of correspondences, every willing and obedient man and woman is able to see that God is one, and that the Lord Jesus Christ, or God in His Divine Humanity, is that one God and the only Being whom men should and whom angels do worship. Then of what unspeakable importance it is that the attention of all clergymen and laymen be speedily called to the writings for the Church of the New Jerusalem which is now descending from God out of heaven!

After practicing medicine for ten or twelve years, and on accepting the chair of "Theory and Practice of Medicine" tendered by the Western Homoeopathic College at Cleveland, Ohio, I commenced, as it were, the study of the practical department of my profession anew, in order to prepare myself for filling the chair profitably to the students and creditably to myself. While preparing forgiving lectures, and especially in after years while away from my active medical practice at Detroit, giving a course of lectures at Cleveland every winter, I began to study and investigate in my leisure hours the causes of diseases. Step by step I pursued my investigations, until I became satisfied that most of the deformities, diseases, and insanity which exist have been caused by the violation of the physical and spiritual laws of our being which could have been avoided in the past, and which can and must be in the future, if our race is to be restored to a state of healthy, symmetrical, and noble manhood. Consequently I came to the conclusion that it is far more important that men, women, and children should be taught the laws of health and to understand the causes of the prevailing deformities and diseases, and how to shun them, than it was for them and their children to get sick, deformed, and suffer, and often to pay their hard-earned money to doctors for the uncertain chance of being cured-in fact, that "an ounce of prevention is worth more than a pound of cure."

As a result of my investigations I wrote a series of articles for the *Detroit Tribune* on the bad habits which cause diseases, insanity, and deformity; and, as opportunity offered, I gave lectures upon such subjects; and finally I wrote a work entitled the "Avoidable Causes of Disease," of 348 pages, of which I printed several editions, the first of which was in 1859, and furnished to different publishers, and advertised to a limited extent; after that it was published for several years by Messrs. Mason Brothers, of New York; after which it came into my hands again. I also wrote a pamphlet of 48 pages on "Marriage and its Violations," which, for a time, was bound separately, but afterward was bound with the "Avoidable Causes of Disease." In all, eleven editions of the work have been printed; the last edition was printed by Messrs Boericke & Tafel, of Philadelphia, who will probably publish any future editions which may be demanded.

I soon found, what my publishers found after me, and other writers and their publishers have found, that it does not pay to advertise books which contain the greatest amount of practical and useful information which is calculated to benefit readers, especially if they call in question the bad habits and evils of life in which so many people indulge; consequently, feeling that a work treating of diseases and their cure, in which I could advertise my first work and call special attention to it, would sell more readily, I wrote a book of 404 pages, entitled "Family Homoeopathy," in which I took great pains to carefully describe in few words the various diseases, and gave as definite and positive instruction as was practicable to guide laymen, so that harmless homoeopathic remedies might take the place of drastic drugs and injurious domestic remedies, which are so frequently used when it is thought not necessary to call a physician, or before his arrival when called. At the end of this volume I inserted a carefully prepared table of the contents of the "Avoidable Causes of Disease," occupying three pages, and referred not unfrequently to that work when treating of various diseases.

With but very slight efforts, and no advertising on my part, "Family Homoeopathy" sold very well-principally through the different homoeopathic pharmacies in our country; and this increased the sale of "The Avoidable Causes of Disease" very materially, as I expected it would. Seventeen editions of "Family Homoeopathy" have been printed and sold, the last edition by Dr. E. R. Ellis, of Detroit, Michigan, who will continue to print and supply applicants as wanted.

SPIRITUAL CAUSES OF DISEASES.

As I continued my investigation into the causes of disease, and especially as I read the writings of Emanuel Swedenborg, I began to see more and more clearly that diseases, to a large extent at least, have a spiritual origin, and that the great obstacles to the removal of their causes lie in the false doctrines of Christian churches. When selfish men who were leaders in the churches desired to exercise their love of rule in spiritual and natural things and to exercise despotic power, when they desired to reduce other men to slavery and to hold them as slaves, or when they desired to gratify other perverted passions and sensual appetites, they all went to the Bible and strove to justify their conduct from its pages, with the expectation of reaching heaven at last; for this purpose it required the invention of special doctrines, and these they taught to their children, and thus the Word of God was made of no effect by the traditions and doctrines of men.

Unfortunately for the Protestant Church, early in its history, instead of "If ye would enter into life, keep the commandments," there was substituted the doctrine of justification by faith alone; which led men, especially the young, to hope that by getting religion and having faith, they could at any time escape the legitimate penalties which are attached by the Lord to evil doing. No young man, religiously brought up, expects to go to hell; but he intends to repent and be converted before he dies; he often thinks he will "sow his wild oats" first, instead of earnestly and faithfully striving to keep the Divine commandments from his youth up. Evil thinking and doing develop an infernal life within him, which often gradually gains strength until he is ruled by his perverted appetites and passions; and day by day his ability to regain his freedom grows less.

When the priesthood of the Roman Catholic Church began to teach men that the punishment which rightly inheres to the doing of evil can be escaped by confessing to the priest, doing penance, and receiving absolution, and that every Catholic priest has from the Lord the power to forgive sins and to grant indulgences, then the hope of escaping the penalties of sin by something short of keeping the Divine Law in everyday life was held out to the young of the Catholic laity, similar to that which the doctrine of faith alone offered to the young of the Protestant world; and the results have been similar. We know, however, that among religious teachers there are many to-day in all of the various sects of Christians who have put away, or are gradually putting away, or materially modifying, the perverted doctrines of the past. As an illustration of the changes which are taking place, I clip the following from an English paper, recently received: —

"The Rev. T. Vincent Tymms, the new Principal of Rawdon College, preaching to his late congregation at Clapham, said: —

> "From the first day I stood in this pulpit until now, I have desired to tear away from every heart that obscuring veil of pagan thought which first attributes a wrathful justice to the Father and a tender mercy to CHRIST, and then represents the Son as dying to soothe the anger and satisfy the relentless demands of the Father. Such unholy and revolting ideas are the leaven of heathenism, not the unleavened bread of Christian truth.'
>
> "This is from the first of 'Three Farewell Sermons,' published by Messrs. James Clarke & Co., Fleet Street, E. C."

More and more, as time progressed, I began to realize that there was very little chance for any radical improvement of our race until the false doctrines which have come down to us from the dark ages were put away; and knowing that in the writings of Emanuel Swedenborg we have a new revelation from the Lord, even the truths of his Second Coming in the clouds of heaven, which are destined to make all things new by leading men back to a life of obedience to the Divine commandments; and, furthermore, believing the most important missionary field to-day in the world to be among the clergy of our country, I wrote an "Address to the Clergy" of 24 pages. This Address I sent to over 50,000 clergymen. A few years before I wrote that Address, the late Mr. L. C. Iungerich, of Philadelphia, through the book publishing firm of J. B. Lippincott & Co., of that city, had offered to clergymen who would order and send the stamps to pay the postage, Swedenborg's "True Christian Religion," and afterward he added the "Apocalypse Revealed;" and the New Church Tract Society added to the above works "Heaven and Hell,"—all to be sent free to clergymen on receipt of postage. Several thousand copies of the above works had been sent when I wrote and sent out my Address. Upon the second page of the cover of my tract was a notice of the above-named gift books; and my aim was to hastily call the attention of clergymen to them, and to give them some idea of the claims of Swedenborg's writings to their attention, and to encourage them to send for and to read the books thus providentially within their reach. As a result of receiving the Address, thousands of clergymen sent for and obtained one or more of the above books.

When I commenced sending the above-named Address to the clergy, I resolved to devote one-tenth of my income to the work of spreading a knowledge of the doctrines of the New Jerusalem and of an orderly life among my fellow-men. I can truly say, and will say for the encouragement of others, that as I have given I have received; for never had I prospered financially as I have since that resolution was made and lived up to. After having secured a competency for myself and family I did not stop at one-tenth of my income.

The result of sending the Address was so satisfactory that I wrote and compiled a work of 260 pages, entitled, "Skepticism and Divine Revelation," with the intention of sending it to the clergy. My aim was to present a hasty view of the application of the science of correspondences in the interpretation of the first chapters of Genesis, and some other parts of the Word, and to meet the arguments of skeptics, and thus to show that the Sacred Scriptures are Divine revelations from God to man, and plenarily inspired, consequently differing as much from the words of man as God's works do from the works of man. In that work the attention of the reader is called to the creation of the world, the creation of man and woman, Eve, the Garden of Eden, its trees and river, the fall of man, the serpent, Cain and Abel, the flood, Noah, Shem, Ham, and Japheth, the flood of waters, the Ark, the Tower of Babel, Sun worship and idolatry, spiritualism, the little reliance to be placed upon communications from spirits, and why. Next, the doctrines of the New Jerusalem-God, the Incarnation, the Divine Trinity, sacrificial worship, the Cross, a true and heavenly life, the end of the world and Second Coming of the Lord, the resurrection, state of infants in the other life, the state and condition of the Heathen and Gentiles in another life, the New Jerusalem-the Church of the Future-the Crown of all Churches, the Divine promise to those who receive the New Jerusalem at the Lord's Second Coming as revealed through Emanuel Swedenborg.

Such were the subjects discussed in the light of the revelations made by the Lord's chosen servant. My aim was to produce the best work I could. Consequently, when I found in the writings of others passages, or even whole sections, in which the ideas that I desired to present were as well or better conveyed than I thought I could present them, I selected them, giving the writers credit for the same, and the sixteenth and twenty-third chapters were written at my request by the Rev. William B. Hayden, who assisted me materially in seeing the work through the press. About one-half of the matter in the volume was selected from other writers.

I commenced to send this work in editions of 10,000 to the clergy of our country, and when I had sent about 50,000, I had the "Address to the Clergy" printed and bound with it, and both were sent to the Catholic clergy, to whom the Address had not previously been sent. From that time both works have been printed and bound in one volume. About 65,000 of the above works, containing a notice of the gift books, named in preceding pages, on the second page of the cover, have been sent to the clergy of America, about 10,000 have been sent to physicians, and as many more have been circulated among laymen. The sending of this book to the clergy immensely increased the orders for the gift books.

The above works have been translated into the German language, and about 48,000 copies sent to German-speaking clergymen in Germany and other parts of Europe, and in our own country. They have been translated into the Swedish language, and about 6000 copies have been sent to the clergy of Sweden and Norway and circulated among the laity; and they have been translated into Italian, and 10,000 sent to and circulated in Italy. And more recently they have been translated into French, and 20,000 printed which are now being sent to the clergy of France and the French-speaking clergy of other European countries, and of our own country.

Then, I have aided materially in sending other works to the clergy of our country, either explaining or containing the doctrines of the New Jerusalem, upon the second page of the covers of which will be found a notice of the gift books offered to clergymen. I aided with money the Swedenborg Publishing Association in sending Rev. Mr. Ravlin's "Progressive Thoughts on Great Subjects" to all the clergy of our country whose names could be had; and, later, I have aided the American Swedenborg Printing and Publishing Society in sending, first, "The New Jerusalem and Its Heavenly Doctrines;" second, "The Doctrine of the Lord;" third, "The Doctrine of Life"—all three Swedenborg's own works-to all the clergy in our country whose names could be readily obtained; in all 82,500. So that almost every clergyman in our country has had an opportunity to acquire some knowledge of the doctrines and revelations made by the Lord through Emanuel Swedenborg for the benefit of men in this new age-doctrines very different from those formulated in the creeds of bygone centuries-and thousands of our clergy are beginning to realize, that we must return to the rational and plain doctrines taught in the Sacred Scriptures, and summed up by the Lord when on earth in the Two Great Commandments, Thou shalt love the Lord with all thy might and strength, and thy neighbor as thyself, and that we must commence the new life by repentance, or by being willing to see our evils and to shun them as sins against God.

As a result of the efforts made by others and myself to make known to the clergy the offer of the gift books, 32,831 clergymen have sent for and obtained "The True Christian Religion," 30,887 have obtained "Heaven and Hell," and 25,522 have obtained "The Apocalypse Revealed," according to the report of the Trustees of the Iungerich fund (May, 1891).

COMMUNION WINE.

For several years after I joined the Church I paid little attention to the subject of communion wine. But at last an article appeared in a New-Church paper, in which the writer claimed that fermented wine was a good and useful article to be used as a beverage, and he tried to justify its use by the teachings of the Church. Such views were so contrary to what I regarded as true, that I immediately commenced a more careful and critical examination of the writings of Swedenborg, to ascertain what is taught therein as to wine. I soon found that he distinctly recognized two kinds of wine, as does the Bible: one kind unfermented, a good and nourishing fluid to which he always gives a good signification when its use is not abused; and the other kind, known by its effects on man when he drinks it to be fermented, to which he has never given a good signification when it is clear from the context that reference is had to fermented wine. And I will here say that my opponents in the Church have done precisely what the advocates of slavery, intoxicating drinks, and skeptics have done in their appeals to the Bible to sustain their views. They find here and there a comparison and passage which, by placing their own construction upon them, they think will justify their views, while they totally ignore a large number of passages which most clearly and positively teach a totally different doctrine; and they ignore scientific facts, the well known effects of drinking fermented wine, and the testimony of ancient writers whenever such testimony does not accord with their own views. Thus they uphold the use of the drunkard's cup as a beverage and even as a sacramental wine; and within my knowledge more than one poor man in our Church who was struggling to reform his life has been led back by partaking of it to drunkenness.

A distinguished clergyman said in a letter to the writer: —

> "I can never forget the experience already related to you when Mr. — —, my wife's brother-in-law, a gentleman of classical education, had become a sober man through my efforts and received the heavenly doctrines… Then came the Lord's Supper and we had fermented California wine. I handed him the cup, he drank, and after church he fled to some place where wine could be had, came home late in the evening drunk, and continued drinking for three months, until he died one evening after being brought home beastly drunk. Unfermented wine is no seducer, and had Mr. — — been given such in the Sacrament, he might be living, a sober man, to-day. Your books on the 'Wine Question' deserve, therefore, all that you have done and expended under the Lord's guidance for their publication and circulation, and God only knows how much good they will yet have to do."

Another clergyman wrote: —

> "I was called to officiate at the funeral of a child. The parents-who were non-professors of religion-became much interested in the New Church. I furnished them suitable reading matter and visited them occasionally. Within a year they united with our Society. The man had formerly been a drinking man, but had ceased entirely. They were regular attendants on our church services. He was a mechanic. His well-behaved life restored public confidence in him, and he soon found constant employment at his trade. After about two years he felt a desire to take the Lord's Supper. I did not dissuade him; for, as he had abstained so long and faithfully, I felt sure he would continue. He presented himself with the communicants. Upon receiving the cup he took a sip and moved to return the cup to me; but suddenly, the old appetite being touched by the alcoholic spark, he returned the cup to his lips-it was about two-thirds full-and nearly drained it, as though urged on by demons. Poor man! Realizing what he had done, and evidently feeling disgraced, he at once arose and left the temple. From that time he returned to drink, and I have been unable to regain sufficient influence over him to effect his return to our services.

"Another man in my Society formerly drank to excess. I dare not encourage him to come to the communion. A majority of our members favor intoxicating wine for the Lord's Supper. How they can do so after witnessing its dreadful effects, I cannot understand. But the light is spreading, and may the Lord hasten the full day."

O Lord! how long? how long shall such evils continue in our churches?

Of course I replied to the article in the New-Church paper alluded to above, and others replied to me, and I to them in return; but it was not long before notice was given that the discussion would cease, and that with three unanswered articles against me in one number of the paper, and that in a paper edited by a clergyman, and published by the General Body of the Church. Well, looking for the welfare of the Church and its members which I loved, I could not stand still and see such false and dangerous views boldly and dogmatically proclaimed in the most extensively circulated periodical of the Church without doing my best to counteract them. Consequently I wrote a reply in a tract form, and sent it to every New-Churchman whose name I could obtain. This was but the beginning. An article appeared in another periodical of the Church to which I was allowed to reply; but the discussion was soon closed, and I was given no chance to reply to the last communication, and a reserved communication which was published afterward. Finding that there was no chance to present the temperance side of the wine question fairly before the readers of these two periodicals, I was led to write several pamphlets in reply to such articles as appeared in favor of the use of fermented wine, in which I endeavored to present fully and fairly, generally in the language of its advocates, their views of the question, and I endeavored to answer them in the light afforded by the Sacred Scriptures, the writings of the Church, ancient history, science, and well-known facts as to the manufacture and preservation of unfermented and fermented wines in all ages.

Several pamphlets were published in reply to the advocates for the use of fermented wine in our New-Church periodicals in the course of five or six years, of which about 10,000 of each were printed and sent to all Newchurchmen whose names I was able to obtain in this country, England, and elsewhere, hoping to reach as far as possible the readers of the writings of my opponents and others. The following are the names of the pamphlets written, printed, and sent, viz: "Pure Wine, Fermented Wine, and Other Alcoholic Drinks," published in 1880; "The Wine Question in the Light of the New Dispensation," in 1882; "Reply to the Academy's Review," in 1883; "Intoxicants, Prohibition, and our New-Church Periodicals," 1885, to which was added "Deterioration of the Puritan Stock," 1884; making in all, with index, 736 pages.

Finally, I had printed an edition of all of the above pamphlets from the plates, and bound in cloth, of which I sent a copy to all New-Church ministers in the world whose names I could get, and to some others.

My controversy with the clergy on the wine question led me to fear that there were other evils gradually creeping into the Church organization which should be exposed, and against which both laymen and clergymen should be warned; therefore, I wrote a tract entitled, "The New Church: its Ministry, Laity, and Ordinances, with an Appendix on Intoxicants and Our New-Church Periodicals," published and sent out in 1886, the latter part to answer some articles which had recently appeared in the Church papers. This tract was sent to about 10,000 or 11,000 Newchurchmen.

Then I wrote and compiled and condensed from my previous writings, including "The Avoidable Causes of Disease," a work of 511 pages, fully presenting the wine question in all its aspects, and the use of tobacco and opium, and the bad habits of women, faulty methods of rearing children, etc., etc., of which in paper covers I sent out over 10,000 to my New-Church brethren, and about 40,000 copies I sent to clergymen of various denominations.

In the year 1883 my attention was seriously called to the signs of deterioration of the Puritan stock in New England, especially in Massachusetts, my native State, where it was shown that in six years, ending in 1881, the deaths among the native population fully equaled, if they did not exceed, the births; whereas, among the people of foreign birth, the births exceeded the deaths by over 87,000. And I found, on visiting my native town in Western Massachusetts, and the school district where I attended, where we used to have about thirty scholars in the winter and twenty in the summer, when I was a boy, and although there are but two families less residing there now than when I was a boy, and all native Americans, still I found that they had but eight or nine scholars during the winter, and not enough to keep up a school in summer.

As a result of my inquiries I wrote a work of 52 pages, calling attention to the spiritual and natural causes of such decline of the native stock, and especially to the bad habits and false ideas of men and women which have produced it. This pamphlet I entitled, "Deterioration of the Puritan Stock, and its Causes," and printed 140,000 copies, which I sent to all the clergymen and physicians in our country whose names I could get, regarding them as the teachers and leaders of the people, and largely responsible for the existence of at least some of the prevailing evils of life.

Within the last few years pamphlets have been written by prominent clergymen of some of the prevailing denominations advocating the use of fermented wine, especially for sacramental purposes, in strong language, and claiming that it is a good and useful fluid. This seemed to aid and comfort distillers, brewers, and saloonists very much. At last one appeared entitled "Communion Wine," in which the advocates for the use of the "Fruit of the Vine," or pure unfermented wine, were assailed in no very gentle language. Several thousand of this pamphlet were sent by a Rev. Doctor of Divinity to clergymen, with a special request from him, to at least some of them, that they should read them and give him their opinion as to its merits. About 285 clergymen responded, most of them in favor of the views contained in the pamphlet, but 22 most decidedly opposed. The arguments in favor of fermented wine were based upon assumptions which were entirely groundless, and which have again and again been exposed. I could but feel that the time had come when a concise statement of the truth upon the wine question should be written and placed in the hands of every clergyman in our country; and as, in the controversy extending over several years, I had had occasion to examine the wine question in all of its various aspects, and to read whatever I could find written on both sides of the question, and had had suggestions from, and the cooperation of, some of the most distinguished scholars upon this question in this country and England, I felt that it was my duty to write a reply, which I did, of 38 pages, which was printed in connection with a short article on "The Holy Supper is Representative," by Mr. J. R. Hoffer, editor of the Mount Joy *Herald*, Mount Joy, Pa. Of this pamphlet over 80,000 were sent by Mr. Hoffer to clergymen in the United States. And of my reply alone, in a tract form, which is based upon the letter of the Sacred Scriptures-the testimony of ancient writers and science-about 50,000 copies have been printed and distributed by Mr. J. N. Stearns, 58 Reade Street, New York, who keeps a supply on hand to fill all orders.

The last pamphlet before this one which I have written is one recently published by "The Swedenborg Publishing Association," of Germantown, Philadelphia, Pa., entitled "The Essential Points of the Wine Question Carefully Examined," which, with an Addendum of 6 pages by W. J. Parsons, son of the late Professor Theophilus Parsons, contained 70 pages. This pamphlet was written for Newchurchmen and based upon the Sacred Scriptures as unfolded by the Science of Correspondences revealed through Swedenborg. This pamphlet was sent only to 10,000 Newchurchmen.

THE RESULTS OF EFFORTS IN BEHALF OF TEMPERANCE.

The reader may reasonably inquire what results have followed all the efforts which I have made to call the attention of the clergy and laity of the New Church, and the clergy of other churches, to the importance of using as a communion wine, the genuine "Fruit of the Vine" as the Lord has organized, ripened, and sweetened it in the grape, instead of a leavened or fermented wine, which, when used as a beverage, causes disease, drunkenness, insanity, and death, in innumerable instances, among the clergy and laity of our churches, and enslaves their children often before their rational faculties are fully developed. I am happy to say that to-day there are quite a number of New-Church clergymen, in this country and England, and a large number of laymen, who, after a careful examination of the subject, are satisfied that the good wine of the Word and the Writings, and the only wine suitable for use as a Communion wine, is always the fruit of the vine, and never fermented wine. Many of these clergymen and church members have not always thought thus, and did not when I commenced writing upon the subject.

At the Annual Meetings of the General Convention of the New Church, when unfermented as well as fermented wine has been permitted to be used, and full notice has been given, nearly or quite one-third of the members present have deliberately partaken of unfermented wine.

I am satisfied, from what I have seen and heard, that one of the most useful works which the Lord has enabled me to do was the writing and sending the reply to "Communion Wine" to over 80,000 clergymen. The clergy of the prevailing organizations are not so difficult to reach upon this subject as are a majority of those of the New Church, for they have not confirmed themselves in favor of fermented wine from the writings for the New Dispensation. It is one thing to see new truths when they are revealed, but it is another step to be willing to see that those truths condemn falses in which we have strongly confirmed ourselves, or evil habits in which we delight, and to avoid confirming ourselves in falses, and to avoid striving to justify evils. To do the latter means to endure and resist temptations, and to engage in a warfare until the old man with his deeds is put off.

The New Church is descending from God out of heaven, and as it progresses, fermented wine is disappearing from the Communion tables of Christian Churches.

"The new wine," says Swedenborg, "is the Divine Truth of the New Testament, and thus of the New Church." (A. R. 316.)

The new wine for the New Christian Church is unfermented wine, pure as it comes from the hands of our Lord and Saviour, Jesus Christ, in the fruit of the vine, and not a leavened wine. And when men return to its exclusive use, multitudes now enslaved, diseased, and insane from leavened wine will be set free, cured and restored to their right mind by the Great Physician-by the inflowing life from Him through this physical representative of His blood.

The New Church is not a new sect or organization, but a new faith and a renewed life resulting from a revelation of Divine Truth, made by the Lord through Emanuel Swedenborg, for the benefit of all sects and all men, that the Christian Church may "revive again" and be reunited in the bonds of Charity, by worshiping the one God whose name is one-even the Lord Jesus Christ-and by striving to live a life according to His commandments.

CHAPTER X.

FINAL APPEAL TO THE CLERGY.

I again appeal to you, as Christian men, to lay aside prejudice and preconceived ideas, if you are troubled with any that have come down to you from darker ages, and to patiently examine the writings of Emanuel Swedenborg.

If you desire and are prepared to read with open eyes and a willing heart, you can but see that the fig-tree is putting forth its leaves, and that we are living in the dawning light and warmth of a new summer. Look at the radical changes which have taken place within the last one hundred and thirty-five years, and are taking place to-day with increasing rapidity, in every department of science, arts, mechanics, medicine, and even in the religious sentiments of the people and in theology, and in civil and ecclesiastical governments, and you may rest assured, that as certain as the Word of the Lord is true, so sure it is that we are now seeing but the beginning of the changes which are yet to be witnessed; for the sure word of prophecy is, "Behold, I make all things new" —New Heavens and a New Earth-old things are to pass away, and we can see that they are passing away.

Swedenborg assures us that he was permitted by the Lord to witness the Last Judgment in 1757, which, like all general judgments, took place in the spiritual world. The Lord when on earth declared, "Now is the judgment of this world, now is the prince of this world cast out." Swedenborg tells us that between the Lord's first coming and His second coming vast societies were organized in the world of spirits, which is intermediate between heaven and hell, from among those who were not fully prepared for either heaven or hell; and they were associated with those of like affections and persuasions in this world. As the First Christian Church became gradually perverted by false doctrines and evils of life, and as its members increased in the spiritual world, their influence was more and more felt among the religious societies in this world, interfering with the inflowing of good and truth from the Lord and His Word into the minds of men, and threatening their ability to see and obey the truth. The judgment consisted in a new influx of Divine truth into such societies, the effects of which were such that those who were really good were received into heaven, and those who were evil joined their like in hell, glad to escape from the new inflowing of heavenly light and life. In this way they were separated from men on the earth and human freedom reestablished. The effects of that judgment are to-day gradually being manifested here on earth.

Swedenborg tells us that he witnessed the downfall of Babylon the great in the spiritual world. By Babylon is meant those who are in the love of spiritual dominion over the souls of men. And also he witnessed the casting down of the Dragon. By the Dragon is meant those who are in the doctrine of salvation by faith and ceremonials alone.

As the above vast organizations in the spiritual world were then removed from contact with men, I will let Swedenborg speak of some of the results which followed that judgment in the spiritual world, and of those which are following and which must follow in the Church on earth.

"After the Last Judgment (in 1757) a new heaven was formed from among Christians, only from those, however, who acknowledged the Lord to be the God of heaven and earth, and also repented in the world of their evil works. From this heaven the New Church on earth, which is the New Jerusalem, descends, and will continue to descend.... And the New Church on earth makes one with the New Heaven." (Preface to A.R.)

"In this new Christian heaven are all those who, from the first formation of the Christian Church, worshiped the Lord and lived according to His commandments in the Word, and were therefore in charity and faith from the Lord through the Word." (A.R. 876.)

Swedenborg tells us that "the slavery and captivity in which the man of the Church was formerly" were removed by the Last Judgment; so that "he can now, from restored liberty, more easily perceive interior truths if he has a desire for them." (L.J. 74.) And again he tells us that, as a result of the Last Judgment, the people of Christendom "would be in a more free state of thinking on matters of faith, that is, on spiritual things which relate to heaven, because spiritual liberty has been restored to them" (L.J. 73); and that consequently "the state of the world and of the Church before the Last Judgment," compared with what it was, or was to be after, "was as evening and night compared with morning and day." (Contin. L. J.)

Now can we not all see that the very changes anticipated in the above quotations are rapidly taking place in the Christian world all around us? Men and women are beginning to cease to be willing to be led blindly by clergymen and creeds, with their understandings under subjection to dogma. Many of our clergy, we see, are not willing to be thus led. Swedenborg tells us that in this New Dispensation men are to be led in freedom according to reason, and that professing to believe doctrines which they neither understand nor perceive to be true is of very little use to men.

As false doctrines are passing away, is it not of vast moment that true and rational doctrines should take their place, that our houses and churches be not left desolate? Somewhat extensively among the clergy, and far more extensively among scientists and intelligent people, is the Divine origin of the Sacred Scriptures being called in question. In the writings of Swedenborg, as has already been stated, you will find this question clearly and distinctly settled, for you are there shown that they are written according to the law of correspondence between natural and spiritual things, and therefore that they contain a connected spiritual sense which causes them to differ from all merely human writings, and demonstrates their Divine origin to all who are willing to examine and to see the truth. The day is not far distant when, in the Christian Church, the Sacred Scriptures will be reverenced as they have never been before; for the coming of the Son of Man in the Clouds of Heaven, or in the literal sense of the Word, is with power and great glory.

Even now in the dawning light old false doctrines are rapidly passing away. Look! What congregation would be willing to sit quietly and hear the doctrine of infant damnation proclaimed? Who is satisfied with the doctrine of election and predestination as taught but a few years ago? That favorite doctrine of my childhood's days, the vicarious atonement as taught then, is trembling in the balance, for it is being found not to accord with the Word of the Lord, nor does it appeal to human reason. The doctrine of a trinity of Divine Persons will soon follow. How few even now believe in the resurrection of the material body! Our church members are rapidly coming to believe with St. Paul that there is a natural body and there is a spiritual body, and that the spiritual body is raised at death, and that flesh and blood cannot inherit the Kingdom of God. The doctrine of a literal hell of fire and brimstone, as taught but a few years ago, is rarely taught to-day.

And now, Christian ministers, as these old doctrines are departing, what have you to substitute for them? You know very well that when extreme views are given up, there is great danger that opposite extreme views will be substituted.

Troublesome questions are arising to-day before the clergy and in our churches, which require to be handled with care by intelligent and wise men, if the Lord and His Word are to be reverenced in our churches as they should be, and men are to be led to live heavenly lives.

The question of probation after death is troubling many clergymen and laymen at this day. They see that men and women often leave this world in a very uncertain state of life, so far as they can judge, ill prepared for either heaven or hell; what is to-become of them is the question. Are they all to put away their false doctrines and evils of life and go to heaven, as some believe; or are some of them to go through purgatory and finally, after being purified, to enter heaven, and the rest go to hell, as others believe? Or again, has a man the same chance of choosing and the same ability to choose between truth and falsehood and good and evil, and of shaping his life there, as he has here?

Upon these questions the New Revelations made by the Lord through Emanuel Swedenborg throw a flood of rational light. They show us that heaven is not a place into which a man can be let as a matter of favor; but that, for a man to enter heaven, heaven must be within him. Heaven consists in loving supremely the Lord and the neighbor, or obedience to the Divine

Commandments. Hell consists in loving self, money, vain show, ruling over others without regard to use, or sensual gratifications supremely. Before a man can become a resident of hell, hell must be within him. Men enter the other world in much the same state as they leave this world; death does not change their essential characters. Good angels appointed by the Lord strive to teach heavenly truths to all, and to lead all into heavenly affections and societies who are willing to be led. But as the Lord respects the freedom of all men in this world and compels no man to love Him, his neighbor, or obedience to the Divine Commandments supremely, He compels no man there. The Lord casts no one into hell, but when our material bodies are put off and we appear among the inhabitants of the spiritual world, our thoughts and intentions can be seen more clearly than in this world; consequently the good and evil necessarily separate; and finally every one sooner or later associates with his like, the good forming heavenly societies and the evil, infernal societies.

It is evident that those who are guided in all they think and do by either love of the Lord, the neighbor, or of obeying the Divine Commandments, need no penal laws or punishments. It is equally evident that men who are actuated by the supreme love of self, vain show, or sensual gratifications must be restrained, in that world as in this, by penal laws and punishments. But we are told that the Lord governs the hells as well as the heavens through His angels, and does not permit vindictive or unjust punishments. All punishments in that world are reformatory, or for the purpose of restraining spirits from evil doing, and protecting others, as all punishments should be in this world. The Lord's tender mercies are around all His creatures in that world as well as in this, and He strives to make all happy. Even the evil man is permitted to enjoy his delight so long as he does not interfere with or harm others or himself.

Here in this state of probation good and evil men dwell together in the same society, so that the evil have good instruction and good examples, and every chance for repentance and reformation; but in hell they dwell among their like, and it would seem that they are not so favorably circumstanced for changing their life's love there as in this world. In the world of spirits into which we enter at death, all who are not fully prepared by their lives here for heaven or hell tarry until their characters are fully developed, when each one goes to his own congenial society either in heaven or hell, according to his ruling love.

Swedenborg, so far as he was permitted, describes what he saw in the spiritual world; but he did not claim to be a prophet-the future, he tells us, is known to the Lord alone, not even to the angels. Some of the readers of his writings, from certain passages contained therein, have come to think that the Lord in His loving kindness may yet so change the inhabitants of hell that they may be received into heavenly societies, as some have drawn from the letter of the Sacred Scriptures a similar conclusion; while a majority of readers, in both cases, have come to a different conclusion. But the future is known to the Lord alone, and He is love itself, and in His hands we may safely leave the inhabitants of hell; especially as our belief one way or the other will not change the final destiny of a single individual one iota; therefore it is not a practical question.

PREVAILING EVILS OF LIFE.

We are living in the midst of prevailing evils of life which should command the special attention of every clergyman and every Christian. Even infants and children are dying on all sides, and those that survive are being contaminated often even in our churches by the example of clergymen and prominent members.

But yesterday, as I was speaking to a very intelligent, well-known citizen of New York, he expressed to me the opinion that gambling and a desire to obtain money or valuables without returning a due equivalent, by purchasing lottery or chance tickets and stock gambling, is a greater evil than selling and drinking intoxicating drinks; and he most earnestly blamed many of our clergy and churches for the prevalence of this great evil; for, as is well known, it is at church fairs that the young and even children frequently take their first lessons, enticed thereto by the hope that they may be able to obtain an article of much value for a trifling sum. In this the work of demoralization commences, and leads naturally to gambling for money, betting on games, horse-racing, buying lottery tickets, and stock gambling, stimulated by the hope of making fortunes by risking small amounts, not stopping to think that what they gain, if successful, others must lose who are probably no better able to lose than they are. How much short of stealing is this? Look at the sad results which follow the practice started in so many of our churches-the poverty, the thieving, the failures, the breaches of trust, the disgrace and loss of character, and the poor wretches in prison, and others who merit punishment. Christian ministers, is not this a most fearful evil which you, if guilty of encouraging it, should put away from your own lives and teach your people to shun as a sin against God?

Again, it is the duty of husbands and wives to reproduce their species or to multiply and replenish the earth, and this is the most important use of life. Yet a vast multitude of women, by tight dressing to gratify vanity, impair health and their ability to bear healthy, well-formed children, and even their ability to nurse such as are born to them; and such deformed women walk into and out of our churches as examples to young girls, without one word of admonition. And some church members deliberately shirk the responsibility of rearing families of children, either because it is not fashionable to have large families, or because children would interfere with their selfish or sensual enjoyment; and this is not the worst which could be said of some.

Now, although it is equally the duty of all husbands and wives to multiply and replenish the earth, yet church members who, either for the want of ability or inclination, have no children, and bachelors and maidens who do not marry, will stand idly by and see the husbands and wives, however poor they may be, who are willing to do their duty, take the entire care of their children until they reach adult age; they deliberately leave the entire responsibility upon the parents of caring for and raising the money required for the support of the children, who are to be the men and women of the next generation. Is this right? It is true that public schools have been established, for all feel that it will not be safe for the children, who are to rule our country a few years hence to grow up in ignorance.

Men and women will roll in their thousands and hundreds of thousands and even millions, and see the toiling, struggling, hard-working brothers and sisters, sometimes even in the same church organization, striving to do faithfully their part in the care of the children who are to people and replenish the earth, without feeling that they have any responsibility or duty to perform in the way of giving a helping hand in this most important work of life. Now I ask you, brethren of the Christian Church, are such things in accordance with the grand and noble precepts of Christianity, in which we profess to believe-thou shalt love thy neighbor as thyself? Of course, husbands and wives who are able are but too glad to take care of their own children; but there are multitudes who need help. If wealthy husbands and wives are not willing or able to have children, or if bachelors and maidens are not willing to marry and have children, have they no duty to perform toward aiding, even financially, and by their own hands if such help is needed, those who do this most important work, and thus add to the number of intelligent and Christian inhabitants of our country? for the want of whom our country is being flooded by multitudes of the most ignorant of other nations, who have comparatively no knowledge of our free institutions and of religious freedom.

It is true that our poorhouses are established at the expense of the public, to which parents who are without means or employment or adequate wages to support their children can go with their children to avoid starvation; but what parents desire to take their children to such institutions? And we have also charitable institutions to which children can be sent to prevent their starving and going naked; but what father or mother likes to part with their children? It is not charity that such need, but the kind, helping hands of Christian brothers and sisters. All things are to be made new. As the light and especially the heat or love of the New Jerusalem descend into the minds of men, hard-hearted selfishness will disappear, and true Christians will love and strive to help one another and all men as they may need.

And now, in conclusion, I appeal to you, Christian ministers, one and all, to diligently read the Revelations made by the Lord at His second coming through His chosen servant, Emanuel Swedenborg, for they will give you new light and, if you are willing, new life. The light is spreading from the East even unto the West, and the day is not far distant when a clergyman, to be acceptable to an intelligent Christian congregation, must be familiar with the grand and rational doctrines and precepts revealed by the Lord for the benefit of the men of our day and the Church of the future.

It must be evident to you even now that many of the clergy and intelligent laymen are steadily drifting in one of two directions; either to a distinct recognition of the Supreme Divinity of the Lord Jesus Christ, of the holiness and Divinity of the Sacred Scriptures and of the life of charity or of obedience to the Divine Commandments as the only way of salvation; or to an ignoring the existence of a personal God, and of course of all revelation from God. There is no middle ground. Choose ye this day whom ye will serve.

Below you will find a notice of a work on the Science of Correspondences, the science in accordance with which all material things were created and the Sacred Scriptures were written. Send for it. It will give you new light.

A REVIEW OF AN ARTICLE ENTITLED "CHRIST AND THE TEMPERANCE QUESTION" IN "THE CHRISTIAN UNION."

In the *Christian Union* for July 11, 1891, will be found an article written by a clergyman which should not be allowed to go unnoticed. The reverend gentleman assumes in that article that "the life and teaching of Jesus Christ constitute a Divine standard for all His followers." And so do I most unequivocally; but I also claim that we should not be blinded by either strong confirmations or sensual appetites in favor of false views and evil habits, so that, having eyes, we see not the truth and consequently cannot lead a life in accordance with the truth. The writer truly says: "Christ is not to be blindly, but intelligently, followed." In other words, I would say the light afforded by science, by well-known facts and ancient history, must be allowed to shine upon such an important question as the one under consideration. Then again, the testimony of distinguished scholars who have devoted years to a careful consideration of the wine question in the light of the Hebrew and Greek Scriptures, of ancient history and science, should not be ignored, and statements made which have repeatedly been shown to have no foundation in truth, but which are contradicted by facts which at this day should be known by every man who attempts to write upon such an important question.

In the consideration of this question the above writer appears to utterly confound good and truth with the evil and false, which, it is manifest, should never be done. His whole argument is based upon assumptions which we shall find, the more carefully we examine them, have no foundation in truth. He assumes that fermented wine is a good and useful article to be used as a beverage, and, after admitting that he thinks the law of Christian love requires a general abstinence at the present day, he says: —

> "But I trust that this necessity belongs simply to the present epoch, and I am not without hope that we shall yet come to a time-though not in my day-when a pure wine can be used by society with no more seriously evil results than now are produced by the use of tea and coffee."

By pure wine he means fermented wine. He apparently thinks that tea and coffee are harmless drinks. Of this more hereafter. Again he says: —

> "Any permanent temperance reform, however great emphasis it may lay on a Christian duty of total abstinence, must draw sharply and maintain stoutly the distinction between total abstinence and temperance, between drunkenness and drinking. It must recognize drunkenness to be everywhere and always a sin, drinking to be made so only by the circumstances; temperance to be always and everywhere a duty, total abstinence to be only a means now to be employed for promoting temperance."

Now let us examine this assumption in the light of science, facts, and history.

First. It is known that all the drunkenness in the world up to the sixth century-and history and even the Bible shows us that there was plenty of it, and this the above writer admits-was caused by drinking fermented wine and other fermented drinks, for the art of distillation was unknown. And almost all of the drunkenness in our country at this day results either directly from men and boys drinking wine, beer, or other fermented drinks, or from the appetite thus formed leading them on to the use of distilled liquors; for it is rarely that they commence by using such liquors. There has never been an age in the world's history when the drinking of fermented wine did not lead large numbers of those who drank it to drunkenness, and it is safe to say that in no age of the world has there ever been more drunkenness among those who drink at all than there is at this day.

As to temperance: That old philosopher, Aristotle, tells us that temperance consists in the moderate use of things good and useful, and total abstinence from things injurious.

Second. Fermented wine is either one of the good gifts of God, to be used as a drink to build up and supply the wants of the human body, and may be used freely as we may use milk, the unfermented juice of grapes, and water, or it is not. Let us examine this question carefully for a few moments. We all know that there are animal, vegetable, and mineral substances which act as poisons when taken into the stomach, and that to thus use them is to violate the laws of health and life and to seriously endanger health, reason, and life; and not a few are destroyed by their use. The Divine commandment in regard to all such we know is, "Thou shall not" use them if they kill or endanger life when used. We know that there are other substances which are useful and necessary to nourish and build up the body and give it strength and health. How are we to distinguish these two classes of substances? By their effects on the body we may distinguish between good and useful substances and poisons. There is a natural appetite for wholesome food, which is satisfied by the usual quantity, and the middle-aged and old do not require any more nor even as much as the young man. But for poisons, unless they are made sweet by other substances, there is no natural appetite, but it has to be cultivated by using the poison; but when the appetite is once developed no other substance in nature will satisfy the appetite for it, and the appetite demands that the quantity taken shall be steadily increased to relieve the craving and diseased symptoms which the poison has caused; and if the natural inclination to increase the quantity or frequency is followed, unrestrained by caution or conscience, the individual comes at last to be able to take a quantity with impunity which would kill more than one person not addicted to its use. We all know that this is notably true in regard to fermented wine and other alcoholic drinks, opium and tobacco.

Again, all poisons, when taken into the stomach in a sufficient quantity and length of time, cause specific diseases characteristic of the poison taken. Healthy food does not do this. You see a man reeling in the streets, or drunk on the sidewalk, or with rum-blossoms on his face; you know that he has been drinking fermented wine or some fluid containing its chief ingredient-alcohol. Now, unfermented wine and other healthy drinks never cause such specific diseases or symptoms, however freely used.

Here then, in the characteristics given above, is a broad gulf, as broad and deep as that between Heaven and Hell, between nourishing, life-giving substances and the poisons named above. Of the one we are to use temperately, but from the latter we are to totally abstain. "Thou shalt not" is clearly written.

In all ages fermented wine has been regarded as a poison. In the Bible it is likened to the poison of dragons and the cruel venom of asps. Solomon tells us not to look upon it, for at last it biteth like a serpent and stingeth like an adder. Clement of Alexandria, who lived at the close of the second century, says: "From its use arise excessive desires and licentious conduct. The circulation is accelerated, and the body inflames the soul." —*Divine Law as to Wines.*

We know by observation that fermented wine is a fluid which fills man when he drinks of it as freely as he may of healthy needed drinks with all manner of uncleanness of both body and soul. How can a clergyman talk of using such a fluid temperately? Can we steal temperately, bear false witness temperately, commit adultery temperately, or murder temperately? Is it right to deliberately do any of these acts temperately? If it is, then it is right to deliberately drink fermented wine temperately, which we know endangers health, freedom, reason and life, and leads men to commit crimes even the most filthy. One glass leads naturally to another, and that to many; just as stealing pennies leads to stealing dollars, and hundreds and thousands of dollars. A perverted appetite or passion can never be fully satisfied, but it leads to sorrow. All such evils must be shunned totally as sins against God.

It would be difficult to find elsewhere in the English language, in so few lines, as many statements so absolutely untrue, dogmatically proclaimed, as in the following from the article in the *Christian Union*: —

> "This notion of two wines, one fermented, the other unfermented, must be dismissed as a pure invention, unsupported by any facts, unsanctioned by any scholarship. There was but one wine known to the ancients-fermented grape-juice. This was the wine Christ made, drank, blessed. There was no other used in His time or known to His day."

First, as to scholarship. Does the writer of the above believe that he is superior as to scholarship to the following distinguished scholars, all of whom believe in "this notion of two wines, one fermented and the other unfermented," several of whom, after a most patient and careful examination of the question, have written one or more volumes upon the subject, and one of them has been twice to the Bible lands for the purpose of carefully investigating the question there and verifying his statements? viz., Moses Stuart, Eliphalet Nott, Alonzo Potter, George Bush, Albert Barns, William M. Jacobus, Taylor Lewis, Geo. W. Sampson, Leon C. Field, F. R. Lees, Norman Kerr, Canon Farrar, Canon Wilberforce, Dawson Burns, Wm. Ritchie, George Duffield, C. H. Fowler, Wm. Patton, Adam Clarke, J. M. Van Buren, S. M. Isaacs, Wm. M. Thayer, John J. Owen; Charles Hartwell, and many other writers I could name, who, after a most critical examination of the question, have written earnestly in favor of the "notion of two wines, one fermented and the other unfermented." In view of the opinion of such men as these, can the above writer say truthfully that the "notion of two wines" is "unsanctioned by any scholarship"? Have we any more distinguished scholars than those I have named? Are not scholars who have for years made a special study of a question like this, in all of its aspects, much more competent to judge correctly than those who have not? It is certain that the writer in the *Christian Union* has never examined both sides of this question with the slightest care; for if he had done so, as an honest Christian man, as I trust he is, he could never have made many of the statements he has made. He says that the "notion of two wines" is unsupported by any facts, and that "there was but one kind of wine known to the ancients-fermented grape-juice." Has he never read the Bible-even the New Testament? I shall first bring the testimony of the Lord Himself against him. He says: —

> "Neither do men put new wine (*oinon neon*) into old bottles; else the bottles break, and the wine runneth out, and the bottles perish; but they put new wine into new bottles, and both are preserved." Matt, ix, 17.

Here we have the fresh, unfermented juice of the grape called wine —"new wine." It could not be put into old bottles and be preserved, for old bottles, especially skin bottles, are sure to contain leaven cells, which would inevitably cause fermentation and burst the bottles, whether they were of skins, glass, or earthenware. We know that fermented wine can be preserved in old bottles, and that it is so preserved without bursting the bottles. Here, then, the fresh, unfermented juice of grapes is called wine by the Lord. Should not our clergy heed His testimony?

There is no difficulty in preserving the juice of grapes, or new wine, unfermented by various methods described by ancient writers. Thus Columella, who lived during the Apostolic days, tells us to fill bottles with fresh grape-juice and seal or cork them carefully and sink them in a well of cold water and fermentation will not ensue. I have tried it successfully; any one can do the same. Next, fill a new or clean bottle with new wine just pressed from the grapes up to its neck, then pour about half an inch of sweet oil on the surface of the wine and cork it carefully, leaving a little space between the cork and oil, and stand the bottle in a cellar, and it will keep. I have three bottles thus preserved free from fermentation for over three years; the cork must not be removed and the bottle must not be shaken. Again, heat the juice to 185 (degrees) Fahr., or to the boiling-point if you please, bottle, cork, and seal it, and it will never ferment.

Now we will turn hastily to the Old Testament. In Isaiah xvi, 10, we read: "The treaders shall tread out no wine (*yayin*) in their presses." Here we have the juice of grapes, as it is trodden from grapes, called wine.

In Jeremiah xl, 10, 12, we read: "But gather ye wine (*yayin*) and summer fruits and oils," and we read that they "gathered wine and summer fruits very much." Here we have the juice of grapes called wine, as it is gathered in with other fruits.

Chapter xlviii, 33: "And I have caused wine (*yayin*) to fail from the wine-presses."

Dr. Adam Clarke says: "The Hebrew, Greek, and Latin words which are rendered 'wine' mean simply the expressed juice of the grape."

This juice, like our cider, may be fermented or unfermented, and it is still called by the same name. Here, then, in both the New and Old Testaments, we have the unfermented juice of grapes distinctly recognized as wine, and called wine; and all admit that the fermented juice of grapes is called wine, consequently there are two wines. And distinguished scholars say: —

> "In all the passages where the good wine is named (in the Bible), there is no lisp of warning, no intimation of danger, no hint of disapprobation, but always of decided approval. How bold and strongly marked is the contrast!
>
> "The *one* the cause of intoxication, of violence, and of woes; "The *other* the occasion of comfort and of peace. "The *one* the cause of irreligion and of self-destruction; "The *other* the devout offering of piety on the altar of God. "The *one* the symbol of the divine wrath; "The *other* the symbol of spiritual blessings. "The *one* the emblem of eternal damnation; "The *other* the emblem of eternal salvation." —*Bible Wines.*

> "The *one* the cause of intoxication, of violence, and of woes;
> "The *other* the occasion of comfort and of peace.
> "The *one* the cause of irreligion and of self-destruction;
> "The *other* the devout offering of piety on the altar of God.
> "The *one* the symbol of the divine wrath;
> "The *other* the symbol of spiritual blessings.
> "The *one* the emblem of eternal damnation;
> "The *other* the emblem of eternal salvation." —*Bible Wines.*

> "The distinction in *quality* between the good and the bad wine is as clear as that between good and bad men, or good and bad wives, or good and bad spirits; for one is the constant subject of warning, designated poison literally, analogically, and figuratively; while the other is commended as refreshing and innocent, which no alcoholic wine is." —*Lees' Appendix*, p. 232.

Tirosh is another Hebrew word that is often used in the Old Testament for grapes and the juice of grapes, like our word must, but it is rarely if ever applied to the juice after fermentation has commenced. We read: "They shall gather together corn and new wine (*tirosh*), they shall eat together and praise Jehovah, and *they who are gathered together shall drink it in the courts of my holiness.*" —Isaiah lxii, 9.

And again, in regard to *tirosh*, we read: "That thou mayest gather in thy corn, thy wine (*tirosh*), and thine oil." (Deut. xi, 14.) "Thus saith the Lord, as the new wine (*tirosh*) is found in the cluster, and *one* saith destroy it not, for a blessing is in it." (Isaiah lxv, 8.) "And thou shalt eat before the Lord thy God in the place He shall choose, the tithe of thy corn and wine (*tirosh*)." (Deut. xiv, 22.) Here we see that *tirosh* was to be eaten.

The word *tirosh* occurs thirty-eight times in the Hebrew Bible.

It is translated into Greek, in the Septuagint, by seventy distinguished Hebrew scholars, about three centuries before the Christian era, as follows: "The LXX renders *tirosh* in every case but two by *oinos* (the Greek word for wine), the generic name for *yayin*."

Now, are we for a moment to suppose that the above seventy distinguished ancient scholars did not understand as well what was included under the name of wine in their day, as does the writer in the *Christian Union* to-day, when they classed the unfermented juice of grapes with wine, and called it wine? How can the above writer say that "there was but one kind of wine known to the ancients-fermented grape juice"? Unfermented wine not known to the ancients, indeed! How utterly contrary to the truth, and to well-known facts, is such a statement. Just look a moment, gentle reader —

> "Aristotle ('Meteorologica,' iv, 9) says of the sweet wine of his day, that it did not intoxicate. And Athenaeus ('Banquet,' ii, 24) makes a similar statement." —*Oinos*.

> "Josephus, the Jewish historian, paraphrasing the dream of Pharaoh's butler, who dreamed that he took clusters of grapes and pressed them into Pharaoh's cup, and gave the cup to Pharaoh, repeatedly calls this grape-juice *wine*. Bishop Lowth, 1778, in his 'Commentary' (Isaiah v, 2) says: 'The fresh juice pressed from the grape' was by Herodotus styled *oinos ampelinos*, that is, wine of the vine." —*Wine of the Word*.

The celebrated Opimian wine, which Pliny (born A. D. 23) tells us (xiv, 4) had in his day, two centuries after it was made, the consistency of honey, was unquestionably an inspissated article. Such was the Taeniotic wine of Egypt, which Athenaeus, in his "Banquet" (i, 25), tells us had such a degree of richness that "it is dissolved little by little when it is mixed with water, just as the Attic honey is dissolved by the same process."

"There is abundance of evidence," says the Rev. Dr. Patton, "that the ancients mixed their wines with water; not because they were so strong with alcohol as to require dilution, but because, being rich syrups, they needed water to prepare them for drinking. The quantity of water was regulated by the richness of the wine and the time of year."

"Aristotle (born about B. C. 384) testifies that the *wines of Arcadia* were so thick that they dried up in goat-skins, and that it was the practice to scrape them off and dissolve the scrapings in water." (Meteorology, iv, 10.) —"Temperance Bible Commentary."

We know very well that these ancient wines, which were called wine in those days, which did not intoxicate, and others that were as thick as honey, were not fermented wines; for fermented wines do intoxicate, and wines as thick as honey cannot be made from fermented wine, for the albuminous and other substances which make condensed wines thick are cast down or out, or destroyed by fermentation. I have four samples of such condensed wines, or grape-juice, which are as thick as honey. One I obtained at Buda-Pesth, Hungary; one in Cairo, Egypt; one in Damascus, Asia; and the fourth was condensed and sent to me by a gentleman then residing in California. I have had these samples now over six years.

Why should the writer in the *Christian Union* quote from another writer, and thus try to make it appear that the ancient condensed wines were nothing but "grape jellies"? Does he not know that they are very different preparations, and prepared by different methods? Condensed wines are prepared by crushing and pressing the juice from the pulp, skins, and seeds, and then boiling or otherwise evaporating the water until the juice is as thick as honey, so that it can be easily preserved from fermentation? whereas grape jellies are made by boiling the grapes until they are well cooked, then rubbing or squeezing all the pulp and skins practicable through a colander, sieve, or coarsely-woven strainer; and then sugar is added to sweeten and aid in forming a jelly. Condensed wines will dissolve in water as we are told the ancient thick wines did, but grape jellies will do so only very imperfectly, for they are composed largely of the pulp of the grape.

The writer in the *Christian Union* tells us, in a passage already quoted, speaking of fermented wine: —

> "This was the wine Christ made, drank, blessed."

And again he says: —

> "He (Christ) commenced His public ministry by making, by a miracle, wine in considerable quantity, and this apparently only to add to the joyous festivities of a wedding. He apparently used wine customarily, if not habitually. When He was about to die, He chose wine as the symbol of His blood, shed for many for the remission of sins, asked His Father's blessing on a cup containing wine, passed it to His disciples with the direction, 'Drink ye all of it.'"

Now, intelligent Christian reader, what are we to think of the above statements? Let us look at these statements in the light of reason, common sense, science, and revelation. Is it probable, is it possible, that at that wedding feast, after the guests had drank freely of an intoxicating wine, that our blessed Lord, guided by love and wisdom, would create a large quantity more of an intoxicating wine for them to drink? It is not possible; and the assumption is flatly contradicted by the Governor of the feast, who pronounced the wine created as the "best wine." Place to the lips of a child of parents who do not use intoxicating drinks, or to a man or woman who never drinks such drinks, two glasses, one containing a well-fermented wine, and the other containing the sweet, delicious juice of good ripe grapes, and there is not the slightest doubt as to which would be chosen and pronounced "best" every time-try it.

Then again, is it possible that, on that occasion, a kind of wine was made of which the Lord has never created a single drop in the fruit of the vine? Fermented wine is a product of leaven or ferment and of man's ingenuity; and its chief and essential constituent, alcohol, for which men drink it, is an effete product, and holds a similar relation to the leaven that urine does to the animal body. As Pasteur says, "ferment eats, as it were," or consumes the nourishing and useful ingredients in the juice of the grapes, decomposes them, and casts out excretions, as man does when he eats grapes. Consequently, fermented wine is an utterly unclean fluid, and it fills man, when he drinks it, with all manner of uncleanness, mentally and physically, from the crown of his head to the soles of his feet, as we well know. It is preeminently a leavened substance, for it is never purified by heat, as is leavened bread. We have an abundance of testimony, which the reverend writer of the article ignores, that the Orthodox Jews have regarded, in all ages, and do to-day as a rule regard, fermented wine as coming under the restrictions placed upon leavened things.

The celebrated Jewish Rabbi, S. M. Isaacs, said in 1869: "The Jews do not use in their feasts for sacred purposes fermented drinks of any kind. The marriage feast is a sacrament with us."

In a recent work (1879) written by a Jewish Rabbi, the Rev. E. M. Myers, entitled "The Jews, their Customs and Ceremonies, with a full account of all their Religious Observances from the Cradle to the Grave," we read that among the strictly orthodox Jews, "During the entire festival (of the Passover) no leavened food nor fermented liquors are permitted to be used, in accordance with Scriptural injunctions." (Ex. xii, 15, 19, 20; Deut. xvii, 3, 4.) This, we think, settles the question so far as the Orthodox Jews are concerned; and their customs, without much question, represent those prevailing at the time of our Lord's advent.

The editor of the London *Methodist Times* lately witnessed the celebration of the Jewish Passover in that city, and at the close of the services said to the Rabbi: "May I ask with what *kind* of wine you have celebrated the Passover this evening?" The answer promptly given was: —

"With a non-intoxicating wine. Jews never use fermented wine in their synagogue services, and must not use it on the Passover, either for synagogue or home purposes. Fermented liquor of any kind comes under the category of 'leaven,' which is proscribed in so many well-known places in the Old Testament. * * * I have recently read the passage in Matthew in which the Paschal Supper is described. There can be no doubt whatever that the wine used upon that occasion was unfermented. Jesus, as an observant Jew, would not only not have drunk fermented wine on the Passover, but would not have celebrated the Passover in any house from which everything fermented had not been removed. I may mention that the wine I use in the service at the synagogue is an infusion of raisins. You will allow me, perhaps, to express my surprise that Christians, who profess to be followers of Jesus of Nazareth, can take what He could not possibly have taken as a Jew-intoxicating wine-at so sacred a service as the Sacrament of the Lord's Supper."

It is utterly impossible that Jesus Christ could have used fermented wine as a symbol of His blood, for in its essential constituents, which are alcohol, vinegar, etc., it bears not the slightest resemblance to blood; whereas unfermented wine, in its essential constituents, which are albumen, sugar, etc., bears the greatest resemblance to blood. This simple fact ought to satisfy every intelligent man.

Then again, our Lord, when He took the cup and blessed and said, "Drink ye all of it," knowing that fermented wine was included under the name of wine, and as if foreseeing that His followers might mistake and use intoxicating wine, carefully avoided the use of the word wine at all, and called it the "fruit of the vine," which unfermented wine is and fermented wine is not. It does seem that these facts should satisfy every intelligent, Christian man. Can there be, my Christian brethren, a greater profanation of a holy ordinance than the use of the drunkard's cup as a communion wine, instead of the fruit of the vine? By the use of fermented wine as a communion wine many a man who was struggling to reform his life has been led back to drunkenness and death. I have known of some sad instances.

It might be well for some of our clergy to hear and heed the warning voice of the Sacred Scriptures: —

"'It is not for kings to drink wine, nor princes strong drink, lest they drink and forget the law and pervert the judgment of the afflicted.' Here is abstinence enjoined, and the reason for it plainly given. Again (Lev. x, 8-11), *it is required of the priests*: 'And the Lord spake unto Aaron, saying, Do not drink wine nor strong drink, thou, nor thy sons with thee, when ye go into the tabernacle of the congregation, lest ye die: it shall be a statute for ever throughout your generations: That ye may put a difference between holy and unholy, and between unclean and clean; and that ye may teach the children of Israel all the statutes which the Lord hath spoken unto them by the hand of Moses.'"

"Wine is a mocker, strong drink is raging: and whosoever is deceived thereby is not wise." —Prov. xx, i.

No one questions that the wine referred to above as unholy and a mocker and unclean, is fermented wine, and no one supposes for a moment that it is unfermented wine. "But they also have erred through wine, and through strong drink are out of the way; the priest and the prophet have erred through strong drink, they are swallowed up of wine, they are out of the way through strong drink, they err in vision, they stumble in judgment. For all tables are full of vomit and filthiness, so that there is no place clean." (Isa. xxviii, 7,8.)

How correctly and literally do the above words represent the effects of drinking fermented wine and strong drinks, seen today as of old. O gentlemen of the clergy! beware! beware! "Woe to him that giveth his neighbor drink; that putteth thy bottle to him." (Hab. ii, 5,15.)

You have young and inexperienced men and women and even boys under your charge. May the Lord protect them!

CANON WILBERFORCE ON SACRAMENTAL WINES.

Canon Wilberforce is reported by the London *Temperance Record* as saying at a recent meeting in England: "He believed if people desired to go back literally and absolutely to the days of the institution of the Sacrament, it would be a most difficult thing, if not impossible, to prove that the particular cup which their Master took in His hand in that solemn crisis of His life when He instituted the Holy Eucharist was fermented at all. There was abundant testimony to prove it was not. Some went back to primitive authorities. He should like to read one or two which might have weight with them. Take for example the testimony of St. Cyprian, who wrote in A. D. 230: —

> "When the Lord gives the name of His body to bread, composed of the union of many particles, He indicates that our people, whose sins He bore, are united. And when He calls wine squeezed out from bunches of grapes His blood, He intimates that our flocks are similarly joined by the varied admixture of a united multitude."

"This distinctly implied, for all he knew, squeezing bunches of grapes. But there was more important testimony from one man who was considered by a certain party in the Church of great value-St. Thomas Aquinas, a great father of the 13th century. He said: —

> " 'The juice of ripe grapes, on the other hand, has already the form of wine; for its sweet taste evidences a mellowing change, which is its completion by natural heat (as it is said in the "Meteorologica," iv, 3, not far from the beginning), and for that reason this Sacrament can be fulfilled by the juice of grapes.' "

While in Egypt in 1884 I visited the American missionaries, and asked them what kind of wine they used as a communion wine in their churches. They told me that almost all of their members were from among the Copts, who are the descendants from the early Christians of Egypt, who have been comparatively isolated and separated from the Christian world for many centuries, and when they told them that the Western Christians used fermented wine, or "shop wine," as they called it, they were horrified at the idea, and would not partake of it; so they steeped or soaked raisins in water, and then pressed the juice from them and used that, as has been done by the Orthodox Jews when they could not obtain pure unfermented wine. I visited the Grand Patriarch of the Coptic Church, and through an interpreter he told me that he did the same, and that it was suitable for use the moment that it was pressed from the raisins. The day is not far distant when the members of the Western Christian churches will be as much horrified at the idea of using fermented wine as a sacramental wine as are the unperverted Christians of Egypt, and this will occur when our clergy and laity cease to be controlled by either strong confirmations or preconceived ideas or by sensual appetites, and can study the Sacred Scriptures and ancient history, and science and well-established facts, in the light of reason and common sense, instead of assuming everything which accords with their desires, and ignoring everything which conflicts therewith.

Again, the writer of the article I am reviewing says: —

> "Drunkenness is always and everywhere a sin; whether drinking is a sin depends upon circumstances; and whether the circumstances are such as to make drinking sinful, each individual must decide for himself, and answer for his decision, not to a priesthood, a society, or a newspaper press, but to his own conscience and his God."

While drunk the drunkard is insane, and when not drunk he is an abject slave. His appetite controls him, soul and body; he will sacrifice his property, his reputation, and the comfort of wife and children to gratify it. If, gentle reader, you have witnessed the struggles which some have witnessed of men striving earnestly to break loose from that habit, you would not be so ready to pronounce drunkenness always a sin; you would hardly dare thus to judge the poor victim. God alone can realize what he suffers. I ask the intelligent reader, in the light of reason and common sense and of the Word of God, which is the greater sinner, the man who, after he has witnessed all the wretchedness, sorrows, drunkenness, and deaths which we see around us, deliberately takes his first glass of the fluid which has caused this misery, or continues to drink after he has once commenced, while he has the ability in freedom to restrain his appetite, or the man who, by thus drinking, has lost his freedom and reason, and then drinks to drunkenness? If either is a sinner, can there be any doubt as to which is the greatest sinner? A far greater number, die from steady drinking than from drunkenness; they die from an inability to withstand the ordinary causes of disease, or to resist diseased action when attacked, and vast multitudes die from diseases caused by so-called temperate drinking, short of drunkenness. The statistics of insurance companies show that the average duration of adult human lives is shortened from seventeen to twenty-four per cent. Is it no sin to enter upon or to continue such a life? Is such deliberate self-murder no sin? And again, no man living who commences and continues drinking can have any assurance that he will not become a drunkard. I well remember when a young man, perhaps eighteen years old, standing on my native New England hills, working upon the highway with a young man three or four years older than myself. I said to him that I thought it was well to make up our minds never to drink intoxicating drinks during health, and to join a temperance society; he differed from me, and he said that when he was tired, or went out in the cold and wet and got chilled, he thought that a little "cider brandy" did him good. "But," he exclaimed with great energy, "the man who cannot restrain his appetite is a fool! If you ever hear of my getting drunk, tell me, and I will quit drinking." I intimated to him that it then might be too late. Alas! alas for that young man! he became a drunkard; he spent the farm left by his father; his wife died; his children were scattered among friends; and years after, when I returned to my native town, I was told that he was a pauper at the poorhouse.

We are told by the reverend gentleman in the *Christian Union* that nature produces alcohol in the juices, as though its production was by a natural and orderly process. The process of fermentation is just as natural as the putrefaction of meat, when not prevented by care, and from an altogether similar cause; and as orderly as the eating of grain by rats if no care is taken to prevent it; and it is a no more natural or orderly process. The writer tells us that: —

> "Whether the community can properly, without infringing on the liberty of the individual, prohibit all manufacture and sale of alcoholic liquors, is a political question, on which the life and teachings of Christ throw no light."

A strange statement, indeed! Is it not right to prohibit theft, highway robbery, and other evil acts? Do Christ's teachings throw no light upon such questions? "Thou shall love thy neighbor as thyself." In our country the government is by the people and for the people, and voters are responsible for the laws made or unmade; and they should be governed by Christ's precepts and not by political cliques. We do not hesitate to enact laws to prohibit druggists and others from selling other well-known poisons to people without the prescription of a physician, for fear they may possibly be used by the purchasers to harm either themselves or others; and I presume the reverend writer does not seriously question the justice and propriety of such laws; yet, strange to say, we license men, and thus give the sanction of the law, to sell fermented wine, beer, and other intoxicating drinks, and allow them to sell tobacco, all deadly poisons, when they know the purchasers will use them to harm themselves and others, and often destroy their lives. Yes, we thus license men to sell when we know that these poisons are sold to men and women who are controlled by an unnatural appetite instead of by reason; when it is known that they have harmed and killed more of the human family than all other poisons put together, and that many of the purchasers, to say the least, will certainly use them to destroy health, reason, and their own lives, and to render their own families and all intimately associated with them unspeakably wretched and unhappy. And yet, exclaims the above writer, whether the community can prohibit such sales of alcoholic liquors or not, without infringing on the liberty of the individual, "is a political question, on which the life and teachings of Christ throw no light." And the inference is that Christians, preachers, and our religious press have nothing to do with this question. "O consistency! thou art a jewel." Let stealing become as universal as the selling of intoxicants, and wives and children thereby be deprived of their means of support as extensively as they are by the selling of intoxicants, would the reverend gentleman stand aloof, and represent that the life and teachings of Christ throw no light upon the question of prohibiting such a violation of the Divine commandments? Shall Christians stand aloof from enacting laws to prohibit stealing for fear of infringing on the liberty of individual thieves? Can crimes be prevented without interfering with the "personal liberty" of criminals to commit crimes?

What is stealing when compared to the selling of intoxicating drinks and tobacco as they are sold in our streets, and all over our own and other lands? Kind Christian parents, which in your estimation would be the greatest crime, and which would you prefer, that a thief should steal from your boy or son, before he is twenty-one years of age, or after you cease to be responsible for him, his money, or that a man should sell cigarettes, beer, fermented wine, or other intoxicants unbeknown to you, and take his money, giving these poisons instead, and thus leading him on step by step, until an unnatural appetite is formed, and he becomes a slave to the use of a poison often before he has reached the age when his rational faculties are fully developed; and when by the use of these poisons the full development of his body is prevented, and his prospects for enjoying good health thereafter and of living to the allotted age of man are most materially lessened. In both instances his money is taken, and we know, by the poverty-stricken men and women and young men we see visiting our saloons, that some of the saloonists, as well as the thief, will take his last penny. Which is the greatest crime, to steal a man's money who is under bondage to a perverted appetite, and consequently comparatively irresponsible for his acts, or to sell him the above named poisons, which so seriously prevent development and endanger his health, reason, and life, and which bring such wretchedness and sorrow to so many homes? In both instances the man's money is gone, his wife and children are deprived of the benefit which might result from its legitimate use; but in the one case the man returns to his family a sober, loving husband and father-in the other, perchance, drunk, or on the direct road that leads to drunkenness.

In reply to his intimation that the Bible permits Christians to use fermented wine, but the Koran does not allow Mohammedans to use it, I would simply intimate to the reverend gentleman that the Lord, in His good Providence, has permitted, through the Koran, the Mohammedans to be protected from the drinking of fermented wine and other intoxicating drinks, as He has attempted to protect Christians directly by the numerous warnings in His Word; but the difference lies right here-the former have heeded the warnings, while the latter have not, and hence the fearful drunkenness prevalent in Christian countries. And we see the people of Christian countries sending their whiskey into heathen or Gentile lands with their missionaries. Alas! alas! Which is better-to be a good heathen or a drunken Christian?

A gentleman whom I desired to see resides at Constantinople. He is an Englishman, and when my wife and myself were there in 1885 he had resided there twenty-two years, and had run the largest flouring mill in Turkey. We visited his mill, which was about two miles up the Golden Horn, and he spent an evening with us at the hotel where we were stopping. During our conversation I said to him: "I would like to know about the Mohammedan Turks: what kind of men are they? In our country you can hardly call a man by a worse name than to call him a Turk." He replied that the Government officials and those who come much in contact with foreigners are apt to be corrupt enough. "But," he exclaimed with great emphasis, "the laboring Turk! the laboring Turk has a great future before him!! If I want a man to row me down the Golden Horn when the weather is rough, or to watch my mills when I am away and asleep, who I know will do his duty faithfully, I always choose a Turk instead of a Christian." He admitted that the fact that they never drink fermented wine or other intoxicating drinks was one of the causes of their greater reliability.

"Hon. Chauncey M. Depew will scarcely be accused of fanaticism on the question of liquor drinking. His opinion as a man of wide observation and knowledge of human nature is valuable even to those who would discount his opinions on the political methods of dealing with the evil. Here is Mr. Depew's experience as stated in a speech before a company of railroad men: —

> "'Twenty-five years ago I knew every man, woman, and child in Peekskill. And it has been a study with me to mark boys who started in every grade of life with myself, to see what has become of them. I was up last fall and began to count them over, and it was an instructive exhibit. Some of them became clerks, merchants, manufacturers, lawyers, doctors. *It is remarkable that every one of those that drank is dead;* not one living of my age. Barring a few who were taken off by sickness, *every one who proved a wreck and wrecked his family did it from rum and no other cause.* Of those who were church-going people, who were steady, industrious, and hard-working men, who were frugal and thrifty, every single one of them, without an exception, owns the house in which he lives and has something laid by, the interest on which, with his house, would carry him through many a rainy day. When a man becomes debased with gambling, rum, or drink, he does not care; all his finer feelings are crowded out. The poor women at home are the ones who suffer-suffer in their tenderest emotions; suffer in their affections for those whom they love better than life.'" —*The Voice*.

I think almost every man who is 75 years old, if he will look back and review carefully his youthful acquaintances, can bear almost if not equally as strong testimony as to the effects of intoxicating drinks on human life.

It is certain that but a small proportion of the drinkers who died prematurely were drunkards; they were simply what is called temperate drinkers.

I fully agree with the reverend writer in the *Christian Union* that we should not judge others to be bad or evil men because they do not speak and act just as we think they should, for we cannot see the motives from which their words and acts spring-they are known to the Lord alone; but should we not judge whether a man's words and acts are true and useful and in accordance with the Divine Commandments, or whether they are false and evil and in violation of the commandments? For instance, when we clearly see that the arguments in favor of fermented wine are all based upon assumptions which the most careful investigations by scholars as competent as any in the world show have no foundation in truth, and when we find from historical records that in all ages its use has caused an immense amount of suffering, wretchedness, drunkenness, and an untold number of premature deaths; and we see the same results following its use all around us at this day; and when science teaches us that its use is entirely unnecessary during health, and a direct violation of the laws of health and life; and when in the Sacred Scriptures fermented wine is likened, as to its effects on man, to the poison of dragons and the cruel venom of asps, and Solomon tells us that at last "it biteth like a serpent and stingeth like an adder;" —is it not clearly our duty to show to our fellow-men, and especially to the young, that to commence drinking fermented wine or beer, or to continue to drink so long as we have the power to resist the inclination to drink, is a violation of the commands, Thou shalt not kill, Thou shalt love the Lord thy God supremely, and not the gratification of a perverted appetite; and should we not as clearly as possible point out the truth, and call men to repentance and to the shunning of such evils as sins against God? How else is the world to be reformed and elevated, and the life of the New Jerusalem to descend from God out of heaven, and find an abiding place among men?

The boy, the young man, and those of all ages, in whom the regenerate life has either not commenced or has barely commenced, cannot be expected to live and act up to the Pauline maxim —"if meat cause my brother to offend," etc. Satisfy such that fermented wine is not the "cup of devils," but that it derives its life from the Lord through heaven instead of through hell, and that it is a good and useful drink, and that it is to be hoped the time will come when it can be safely drank, can they want any greater license for commencing and for continuing the life which leads to drunkenness? No one ever intends to become a drunkard or to destroy his life by drinking. He only drinks enough to satisfy his perverted appetite and to make him feel good; that is all.

Now, dear Christian reader, what can be more unfortunate for the Christian Church than for clergymen standing high in the Church, as do several who have written in favor of fermented wine, to write when they possess *only* such an extremely superficial knowledge of the wine question, in its Biblical, historical, scientific, and medical aspects, as is manifested in the article under review, and several others which have been printed and circulated within a few years? And how unfortunate that such articles should ever be published in religious periodicals that enter the homes where dwell children, and the young and innocent as well as drinkers! I thank the Lord that no religious paper bearing such seductive messages ever entered my father's house as I approached manhood.

The greatest obstacle which the grand temperance reformation has to encounter to-day is the stand publicly taken by so many of our clergy and religious periodicals in favor of fermented wine as a good and useful drink, and the use of intoxicating wine as a communion wine in so many of our churches. But the True Light has come into the world, and it will shine more and more until the perfect day.

As to tea and coffee, while they can hardly be compared with intoxicating drinks, tobacco, and opium, as to their injurious effects on man when he uses them, yet they are very far from being harmless; for, like the other poisons named, their use begets an unnatural appetite which healthy fluids will not satisfy, and they cause symptoms and diseases characteristic of the fluid taken. Tea causes sleeplessness, palpitation of the heart, and other symptoms, while coffee causes the "coffee headache," often destroys the morning appetite; if given to children, interferes with their development, interferes with digestion, and causes a variety of nervous symptoms about the chest and stomach. Parents make a great mistake and do their children great injustice when they allow them to taste of tea or coffee before they are twenty-one years of age, or until they have passed out from their control. If the young can be kept from becoming enslaved by such habits, and consequently remain in freedom, until their rational faculties are fully developed, in the increasing light of this new day, it will not be difficult for them to see that all such substances should be avoided. They do not add to one's enjoyment, for they, like intoxicants, tobacco, and all stimulating condiments, destroy or seriously impair the natural delicacy of taste with which the Lord has endowed us, when we eat or drink wholesome and needed articles of food. I am seventy-six years of age, yet I never had a better appetite, and food never tasted better than it does to-day; and I attribute this to my having so generally avoided improper articles of food and drink. After a most patient and careful examination of both sides of the wine question in the light of Divine Revelation, ancient history and of science, for many years, and after having witnessed the fearful demoralization, the wretchedness and sorrow, the diseases and deaths which result from drinking fermented wine and other intoxicants, nothing so surprises me, and discourages me, in regard to the immediate future of the American people, as the pertinacity and persistency with which so many of the clergy of our country, without any careful examination of both sides of this question, are striving to justify the use of fermented wine as a beverage and even as a Communion wine. Instead of assuming and ignoring everything, let the advocates of fermented wine answer the following inquiry by the Rev. Dr. Eliphalet Nott, President of Union College: "Can the same thing, in the same state, be good and bad; a symbol of wrath and a symbol of mercy; a thing to be sought after and a thing to be avoided? Certainly not. And is the Bible, then, inconsistent with itself? No, certainly."

Footnotes

1. For the same object the experienced allopath delights to invent a fixed name, by preference a Greek one, for the malady, in order to make the patient believe that he has long
known this disease as an old acquaintance, and hence is the fitted person to cure it.

2. Homoeopathy sheds not a drop of blood, administers no emetics, purgatives, laxatives
or diaphoretics, drives off no external affection by external means, prescribes no hot or
unknown mineral baths or medicated clysters, applies no Spanish flies or mustard plasters, no setons, no issues, excites no ptyalism, burns not with moxa or red-hot iron to
the very bone, and so forth, but gives with its own hand its own preparations of simple uncompounded medicines, which it is accurately acquainted with, never subdues
pain by opium, etc.

3. Filix Mas-Aspidium

4. His mission is not, however, to construct so-called systems, by interweaving empty
speculations and hypotheses concerning the internal essential nature of the vital
processes and the mode in which diseases originate in the interior of the organism,
(whereon so many physicians have hitherto ambitiously wasted their talents and their
time); nor is it to attempt to give countless explanations regarding the phenomena
in diseases and their proximate cause (which must ever remain concealed), wrapped
in unintelligible words and an inflated abstract mode of expression, which should
sound very learned in order to astonish the ignorant – whilst sick humanity sighs in
vain for aid. Of such learned reveries (to which the name of theoretic medicine is
given, and for which special professorships are instituted) we have had quite enough,
and it is now high time that all who call themselves physicians should at length
cease to deceive suffering mankind with mere talk, and begin now, instead, for once
to act, that is, really to help and to cure.

5. I know not, therefore, how it was possible for physicians at the sick-bed to allow
themselves to suppose that, without most carefully attending to the symptoms and
being guided by them in the treatment, they ought to seek and could discover, only in
the hidden and unknown interior, what there was to be cured in the disease, arrogantly
and ludicrously pretending that they could, without paying much attention to the
symptoms, discover the alteration that had occurred in the invisible interior, and set
it to rights with (unknown!) medicines, and that such a procedure as this could alone
be called radical and rational treatment.

6. It is not necessary to say that every intelligent physician would first remove this where
it exists; the indisposition thereupon generally ceases spontaneously. He will remove
from the room strong-smelling flowers, which have a tendency to cause syncope and
hysterical sufferings; extract from the cornea the foreign body that excites inflammation of the eye; loosen the over-tight bandage on a wounded limb that threatens
to cause mortification, and apply a more suitable one; lay bare and put ligature on
the wounded artery that produces fainting; endeavour to promote the expulsion by
vomiting of belladonna berries etc., that may have been swallowed; extract foreign
substances that may have got into the orifices of the body (the nose, gullet, ears, ure-
thra, rectum, vagina); crush the vesical calculus; open the imperforate anus of the
newborn infant, etc.

7. In all times, the old school physicians, not knowing how else to give relief, have sought
to combat and if possible to suppress by medicines, here and there, a single symptom
from among a number in diseases – a one-sided procedure, which, under the name of

symptomatic treatment, has justly excited universal contempt, because by it, not only was nothing gained, but much harm was inflicted. A single one of the symptoms present is no more the disease itself than a foot is the man himself. This procedure was so much the more reprehensible, that such a single symptom was only treated by an antagonistic remedy (therefore only in an enantiopathic and palliative manner), whereby, after a slight alleviation, it was subsequently only rendered all the worse.

8. When a patient has been cured of his disease by a true physician, in such a manner that no trace of the disease, no morbid symptom, remains, and all the signs of health have permanently returned, how can anyone, without offering an insult to common sense, affirm in such an individual the whole bodily disease still remains interior? And yet the chief of the old school, Hufeland, asserts this in the following words: "Homoeopathy can remove symptoms, but the disease remains." (Vide Homoopathie, p.27, 1, 19.) This he maintains partly from mortification at the progress made by homoeopathy to the benefits of mankind, partly because he still holds thoroughly material notions respecting disease, which he is still unable to regard as a state of being of the organism wherein it is dynamically altered by the morbidly deranged vital force, as an altered state of health, but he views the disease as a something material, which after the cure is completed, may still remain lurking in some corner in the interior of the body, in order, some day during the most vigorous health, to burst forth at its pleasure with its material presence! So dreadful is still the blindness of the old pathology! No wonder that it could only produce a system of therapeutics which is solely occupied with scouring out the poor patient.

9. It is dead, and only subject to the power of the external physical world; it decays, and is again resolved into its chemical constituents.

10. Materia peccans!

11. What is dynamic influence, – dynamic power? Our earth, by virtue of a hidden invisible energy, carries the moon around her in twenty-eight days and several hours, and the moon alternately, in definite fixed hours (deducting certain differences which occur with the full and new moon) raises our northern seas to flood tide and again correspondingly lowers them to ebb. Apparently this takes place not through material agencies, not through mechanical contrivances, as are used for products of human labor; and so we see numerous other events about us as results of the action of one substance on another substance without being able to recognize a sensible connection between cause and effect. Only the cultured, practised in comparison and deduction, can form for himself a kind of supra-sensual idea sufficient to keep all that is material or mechanical in his thoughts from such concepts. He calls such effects dynamic, virtual, that is, such as result from absolute, specific, pure energy and action of he one substance upon the other substance.

12. How the vital force causes the organism to display morbid phenomena, that is, how it produces disease, it would be of no practical utility to the physician to know, and will forever remain concealed from him; only what it is necessary for him to know of the disease and what is fully sufficient for enabling him to cure it, has the Lord of life revealed to his senses

13. Most severe disease may be produced by sufficient disturbance of the vital force through the imagination and also cured by the same means.

14. A warning dream, a superstitious fancy, or a solemn prediction that death would occur at a certain day or at a certain hour, has not unfrequently produced all the signs of commencing and increasing disease, of approaching death and death itself at the hour

announced, which could not happen without the simultaneous production of the inward change (corresponding to the state observed internally); and hence in such cases all the morbid signs indicative of approaching death have frequently been dissipated by an identical cause, by some cunning deception or persuasion to a belief in the contrary, and health suddenly restored, which could not have happened without the removal, by means of this mortal remedy, of the internal and external morbid change that threatened death.

15.   It is only thus that God the preserver of mankind, could reveal His wisdom and goodness in reference to the cure of the disease to which man is liable here below, by showing to the physician what he had to remove in disease in order to annihilate them and thus re-establish health. But what would we think of His wisdom and goodness if He has shrouded in mysterious obscurity that which was to be cured in diseases (as is asserted by the dominant school of medicine, which affects to possess a supernatural insight into the nature of things), and shut it up in the hidden interior, and thus rendered it impossible for man to know the malady accurately, consequently impossible for him to cure it?

16.   The other possible mode of employing medicines for diseases besides these two is the allopathic method, in which medicines are given, whose symptoms have no direct pathological relation to the morbid state, neither similar nor opposite, but quite heterogeneous to the symptoms of the disease. This procedure plays, as I have shown elsewhere, an irresponsible murderous game with the life of the patient by means of dangerous, violent medicines, whose action is unknown and which are chosen on mere conjectures and given in large and frequent doses. Again, by means of painful operations, intended to lead the disease to other regions and taking the strength and vital juices of the patient, through evacuations above and below, sweat or salivation, but especially through squandering the irreplaceable blood, as is done by the reigning routine practice, used blindly and relentlessly, usually with the pretext that the physician should imitate and further the sick nature in its efforts to help itself, without considering how irrational it is, to imitate and further these very imperfect, mostly inappropriate efforts of the instinctive unintelligent vital energy which is implanted in our organism, so long as it is healthy to carry on life in harmonious development, but not to heal itself in disease. For, were it possessed of such a model ability, it would never have allowed the organism to get sick. When made ill by noxious agents, our life principle cannot do anything else than express its depression caused by disturbance of the regularity of its life, by symptoms, by means of which the intelligent physician is ask for aid. If this is not given, it strives to save by increasing the ailment, especially through violent evacuations, no matter what this entails, often with the largest sacrifices or destruction of life itself.

17.   I do not mean that sort of experience of which the ordinary practitioners of the old school boast, after they have for years worked away with a lot of complex prescriptions on a number of diseases which they never carefully investigate, but which, faithful to their school, they consider as already described in works of systematic pathology, and dreamed that they could detect in them some imaginary morbific matter, or ascribe to them some other hypothetical internal abnormality. They always saw something in them, but knew not what it was they saw, and they got results, from the complex forces acting on an unknown object, that no human being but only a God could have unravelled – results from which nothing can be learned, no experience gained. Fifty years' experience of this sort is like fifty years of looking into a kaleidoscope filled with unknown colored objects, and perpetually turning round; thousands of ever changing figures and no accounting for them!

18.   Thus are cured both physical affections and moral maladies. How is it that in the early dawn the brilliant Jupiter vanishes from the gaze of the beholder? By a stronger very similar power acting on his optic nerve, the brightness of approaching day! – In situations replete with foetid odors, wherewith is it usual to soothe effectually the offended olfactory nerves? With snuff, that affects the sense of smell in a similar but stronger manner! No music, no sugared cake, which act on the nerves of other senses, can cure this olfactory disgust. How does the soldier cunningly stifle the piteous cries of him who runs the gauntlet from the ears of the compassionate bystanders? By the shrill notes of the fife commingled with the roll of the noisy drum! And the distant roar of the enemy's cannon that inspires his army with fear? By the loud boom of the big drum! For neither the one nor the other would the distribution of a brilliant piece of uniform nor a reprimand to the regiment suffice. In like manner, mourning and sorrow will be effaced from the mind by the account of another and still greater cause for sorrow happening to another, even though it be a mere fiction. The injurious consequences of too great joy will be removed by drinking coffee, which produces an excessive joyous state of mind. Nations like the Germans, who have for centuries been gradually sinking deeper and deeper in soulless apathy and degrading serfdom, must first be trodden still deeper in the dust by the Western Conqueror, until their situation became intolerable; their mean opinion of themselves was thereby over-strained and removed; they again became alive to their dignity as men, and then, for the first time, they raised their heads as Germans.

19.   The short duration of the action of the artificial morbific forces, which we term medicines, makes it possible that, although they are stronger than the natural diseases, they can yet be much more easily overcome by the vital force than can the weaker natural diseases, which solely in consequence of the longer, generally lifelong, duration of their action (psora, syphilis, sycosis), can never be vanquished and extinguished by it alone, until the physician affects the vital force in a stronger manner by an agent that produces a disease very similar, but stronger to wit a homoeopathic medicine. The cures of diseases of many years' duration (46), by the occurrence of smallpox and measles (both of which run a course of only a few weeks), are processes of a similar character.

20.   When I call a disease a derangement of man's state of health, I am far from wishing thereby to give a hyperphysical explanation of the internal nature of disease generally, or of any case of disease in particular. It is only intended by this expression to intimate, what it can be proved diseases are not and cannot be, that they are not mechanical or chemical alterations of material substance of the body, and not dependant on a material morbific substance, but that they are merely spirit-like (conceptual) dynamic derangements of the life.

21.   A striking fact in corroboration of this is, that whilst previously to the year 1801, when the smooth scarlatina of Sydenham still occasionally prevailed epidemically among children, it attacked without exception all children who had escaped it in a former epidemic; in a similar epidemic which I witnessed in Konigslutter, on the contrary, all the children who took in time a very small dose of belladonna remained unaffected by this highly infectious infantile disease. If medicines can protect from a disease that is raging around, they must possess a vastly superior power of affecting our vital force.

22.   "Memoires et Observations," in the Description de l' Egpte, tom. i.

23.   But if treated with violent allopathic remedies, other diseases will be formed in its place which are more difficult and dangerous to life.

24.   Obs., lib. I, obs. 8.

25.   In Hufeland's Journal, xv, 2.

26.   Chevalier, in Hufeland's Neuesten Annalen der franzosichen Heikunde, ii, p.192.

27.   Mania phthisi superveniens eam cum omnibus suis phaenomenis auffert, verum mox redit phthisis et occidit, abeunte mania. Reil Memorab., fasc. iii, v, p.171.

28.   In the Edinb. Med. Comment., pt. i, 1.

29.   John Hunter, On the veneral Disease, p.5.

30.   Rainey, in the Edinb. Med. Comment., iii, p.480.

31.   Very accurately described by Withering and Plenciz, but differing greatly from the purpura (or Roodvonk), which is often erroneously denominated scarlet fever. It is only of late year that the two, which were originally very different diseases, have come to resemble each other in their symptoms.

32.   Jenner, in Medicinische Annalen, August, 1800, p.747.

33.   In Hufeland's Journal der praktischen Arzneikunde, xx, 3, p.50.

34.   Loc. cit.

35.   Obs. phys. med., lib. ii, obs, 30.

36.   From careful experiments and cures of complex diseases of this kind, I am now firmly convinced that no real amalgamation of the two takes place, but that in such cases the one exists in the organism besides the other only, each in pairs that are adapted for it, and their cure will be completely effected by a judicious alternation of the best mercurial preparation, with the remedies specific for the psora, each given in the most suitable dose and form.

37.   Vide Transactions of a Society for the Improvement of Med. and Chir. Knowledge, ii.

38.   In Edinb. Med and Phys. Journ., 1805.

39.   In Med. and Phys. Journ., 1805.

40.   Opera, ii, p.i, cap. 10.

41.   In hufeland's Journal, xvii. 42. For mercury, besides the morbid symptoms which by virtue of similarity can cure the venereal disease homoeopathically, has among its effects many others unlike those of syphilis, for instance, swelling and ulceration of bones, which, if it be employed in large doses, causes new maladies and commit great ravages in the body, especially when complicated with psora, as is so frequently the case.

42.   Vide, supra, 26, note.

43.   Just as the image of a lamp's flame is rapidly overpowered and effaced from our retina by the stronger sunbeam impinging on the eye.

44.   Traite de l'inoculation, p.189.

45.   Heilkunde fur Mutter, p.384.

46.   Interpres clinicus, p.293.

47.   Neue Heilart der Kinderpocken. Ulm, 1769, p.68; and Specim., obs. No. 18.

48.   Op. cit.

49.   Nov. Act. Nat. cur., vol, I, obs. 22.

50.   Nachricht Von dem Krankeninstitut zu Erlangen, 1783.

51.   A new footnote is added here in the Sixth Edition, as follows: This seems to be the
       reason for this beneficial remarkable fact namely that since the general distribution of
       Janner's Cow-pox vaccination, human small-pox never again appeared as epidemically
       or virulently as 40-45 years before when one city visited lost at least one-half and often
       three-quarters of its children by death of this miserable pestilence.

52.   Willian, Ueber die Kuhpockenimpfung, aus dem Engl., mit Zusatzen G.P. Muhry,
       Gottingen, 1808.

53.   Especially Clavier, Hurel and Desmormeaux, in the Bulletin des sciencs medicales,
       publie par les membres de l' Eure, 1808, also in the Journal de medicine continue,
       vol. xv, p.206.

54.   Balhorn, in Hufeland's Journal, 10, ii.

55.   Stevenson, in Duncan's Annals of Medicine, lustr. 2, vol. I, pt. 2, No. 9.

56.   In Hufeland's Journal, xxiii.

57.   On the Veneral Disease, p.4.

58.   Cullen's Elements of Practical Medicine, pt. 2, I, 3, ch. vii.

59.   Or at least that symptom was removed.

60.   In Hufeland's Journal, xx, 3, p.50.

61.   Rau, Ueber d. Werth des hom. Heidelb., 1824, p.85.

62.   And the exanthematous contagious principle present in the cow-pox lymph.

63.   Namely, small-pox and measles.

64.   As if the establishment of a science, based only on observation of nature and pure
       experiment and experience idle speculation and scholastic vaporings could have a place.

65.   Up to the most recent times what is curable in sickness was supposed to be material
       that had to be removed since no one could conceive of a dynamic effect (11 note) of
       morbific agencies, such as medicines exercise upon the life of the animal organism.

66.   To fill the measure of self infatuation to overflowing here were mixed (very learnedly)
       constantly more, indeed, many different medicines in so-called prescriptions to be
       administered in frequent and large doses and thereby the precious, easily-destroyed
       human life was endangered in the hands of these perverted ones. Especially so with
       seton, venesection, emetics, purgatives, plasters, fontanelles and cauterization.

67.   A third mode of employing medicines in diseases has been attempted to be created by
       means of Isopathy, as it is called – that is to say, a method of curing a given disease
       by the same contagious principle that produces it. But even granting this could be
       done, yet, after all, seeing that the virus is given to the patient highly potentized,
       and consequently, in an altered condition, the cure is effected only by opposing a
       simillimum to a simillimum.

68.   Little as physicians have hitherto been in the habit of observing accurately, the aggrava-
       tion that so certainly follows such palliative treatment could not altogether escape their
       notice. A striking example of this is to be found in J. H. Schulze's Diss. qua corporis
       humani momentanearum alterationum specimina quoedam expenduntur, Hale, 1741,

28. Willis bears testimony to something similar (Pharm. rat., 7, cap. I, p.298): "Opi-
ata dolores atroscissimos plerumque sedant atque indolentiam – procurant, camque –
aliquamdiu et pro stato quodam tempore continuant, quo spatio elapso dolores mox
recrusescunt et brevi ad sol itam ferociam augentur." And also at page 295: "Exac-
tis opii viribus illico redeunt tormina, nec atrocitatem suam remittunt, nisi dum ab
eodem pharmaco rursus incantuntur." In like manner J. Hunter (On the Venereal Disease, p.13) says that wine and cordials given to the weak increase the action without
giving real strength, and the powers of the body are afterwards sunk proportionally as
they have been raised, by which nothing can be gained, but a great deal may be lost.

69.   Vide Introduction.

70.   Vide Hufeland, in his pamphlet, Die Homoopathie, p.20.

71.   All usual palliatives given for the suffering of the sick have (as is seen here) as after-
effects an increase of the same suffering and the older physicians had to repeat them
in ever stronger doses in order to achieve a similar modification, which however, was
never permanent and never sufficient to prevent an increased recurrence of the ailment. But Brousseau, who twenty-five years before contended against the senseless
mixing of different drugs in prescription and thereby ending its reign in France, (for
which mankind is grateful to him) introduced his so-called physiological system (without taking note of the homoeopathic method then already established), a method of
treatment, while effectively lessening and permanently preventing the return of all the
sufferings, was applicable to all diseases of mankind; a thing that the palliatives then
in use were not capable of affecting.

72.   Only in the most urgent cases, where danger to life and imminent death allow no
time for the action of a homoeopathic remedy – not hours, sometimes not even quar-
ter-hours, and scarcely minutes – in sudden accidents occurring to previously healthy
individuals – for example, in asphyxia and suspended animation from lightning, from
suffocation, freezing, drowning, etc. – is it admissible and judicious, at all events as a
preliminary measure to stimulate the irritability and sensibility (the physical life) with
a palliative, as for instance, with gentle electrical shocks, with clysters of strong coffee,
with a stimulating odor, gradual application of heat, etc. When this stimulation is
effected, the play of the vital organs again goes on in its former healthy manner, for
there is here no disease* to be removed, but merely an obstruction and suppression of
the healthy vital force. To this category belong various antidotes to sudden poisoning:
alkalies from mineral acids, hepar sulphuris for metallic poisons, coffee and camphora
(and ipecacuanha) for poisoning by opium, etc.
It does not follow that a homoeopathic medicine has been ill selected for a case of disease because some of the medicinal symptoms are only antipathic to some of the less
important and minor symptoms of the disease; if only the others, the stronger well-
marked (characteristic), and peculiar symptoms of the disease are covered and matched
by the same medicine with similarity of symptoms – that is to say, overpowered, destroyed and extinguished; the few opposite symptoms also disappear of themselves
after the expiry of the term of action of the medicament, without retarding the cure
in the least.
* And yet the new sect that mixes the two systems appeals (though in vain) to this
observation, in order that they may have an excuse for encountering everywhere such
exceptions to the general rule in diseases, and to justify their convenient employment
of allopathic palliatives, and of other injurious allopathic trash besides, solely for the
sake of sparing themselves the trouble of seeking for the suitable homoeopathic remedy for each case of disease – and thus conveniently appear as homoeopathic physicians,

without being such. But their performances are on a par with the system they pursue; they are corrupting.

73.   In the living human being no permanent neutralization of contrary or antagonistic sensations can take place, as happens with substances of opposite qualities in the chemical laboratory, where, for instance, sulphuric acid and potash unite to form a perfectly different substance, a neutral salt, which is now no longer either acid or alkali, and is not decomposed even by heat. Such amalgamations and thorough combinations to form something permanently neutral and indifferent do not, as has been said, ever take place with respect to synamic impressions of an antagonistic nature in our sensific apparatus. Only a semblance of neutralization and mutual removal occurs in such cases at first, but the antagonistic sensations do not permanently remove one another. The tears of the mourner will be dried for but a short time by a laughable play; the jokes are, however, soon forgotten, and his tears then flow still more abundantly than before.

74.   Plain as this proposition is, it has been misunderstood, and in opposition to it some have asserted "that the palliative in its secondary action, would then be similar to the disease present, must be capable of curing just as well as a homoeopathic medicine does by its primary action." But they did not reflect that the secondary action is not a product of the medicine, but invariably of the antagonistically acting vital force of the organism; that therefore this secondary action resulting from the vital force on the employment of a palliative is a state similar to the symptoms of the disease which the palliative left uneradicated, and which the reaction of the vital force against the palliative consequently increased still more.

75.   As when in a dark dungeon, where the prisoner could with difficulty recognize objects close to him, alcohol is suddenly lighted, everything is instantly illuminated in a most consolatory manner to the unhappy wretch; but when it is extinguished, the brighter the flame was previously the blacker is the night which now envelopes him, and renders everything about him much more difficult to be seen than before.

76.   The homoeopathic physician, who does not entertain the foregone conclusion devised by the ordinary school (who have fixed upon a few names of such fevers, besides which mighty nature dare not produce any others, so as to admit of their treating these disease according to some fixed method), does not acknowledge the names goal fever, bilious fever, typhus fever, putrid fever, nervous fever or mucous fever, but treats them each according to their several peculiarities.

77.   Subsequently to the year 1801 a kind of pupura miliaris (roodvonk), which came from the West, was by physicians confounded with the scarlet fever, notwithstanding that they exhibited totally different symptoms, that the latter found its prophylatic and curative remedy in belladonna, the former in aconite, and that the former was generally merely sporadic, while the latter was invariable epidemic. Of late years it seems as if the two occasionally joined to form an eruptive fever of a peculiar kind, for which neither the one nor the other remedy, alone, will be found to be exactly homoeopathic.

78.   The only possible case of plethora shows itself with the healthy woman, several days before her monthly period, with a feeling of a certain fullness of womb and breasts, but without inflammation.

79.   Among all imaginable methods for the relief of sickness, no greater allopathic, irrational or inappropriate one can be thought of than this Brousseauic, debilitating treatment by means of venesection and hunger diet, which for many years has spread over a large part of the earth. No intelligent man can see in it anything medical, or medically helpful, whereas real medicines, even if chosen blindly and administered to a patient, may at times prove of benefit in a given case of sickness because they may

accidentally have been homoeopathic to the case. But from venesection, healthy common sense can expect nothing more than certain lessening and shortening of life. It is a sorrowful and wholly groundless fallacy that most and indeed all diseases depend on local inflammation. Even for true local inflammation, the most certain and quickest cure is found in medicines capable of taking away dynamically the arterial irritation upon which the inflammation is based and this without the least loss of fluids and strength. Local venesections, even from the affected part, only tend to increase renewed inflammation of these parts. And precisely so it is generally inappropriate, aye, murderous to take away many pounds of blood from the veins in inflammatory fevers, when a few appropriate medicines would dispel this irritated arterial state, driving the hitherto quiet blood together with the disease in a few hours without the least loss of fluids and strength. Such great loss of blood is evidently irreplaceable for the remaining continuance of life, since the organs intended by the Creator for bloodmaking have thereby become so weakened that while they may manufacture blood in the same quantity but not again of the same good quality. And how impossible is it for this imagined plethora to have been produced in such remarkable rapidity and so to drain it off by frequent venesections when yet an hour before the pulse of this heated patient (before the fever and chill stage) was so quiet. No man, no sick person has ever too much blood or too much strength. On the contrary, every sick man lacks strength, otherwise his vital energy would have prevented the development of the disease. Thus it is irrational and cruel to add to this weakened patient, a greater, indeed the most serious source of debility that can be imagined. It is a murderous malpractice irrational and cruel based on a wholly groundless and absurd theory instead of taking away his disease which is ever dynamic and only to be removed by dynamic potencies.

80.   If the patient succumbs, the practiser of such a treatment is in the habit of pointing out to the sorrowing relatives, at the post-mortem examination, these internal organic disfigurements, which are due to his pseudo-art, but which he artfully maintains to be the original incurable disease (see my book, Die Alloopathie, ein Wort deh Warnung an Kranke jeder Art, Leipzig, bei Baumgartner (translated in Lesser Writings)). Those deceitful records, the illustrated works on pathological anatomy, exhibit the products of such lamentable bungling. Deceased people from the country and those from the poor of cities who have died without such bungling with hurtful measures are not opened up through pathological anatomy as a rule. Such corruption and deformities would not be found in their corpses. From this fact can be judged the value of the evidence drawn from these beautiful illustrations as well as of the honesty of these authors and book makers.

81.   During the flourishing years of youth and with the commencement of regular menstruation joined to a mode of life beneficial to soul, heart and body, they remain unrecognized for years. Those afflicted appeal in perfect health to their relatives and acquaintances and the disease that was received by infection or inheritance seems to have wholly disappeared. But in later years, after adverse events and conditions of life, they are sure to appear anew and develop the more rapidly and assume a more serious character in proportion as the vital principle has become disturbed by debilitating passions, worry and care, but especially when disordered by inappropriate medicinal treatment.

82.   I spent twelve years in investigating the source of this incredibly large number of chronic affections, in ascertaining and collecting certain proofs of this great truth, which had remained unknown to all former or contemporary observers, and in discovering at the same time the principal (antipsoric) remedies, which collectively are nearly a match for this thousand-headed monster of disease in all its different developments and forms. I have published my observations on this subject in the book entitled The

Chronic Diseases (4 vols., Dresden, Arnold. (2nd edit., Dusseldorf, Schaub.)) before I had obtained this knowledge I could only treat the whole number of chronic diseases as isolated, individual maladies, with those medicinal substances whose pure effects had been tested on healthy persons up to that period, so that every case of chronic disease was treated by my disciples according to the group of symptoms it presented, just like an idiopathic disease, and it was often so for cured that sick mankind rejoiced at the extensive remedial treasures already amassed by the new healing art. How much greater cause is there now for rejoicing that the desired goal has been so much more nearly attained, inasmuch as the recently discovered and far more specific homoeopathic remedies for chronic affections arising from psora (properly termed antipsoric remedies) and the special instructions for their preparation and employment have been published; and from among them the true physician can now select for his curative agents those whose medicinal symptoms correspond in the most similar (homoeopathic) manner to the chronic disease he has to cure; and thus, by the employment of (antipsoric) medicines more suitable for this miasm, he is enabled to render more essential service and almost invariably to effect a perfect cure.

83. Some of these causes that exercise a modifying influence on the transformation of psora into chronic diseases manifestly depend sometimes on the climate and the peculiar physical character of the place of abode, sometimes on the very great varieties in the physical and mental training of youth, both of which may have been neglected, delayed or carried to excess, or on their abuse in the business or conditions of life, in the matter of diet and regimen, passions, manners, habits and customs of various kinds.

84. How many improper ambiguous names do not these works contain, under each of which are included excessively different morbid conditions, which often resemble each other in one single symptom only, as ague, jaundice, dropsy, consumption, leucorrhoea, haemorrhoids, rheumatism, apoplexy, convulsions, hysteria, hypochondriasis, melancholia, mania, quinsy, palsy, etc., which are represented as diseases of a fixed and unvarying character, and are treated, on account of their name, according to a determinate plan! How can the bestowal of such a name justify an identical medical treatment? And if the treatment is not always to be the same, why make use of an identical name which postulates an identity of treatment? "Nihil sane in artem medicam pestiferum magis unquam irrepsit malum, quam generalia quaedam medicinam," says Huxham, a man as clear-sighted as he was estimable on account of his conscientiousness (Op. phys. med., tom. I.). And in like manner Frittze laments (Annalen, I, p.80) "that essentially different diseases are designated by the same name." Even those epidemic diseases, which undoubtedly may be propagated in every separate epidemic by a peculiar contagious principle which remains unknown to us, are designated, in the old school of medicine by particular names, just as if they were well-known fixed diseases that invariably recurred under the same form, as hospital fever, goal fever, camp fever, putrid fever, bilious fever, nervous fever, mucous fever, although each epidemic of such roving fevers exhibits itself at every occurrence as another, a new disease, such as it has never before appeared in exactly the same form, differing very much, in every instance, in its course, as well as in many of its most striking symptoms and its whole appearance. Each is so for dissimilar to all previous epidemics, whatever names they may bear, that it would be dereliction of all logical accuracy in our ideas of things were we to give to these maladies, that differ so much among themselves, one of those names we meet with in pathological writings, and treat them all medicinally in conformity with this misused name. The candid Sydenham alone perceived this, when he (Obs. med., cap. ii, De morb, epid.) insists upon the necessity of not considering any epidemic disease as having occurred before and treating it in the same way as another, since all that occur successively, be they ever so numerous, differ from one another: "Nihil quic-

quam (opinor,) animum universae qua patet medicinae pomoeria perlustrantem, tanta admiratione percellet, quam discolor illa et sui plane dissimilis morborum Epidemicorum facies; non tam qua varias ejusdem anni tempestates, quam qua discrepantes divewrsorum ab invicem annorum constitutiones referunt, ab iisque dependent. Quae tam aperta praedictorum morborum diversitas tum propriis ac sibi peculiaribus symptomatis, tum etiam medendi ratione, quam hi ab illis disparem prorsus sibi vendicant, satis illucescit. Ex quibus constat morbus hosce, ut ut externa quadantenus specie, er symptomatis aliquot utrisque pariter super venientibus, convenire paulo incautioribus videantur, re tamen ipsa (si bene adverteris animum), alienae admondum esse indolis, et distare ut aera lupinis."

85.   Hence the following directions for investigating the symptoms are only partially applicable for acute diseases.

86.   Every interruption breaks the train of thought of the narrators, and all they would have said at first does not again occur to them in precisely the same manner after that.

87.   For instance the physician should not ask, Was not this or that circumstance present? He should never be guilty of making such suggestions, which tend to seduce the patient into giving a false answer and a false account of his symptoms.

88.   For example what was the character of his stools? How does he pass his water? How is it with his day and night sleep? What is the state of his disposition, his humor, his memory? How about the thirst? What sort of taste has he in his mouth? What kinds of food and drink are most relished? What are most repugnant to him? Has each its full natural taste, or some other unusual taste? How does he feel after eating or drinking? Has he anything to tell about the head, the limbs or the abdomen?

89.   For example, how often are his bowels moved? What is the exact character of the stools? Did the whitish evacuation consist of mucus or faeces? Had he or had he not pains during the evacuation? What was their exact character, and where were they seated? What did the patient vomit? Is the bad taste in the mouth putrid, or bitter, or sour, or what? before or after eating, or during the repast? At what period of the day was it worst? What is the taste of what is eructated? Does the urine only become turbid on standing, or is it turbid when first discharged? What is its color when first emitted? Of what color is the sediment? How does he behave during sleep? Does he whine, moan, talk or cry out in his sleep? Does he start during sleep? Does he snore during inspiration, or during expiration? Does he lie only on his back, or on which side? Does he cover himself well up, or can he not bear the clothes on him? Does he easily awake, or does he sleep too soundly? How often does this or that symptom occur? What is the cause that produces it each time it occurs? does it come on whilst sitting, lying, standing, or when in motion? only when fasting, or in the morning, or only in the evening, or only after a meal, or when does it usually appear? When did the rigor come on? was it merely a chilly sensation, or was he actually cold at the same time? if so, in what parts? or while feeling chilly, was he actually warm to the touch? was it merely a sensation of cold, without shivering? was he hot without redness of the face? what parts of him were hot to the touch? or did he complain of heat without being hot to the touch? How long did the chilliness last? how long the hot stage? When did the thirst come on – during the cold stage? during the heat? or previous to it? or subsequent to it? How great was the thirst, and what was the beverage desired? When did the sweat come on – at the beginning or the end of the heat? or how many hours after the heat? when asleep or when awake? How great was the sweat? was it warm or cold? on what parts? how did it smell? What does he complain of before or during the cold stage? what during the hot stage? what

after it? what during or after the sweating stage? In women, note the character of menstruation and other discharges, etc.

90.   For example, how the patient behaved during the visit – whether he was morose, quarrelsome, hasty, lachrymose, anxious, despairing or sad, or hopeful, calm etc. Whether he was in a drowsy state or in any way dull of comprehension; whether he spoke hoarsely, or in a low tone, or incoherently, or how other wise did he talk? what was the color of his face and eyes, and of his skin generally? what degree of liveliness and power was there in his expression and eyes? what was the state of his tongue, his breathing, the smell from his mouth, and his hearing? were his pupils dilated or contracted? how rapidly and to what extent did they alter in the dark and in the light? what was the character of the pulse? what was the condition of the abdomen? how moist or hot, how cold or dry to the touch, was the skin of this or that part or generally? whether he lay with head thrown back, with mouth half or wholly open, with the arms placed above the head, on his back, or in what other position? what effort did he make to raise himself? and anything else in him that may strike the physician as being remarkable.

91.   Any causes of a disgraceful character, which the patient or his friends do not like to confess, at least not voluntarily, the physician must endeavor to elicit by skilfully framing his questions, or by private information. To these belong poisoning or attempted suicide, onanism, indulgence in ordinary or unnatural debauchery, excess in wine, cordials, punch and other ardent beverages, or coffee, – over-indulgence in eating generally, or in some particular food of a hurtful character, – infection with venereal disease or itch, unfortunate love, jealousy, domestic infelicity, worry, grief on account of some family misfortune, ill-usage, balked revenge, injured pride, embarrassment of a pecuniary nature, superstitious fear, – hunger, – or an imperfection in the private parts, a rupture, a prolapse, and so forth.

92.   In chronic diseases of females it is specially necessary to pay attention to pregnancy, sterility, sexual desire, accouchements, miscarriages, suckling, and the state of the menstrual discharge. With respect to the last-named more particularly, we should not neglect to ascertain if it recurs at too short intervals, or is delayed beyond the proper time, how many days it lasts, whether its flow is continuous or interrupted, what is its general quality, how dark is its color, whether there is leucorrhoea before its appearance or after its termination, but especially by what bodily or mental ailments, what sensations and pains, it is preceded, accompanied or followed; if there is leucorrhoea, what is its nature, what sensations attend its flow, in what quantity it is, and what are the conditions and occasions under which it occurs?

93.   A pure fabrication of symptoms and sufferings will never be met with in hypochondriacs, even in the most impatient of them – a comparison of the sufferings they complain of at various times when the physician gives them nothing at all, or something quite unmedical, proves this plainly; – but we must deduct something from their exaggeration, at all events ascribe the strong character of their expressions to their expressions when talking of their ailments becomes of itself an important symptom in the list of features of which the portrait of the disease is composed. The case is different with insane persons and rascally feigners of disease.

94.   The physician who has already, in the first cases, been able to choose a remedy approximating to the homoeopathic specific, will, from the subsequence cases, be enabled either to verify the suitableness of the medicine chosen, or to discover a more appropriate, the most appropriate homoeopathic remedy.

95.   The old school physician gave himself very little trouble in this matter in his mode of treatment. He would not listen to any minute detail of all the circumstances of his case by the patient; indeed, he frequently cut him short in his relation of his sufferings, in order that he might not be delayed in the rapid writing of his prescription, composed of a variety of ingredients unknown to him in their true effects. No allopathic physician, as has been said, sought to learn all the circumstances of the patient's case, and still less did he make a note in writing of them. On seeing the patient again several days afterwards he recollected nothing concerning the few details he had heard at the first visit (having in the meantime seen so many other patients laboring under different affections); he had allowed everything to go in at one ear and out at the other. At subsequent visits he only asked a few general questions, went through the ceremony of feeling the pulse at the wrist, looked at the tongue, and at the same moment wrote another prescription, on equally irrational principles, or ordered the first one to be continued (in considerable quantities several times a day), and, with a graceful bow, he hurried off to the fiftieth or sixtieth patient he had to visit, in this thoughtless way, in the course of that forenoon. The profession which of all others requires actually the most reflection, a conscientious, careful examination of the state of each individual patient and a special treatment founded thereon, was conducted in this manner by persons who called themselves physicians, rational practitioners. The result, as might naturally be expected, was almost invariably bad; and yet patients had to go to them for advise, partly because there were none better to be had, partly for fashion's sake.

96.   Not one single physician, as far as I know, during the previous two thousand five hundred years, thought of this so natural, so absolutely necessary and only genuine mode of testing medicines for their pure and peculiar effects in deranging the health of man, in order to learn what morbid state each medicine is capable of curing, except the great and immoral Albrecht von Haller. He alone, besides myself, saw the necessity of this (vide the Preface to the Pharmacopoeia Helvet, Basil, 1771, fol., p.12); Nempe primum in corpore sano medela tentanda est, sine peregrina ulla miscela; odoreque et sapore ejus exploratis, exigua illiu dosis ingerenda et ad ommes, quae inde contingunt, affectiones, quis pulsus, qui calor, quae respiratia, quaenam excretiones, attendum. Inde ad ductum phaenomenorum, in sano obviorum, transeas ad experimenta in corpore aegroro," etc. But no one, not a single physician, attended to or followed up this invaluable hint.

97.   It is impossible that there can be another true, best method of curing dynamic diseases (i.e., all diseases not strictly surgical) besides homoeopathy, just as it is impossible to draw more than one straight line betwixt two given points. He who imagines that there are other modes of curing diseases besides it could not have appreciated homoeopathy fundamentally nor practised it with sufficient care, nor could he ever have seen or read cases of properly performed homoeopathic cures; nor, on the other hand, could he have discerned the baselessness of all allopathic modes of treating diseases and their bad or even dreadful effects, if, with such lax indifference, he places the only true healing art on an equality with those hurtful methods of treatment, or alleges the latter to be auxiliaries to homoeopathy which it could not do without! My true, conscientious followers, the pure homoeopathists, with their successful, almost never-failing treatment, might teach these persons better.

98.   The first fruits of these labors, as perfect as they could be at that time, I recorded in the Fragmenta de viribus medicamentorum positivis, sive in sano corpore humano observatis, pts. I, ii, Lipsiae, 8, 1805, ap. J. A. Barth; the more mature fruits in the Reine Arzneimittellebre, I Th., dritte Ausg.; II Th., dritte Ausg., 1833; III Th., zweite Ausg., 1825; IV Th., zw. Ausg., 1827 (English translation, Materia Medica Pura, vols I and ii); and in the second, third, and fourth parts of Die chronischen Krankheiten,

1828, 1830, Dresden bei Arnold (2nd edit., with a fifth part, Dusseldorf bei Schaub, 1835, 1839).

99. See what I have said on this subject in the "Examination of the Sources of the Ordinary Materia Medica," prefixed to the third part of my Reine Arzneimittellebre (translated in the Materia Medica Pura, vol. ii).

100. Some few persons are apt to faint from the smell of roses and to fall into many other morbid, and sometimes dangerous states from partaking of mussels, crabs or the roe of the barbel, from touching the leaves of some kinds of sumach, etc.

101. Thus the Princess Maria Porphyroghnita restored her brother, the Emperor Alexius, who suffered from faintings, by sprinkling him with rose water in the presence of his aunt Eudoxia (Hist. byz. Alexias, lib. xv, p. 503, ed. Posser); and Horstius (Oper., iii, p.59) saw great benefit from rose vinegar in cases of syncope.

102. This fact was also perceived by the estimable A. v. Haller, who says (Preface to his Hist. stirp. helv.): "Latet immensa virium diversitas in iis ipsis plantis, quarum facies externas dudum novimus, animas quasi et quodcunque caelestius habent, nondum perspeximus."

103. Anyone who has a thorough knowledge of, and can appreciate the remarkable difference of, effects on the health of man of every single substance from those of every other, will readily perceive that among them there can be, in a medical point of view, no equivalent remedies whatever, no surrogates. Only those who do not know the pure, positive effects of the different medicines can be so foolish as to try to persuade us that one can serve in the stead of the other, and can in the same disease prove just as serviceable as the other. Thus do ignorant children confound the most essential different things, because they scarcely know their external appearances, far less their real value, their true importance and their very dissimilar inherent properties.

104. If this be pure truth, as it undoubtedly is, then no physician who would not be regarded as devoid of reason, and who would not act contrary to the dictates of his conscience, the sole arbiter of real worth, can employ in the treatment of diseases any medicinal substance but one with whose real significance he is thoroughly and perfectly conversant, i.e., whose positive action on the health of healthy individuals he has so accurately tested that he knows for certain that it is capable of producing a very similar morbid state, more similar than any other medicine with which he is perfectly acquainted, to that presented by the case of disease he intends to cure by means of it; for, as has been shown above, neither man, nor mighty Nature herself, can effect a perfect, rapid and permanent cure otherwise than with a homoeopathic remedy. Henceforth no true physician can abstain from making such experiment, in order to obtain this most necessary and only knowledge of the medicines that are essential to cure, this knowledge which has hitherto been neglected by the physicians in all ages. In all former ages – posterity will scarcely believe it – physicians have hitherto contented themselves with blindly prescribing for diseases medicines whose value was unknown, and which had never been tested relative to their highly important, very various, pure dynamic action on the health of man; and, moreover, they mingled several of these unknown medicines that differed so vastly among each other in one formula, and left it to chance to determine what effects should thereby be produced on the patient. This is just as if a madman should force his way into the workshop of an artisan, seize upon handfuls of very different tools, with the uses of all of which he is quite unacquainted, in order, as he imagines, to work at the objects of art he sees around him. I need hardly remark that these would be destroyed, I may say utterly ruined, by his senseless operations.

105.   Young green peas, green French beans ('boiled potatoes' in the Sixth Edition) and in all cases carrots are allowable, as the least medicinal vegetables.

106.   The subject of experiment must either be not in the habit of taking pure wine, brandy, coffee or tea, or he must have totally abstained for a considerable time previously from the use of these injurious beverages, some of which are stimulating, others medicinal.

107.   He who makes known to the medical world the results of such experiments becomes thereby responsible for the trustworthiness of the person experimented on and his statements, and justly so, as the weal of suffering humanity is here at stake.

108.   Those trials made by the physician on himself have for him other and inestimable advantages. In the first place, the great truth that the medicinal virtue of all drugs, whereon depends their curative power, lies in the changes of health he has himself undergone from the medicines he has proved, and the morbid states he has himself experienced from them, becomes for him an incontrovertible fact. Again by such note-worthy observations on himself he will be brought to understand his own sensations, his mode of thinking and his disposition (the foundation of all true wisdom), and he will be also trained to be, what every physician ought to be, a good observer. All our observations on others are not nearly so interesting as those made on ourselves. The observer of others must always dread lest the experimenter did not feel exactly what he said, or lest he did not describe his sensations with the most appropriate expressions. He must always remain in doubt whether he has not been deceived, at least to some extent. These obstacles to the knowledge of the truth, which can never be thoroughly surmounted in our investigations of the artificial morbid symptoms that occur in others from the ingestion of medicines, cease entirely when we make the trials on ourselves. He who makes these trials on himself knows for certain what he has felt, and each trial is a new inducement for him to investigate the powers of other medicines. He thus becomes more and more practised in the art of observing, of such importance to the physician, by continuing to observe himself, the one on whom he can most rely and who will never deceive him; and this he will do all the more zeal-ously as these experiments on himself promise to give him a reliable knowledge of the true value and significance of the instruments of cure that are still to a great degree unknown to our art. Let it not be imagined that such slight indispositions caused by taking medicines for the purpose of proving them can be in the main injurious to the health. Experience shows on the contrary, that the organism of the prover be-comes, by these frequent attacks on his health, all the more expert in repelling all external influences inimical to his frame and all artificial and natural morbific noxious agents, and becomes more hardened to resist everything of an injurious character, by means of these moderate experiments on his own person with medicines. His health becomes more unalterable; he becomes more robust, as all experience shows.

109.   Symptoms which, during the whole course of the disease, might have been observed only a long time previously, or never before, consequently new ones, belonging to the medicine.

110.   Latterly it has been the habit to entrust the proving of medicines to unknown persons at a distance, who were paid for their work, and the formation so obtained was printed. But by so doing, the work which is of all others the most important, which is to form the basis of the only true healing art, and which demands the greatest moral certainty and trustworthiness seems to me, I regret to say, to become doubtful and uncertain in its results and to lose all value.

111.   At first, about forty years ago, I was the only person who made the provings of the pure powders of medicines the most important of his occupations. Since then I have

been assisted in this by some young men, who instituted experiments on themselves, and whose observations I have critically revised. Following these some genuine work of this kind was done by a few others. But what shall we not be able to effect in the way of curing in the whole extent of the infinitely large domain of disease, when numbers of accurate and trustworthy observers shall have rendered their services in enriching this, the only true materia medica, by careful experiments on themselves! The healing art will then come near the mathematical sciences in certainty.

112.   See the second note to 109.

113.   But this laborious, sometimes very laborious, search for and selection of the homoeopathic remedy most suitable in every respect to each morbid state, is an operation which, notwithstanding all the admirable books for facilitating it, still demands the study of the original sources themselves, and at the same time a great amount of circumspection and serious deliberation, which have their best rewards in the consciousness of having faithfully discharged our duty. How could his laborious, care-demanding task, by which alone the best way of curing diseases is rendered possible, please the gentlemen of the new mongrel sect, who assume the honorable name of homoeopathists, and even seem to employ medicines in form and appearance homoeopathic, but determined upon by them anyhow (quidquid in buccam venit), and who, when the unsuitable remedy does not immediately give relief, in place of laying the blame on their unpardonable ignorance and laxity in performing the most and important and serious of all human affairs, ascribe it to homoeopathy, which they accuse of great imperfection (if the truth be told, its imperfection consists in this, that the most suitable homoeopathic remedy for each morbid condition does not spontaneously fly into their mouths like roasted pigeons, without any trouble on their own part). They know, however, from frequent practice, how to make up for the inefficiency of the scarcely half homoeopathic remedy by the employment of allopathic means, that come much more handy to them, among which one or more dozens of leeches applied to the affected part, or little harmless venesections to the extent of eight ounces, and so forth, play an important part; and should the patient, in spite of all this, recover, they extol their venesections, leeches, etc., alleging that, had it not been for these, the patient would not have been pulled through, and they give us to understand, in no doubtful language, that these operations, derived without much exercise of genius from the pernicious routine of the old school, in reality contributed the best share towards the cure. But if the patient die under the treatment, as not unfrequently happens, they seek to console the friends by saying that "they themselves were witnesses that everything conceivable had been done for the lamented deceased". Who would do this frivolous and pernicious tribe the honour to call them, after the name of the very laborious but salutary art, homoeopathic physicians? May the just recompense await them, that, when taken ill, they may be treated in the same manner!

114.   Dr. von Bonninghausen, by the publication of the characteristic symptoms of homoeopathic medicines and his repertory has rendered a great service to Homoeopathy as well as Dr. J.H.G. Jahr in his handbook of principal symptoms.

115.   This exaltation of the medicinal symptoms over those disease symptoms analogous to them, which looks like an aggravation, has been observed by other physicians also, when by accident they employed a homoeopathic remedy. When a patient suffering from itch complains of an increase of the eruption after sulphur, his physician who knows not the cause of this, consoles him with the assurance that the itch must first come out properly before it can be cured; he knows not, however, that this is a sulphur eruption, that assumes the appearance of an increase of the itch. "The facial eruption which the viola tricolor cured was aggravated by it at the commencement of

its action," Leroy tells us (Heilk, fur Mutter, p.406), but he knew not that the apparent aggravation was owing to the somewhat too large dose of the remedy, which in this instance was to a certain extent homoeopathic. Lysons says (Med. Transact., vol ii, London, 1772), "The bark of the elm cures most certainly those skin diseases which it increases at the beginning of its action." Had he not given the bark in the monstrous doses usual in the allopathic system, but in the quite small doses requisite when the medicine shows similarity of symptoms, that is to say, when it is used homoeopathically, he would have effected a cure without, or almost without, seeing this apparent increase of the disease (homoeopathic aggravation).

116. When they were not caused by an important error in regimen, a violent emotion, or a tumultuous revolution in the organism, such as the occurrence or cessation of the menses, conception, childbirth, and so forth.

117. In cases where the patient (which, however, happens excessively seldom in chronic, but not infrequently in acute, diseases) feels very ill, although his symptoms are very indistinct, so that this state may be attributed more to the benumbed state of the nerves, which does not permit the patient's pains and sufferings to be distinctly perceived, this torpor of the internal sensibility is removed by opium, and in its secondary action the symptoms of the disease become distinctly apparent.

118. One of the many great and pernicious blunders of the old school.

119. Foot-note in Fifth Edition only. As, for instance, aconite, rhus, belladonna, mercury, etc.

120. Recent itch eruption, chancre, condylomata, as I have indicated in my book of Chronic Diseases.

121. As was the case before my time with the remedies for the condylomatous disease (and the antipsoric medicines).

122. The issues of the old-school do something similar; as artificial ulcers on external parts, they silence some internal chronic diseases, but only for a short time, as long as they cause a painful irritation to which the sick organism is not used, without being able to cure them; but, on the other hand, they weaken and destroy the general health much more than is done by most of the metastases effected by the instinctive vital force.

123. For any medicines that might at the same time be given internally served but to aggravate the malady, as these remedies possessed no specific power of curing the whole disease, but assailed the organism, weakened it and inflicted on it, in addition, other chronic medicinal diseases.

124. I cannot therefore advise, for instance, the local extirpation of the so-called cancer of the lips and face (the product of highly developed psora, not infrequently in conjunction with syphilis) by means of the arsenical remedy of Frere Cosme, not only because it is excessively painful and often fails, but more for this reason, because, if this dynamic remedy should indeed succeed in freeing the affected part of the body from the malignant ulcer locally, the basic malady is thereby not diminished in the slightest, the preserving vital force is therefore necessitated to transfer the field of operation of the great internal malady to some more important part (as it does in every case of metastasis), and the consequence is blindness, deafness, insanity, suffocative asthma, dropsy, apoplexy, etc. But this ambiguous local liberation of the part from the malignant ulcer by the topical arsenical remedy only succeeds, after all, in those cases where the ulcer has not yet attained any great size, and when the vital force is still very energetic; but it is just in such a state of things that the complete internal

cure of the whole original disease is also still practicable. The result is the same without previous cure of the inner miasm when cancer of the face or breast is removed by the knife alone and when encysted tumors are enucleated; something worse ensues, or at any rate death is hastened. This has been the case times without number, but the old school still goes blindly on in the same way in every new case, with the same disastrous results.

125.   Itch eruption, chancre (bubo), condylomata.

126.   In investigations of this nature we must not allow ourselves to be deceived by the assertions of the patients of their friends, who frequently assign as the cause of chronic, even of the severest and most inveterate diseases, either a cold caught (a thorough wetting, drinking cold water after being heated) many years ago, or a former fright, a sprain, a vexation (sometimes even a bewitchment), etc. These causes are much too insignificant to develop a chronic disease in a healthy body, to keep it up for years, and to aggravate it year by year, as is the case with all chronic diseases from developed psora. Causes of a much more important character than those remembered noxious influences must lie at the root of the initiation and progress of a serious, obstinate disease of long standing; the assigned causes could only rouse into activity the latent chronic miasm.

127.   How often, for instance, do we not meet with a mild, soft disposition in patients who have for years been afflicted with the most painful diseases, so that the physician feels constrained to esteem and compassionate the sufferer! But if he subdue the disease and restore the patient to health – as is frequently done in homoeopathic practice – he is often astonished and horrified at the frightful alteration in his disposition. He often witnesses the occurrence of ingratitude, cruelty, refined malice and propensities most disgraceful and degrading to humanity, which were precisely the qualities possessed by the patient before he grew ill. Those who were patient when well often become obstinate, violent, hasty, or even intolerant and capricious, or impatient or disponding when ill; those formerly chaste and modest often frequently become lascivious and shameless. A clear-headed person not infrequently becomes obtuse of intellect, while one ordinarily weak-minded becomes more prudent and thoughtful; and a man slow to make up his mind sometimes acquires great presence of mind and quickness of resolve, etc.

128.   Thus aconite will seldom or never effect a rapid or permanent cure in a patient of a quiet, calm, equable disposition; and just as little will nux vomica be serviceable where the disposition is mild and phlegmatic, pulsatilla where it is happy, gay and obstinate, or ignatia where it is imperturbable and disposed neither to be frightened nor vexed.

129.   It very rarely happens that a mental or emotional disease of long standing ceases spontaneously (for the internal dyscrasia transfers itself again to the grosser corporeal organs); such are the few cases met with now and then, where a former inmate of a madhouse has been dismissed apparently recovered. Hitherto, moreover, all madhouses have continued to be chokefull, so that the multitude of other insane persons who seek for admission into such institutions could scarcely find room in them unless some of the insane in the house died. Not one is ever really and permanently cured in them! A convincing proof, among many others, of the complete nullity of the non-healing art hitherto practised, which has been ridiculously honored by allopathic ostentation with the title of rational medicine. How often, on the other hand, has not the true healing art, genuine pure homoeopathy, been able to restore such unfortunate beings to the possession of their mental and corporeal health, and so give them back again to their delighted friends and to the world!

130.   It would seem as though the mind, in these cases, felt with uneasiness and grief the truth of these rational representations and acted upon the body as it wished to restore the lost harmony, but that the body, by means of its disease, reacted upon the organs of the mind and disposition and put them in still greater disorder by a fresh transference of its sufferings on to them.

131.   It is impossible to marvel at the hard-heartedness and indiscretion of the medical men in many establishments for patients of this kind, who, without attempting to discover the true and only efficacious mode of curing such disease, which is by homoeopathic medicinal (antipsoric) means, content themselves with torturing these most pitiable of all human beings with the most violent blows and other painful torments. By this unconscientious and revolting procedure they debase themselves beneath the level of the turnkeys in a house of correction, for the latter inflict such chastisement as the duty devolving on their office, and on criminals only, whilst the former appear, from a humiliating consciousness of their uselessness as physicians, only to vent their spite at the supposed incurability of mental diseases in harshness towards the pitiable, innocent sufferers, for they are too ignorant to be of any use and too indolent to adopt a judicious mode of treatment.

132.   Two or three states may alternate with one another. Thus, for instance, in the case of double alternating diseases, certain pains may occur persistently in the legs, etc., immediately on the disappearance of a kind of ophthalmia, which latter again appears as soon as the pain in the limbs has gone off for the time – convulsions and spasms may alternate immediately with any other affection of the body or some part of it – in a case of threefold alternating states in a common indisposition, periods of apparent increase of health and unusual exaltation of the corporeal and mental powers (extravagant gaiety, extraordinary activity of the body, excess of comfortable feeling, inordinate appetite, etc.) may occur, after which, and quite unexpectedly, gloomy, melancholy humor, intolerable hypochondriacal derangement of the disposition, with disorder of several of the vital operations, the digestion, sleep, etc., appear, which again, and just as suddenly, give place to the habitual moderate ill-health; and so also several and very various alternating states. When the new state makes its appearance, there is often no perceptible trace of the former one. In other cases only slight traces of the former alternating state remain when the new one occurs; few of the symptoms of the first state remain on the appearance and during the continuance of the second. Sometimes the morbid alternating states are quite of opposite natures, as for instance, melancholy periodically alternating with gay insanity or frenzy.

133.   The pathology hitherto in vogue, which is still in the stage of irrational infancy, recognizes but one single intermittent fever, which it likewise termed ague, and admits of no varieties but such as are constituted by the different intervals at which the paroxysms recur, quotidian, tertian, quartan etc. But there are much more important differences among them than what are marked by the periods of their recurrence; there are innumerable varieties of these fevers, some of which cannot even be denominated ague, as their fits consist solely of heat; others, again, are characterised by cold alone, with or without subsequent perspiration; yet others which exhibit general coldness of the surface, with a sensation on the patient's part, or whilst the body feels externally hot, the patient feels cold; others, again, in which one paroxysm consists entirely of a rigor or simple chilliness followed by an interval of health, while the next consists of heat alone, followed or not by perspiration; others, again, in which the heat comes first and the cold stage not till that is gone; others, again, wherein after a cold or hot stage apyrexia ensues, and then perspiration comes on like a second fit, often many hours subsequently; others, again, in which no perspiration at all comes on, and yet others in which the whole attack consists of perspiration alone, without any cold or hot stage,

or in which the perspiration is only present during the heat; and there are innumerable other differences, especially in regard to the accessory symptoms, such as headache of a peculiar kind, bad taste of the mouth, nausea, vomiting, diarrhoea, want of or excessive thirst, peculiar pains in the body or limbs, disturbed sleep, deliria, alterations of temper, spasms, etc., before, during or after the sweating stage, and countless other varieties. All these are manifestly intermittent fevers of very different kinds, each of which, as might naturally be supposed, requires a special (homoeopathic) treatment. It must be confessed that they can almost all be suppressed (as is often done) by enormous doses of bark and of its pharmaceutical preparation, the sulphate of quinine; that is to say, their periodical recurrence (their typus) may be extinguished by it, but the patients who suffered from intermittent fevers for which cinchona bark is not suitable, as is the case with all those epidemic intermittent fevers that traverse whole countries and even mountainous districts, are not restored to health by the extinction of the typus; on the contrary, they now remain ill in another manner, and worse, often much worse, than before; they are affected by peculiar, chronic bark dyscrasias, and can scarcely be restored to health even by a prolonged treatment by the true system of medicine – and yet that is what is called curing, forsooth!

134.   Dr. von Bonninghausen, who has rendered more services to our beneficent system of medicine than any other of my disciples, has best elucidated this subject, which demands so much care, and has facilitated the choice of the efficient remedy for the various epidemics of fever, in his work entitled Versuch einer homoopathischen Therapie der Wechselfieber, 1833, Muster bi Regensberg.

135.   This is observed in the fatal cases, by no means rare, in which a moderate dose of opium given during the cold stage quickly deprived the patients of life.

136.   Large, oft-repeated doses of cinchona bark, as also concentrated cinchona remedies, such as the sulphate of quinine, have certainly the power of freeing such patients from the periodical fits of the marsh ague; but those thus deceived into the belief that they are cured remain diseased in another way, frequently with an incurable Quinin intoxication (see 276 note.)

137.   What I said in the fifth edition of the organon, in a long note to this paragraph in order to prevent these undesirable reactions of the vital energy, was all the experience I then had justified. But during the last four or five years, however, all these difficulties are wholly solved by my new altered but perfected method. The same carefully selected medicine may now be given daily and for months, if necessary in this way, namely, after the lower degree of potency has been used for one or two weeks in the treatment of chronic disease, advance is made in the same way to higher degrees, (beginning according to the new dynamization method, taught herewith with the use of the lowest degrees).

138.   We ought not even with the best chosen homoeopathic medicine, for instance one pellet of the same potency that was beneficial at first, to let the patient have a second or third dose, taken dry. In the same way, if the medicine was dissolved in water and the first dose proved beneficial, a second or third and even smaller dose from the bottle standing undisturbed, even in intervals of a few days, would prove no longer beneficial, even though the original preparation had been potentized with ten succussions or as I suggested later with but two succussions in order to obviate this disadvantage and this according to above reasons. But through modification of every dose in its dynamiztion degree, as I herewith teach, there exists no offence, even if the doses be repeated more frequently, even if the medicine be ever so highly potentized with ever so many succussions. It almost seems as if the best selected homoeopathic remedy

could best extract the morbid disorder from the vital force and in chronic disease to extinguish the same only if applied in several different forms.

139.   Made in 40, 30, 20, 15 or 8 tablespoons of water with the addition of some alcohol or a piece of charcoal in order to preserve it. If charcoal is used, it is suspended by means of a thread in the vial and is taken out when the vial is succussed. The solution of the medicinal globule (and it is rarely necessary to use more than one globule) of a thoroughly potentized medicine in a large quantity of water can be obviated by making a solution in only 7-8 tablespoons of water and after thorough succussion of the vial take from it one tablespoon and put it in a glass of water (containing about 7 to 8 spoonfuls), this stirred thoroughly and then given a dose to the patient. If he is unusually excited and sensitive, a teaspoon of this solution may be put in a second glass of water, thoroughly stirred and teaspoonful doses or more be given. There are patients of so great sensitiveness that a third or fourth glass, similarly prepared, may be necessary. Each such prepared glass must be made fresh daily. the globule of the high potency is best crushed in a few grains of sugar of milk which the patient can put in the vial and be dissolved in the requisite quantity of water.

140.   As all experience shows that the dose of the specially suited homoeopathic medicine can scarcely be prepared too small to effect perceptible amelioration in the disease for which it is appropriate (275-278), we should act injudiciously and hurtfully were we when no improvement, or some, though it be even slight, aggravation ensues, to repeat or even increase the dose of the same medicine, as is done in the old system, under the delusion that it was not efficacious on account of its small quantity (its too small dose). Every aggravation by the production of new symptoms – when nothing untoward has occurred in the mental or physical regimen – invariably proves unsuitableness on the part of the medicine formerly given in the case of disease before us, but never indicates that the dose has been too weak.

141.   The well informed and conscientiously careful physician will never be in a position to require an antidote in his practice if he will begin, as he should, to give the selected medicine in the smallest possible dose. Like minute doses of a better chosen remedy will re-establish order throughout.

142.   As I have more particularly described in the introduction to "Ignatia" (in the first volume of the Materia Medica Pura).

143.   The signs of improvement in the disposition and mind, however, may be expected only soon after the medicine has been taken when the dose has been sufficiently minute (i.e., as small as possible), an unnecessary large dose of even the most suitable homoeopathic medicine acts too violently, and at first produces too great and too lasting a disturbance of the mind and disposition to allow us soon to perceive the improvement in them. I must here observe that this so essential rule is chiefly transgressed by presumptuous tryos in homoeopathy, and by physicians who are converted to homoeopathy from the ranks of the old school. From old prejudices these persons abhor the smallest doses of the lowest dilutions of medicine in such cases, and hence they fail to experience the great advantages and blessings of that mode of proceeding which a thousandfold experience has shown to be the most salutary; they cannot effect all that homoeopathy is capable of doing, and hence they have no claim to be considered its adherents.

144.   The softest tones of a distant flute that in the still midnight hours would inspire a tender heart with exalted feelings and dissolve it in religious ecstasy, are inaudible and powerless amid discordant cries and the noise of day.

145.   Coffee; fine Chinese and other herb teas; beer prepared with medicinal vegetable substances unsuitable for the patient's state; so-called fine liquors made with medicinal

spices; all kinds of punch; spiced chocolate; odorous waters and perfumes of many kinds; strong-scented flowers in the apartment; tooth powders and essences and perfumed sachets compounded of drugs; highly spiced dishes and sauces; spiced cakes and ices; crude medicinal vegetables for soups; dishes of herbs, roots and stalks of plants possessing medicinal qualities; asparagus with long green tips, hops, and all vegetables possessing medicinal properties, celery, onions; old cheese, and meats that are in a state of decomposition, or that passes medicinal properties (as the flesh and fat of pork, ducks and geese, or veal that is too young and sour viands), ought just as certainly to be kept from patients as they should avoid all excesses in food, and in the use of sugar and salt, as also spirituous drinks, undiluted with water, heated rooms, woollen clothing next the skin, a sedentary life in close apartments, or the frequent indulgence in mere passive exercise (such as riding, driving or swinging), prolonged suckling, taking a long siesta in a recumbent posture in bed, sitting up long at night, uncleanliness, unnatural debauchery, enervation by reading obscene books, reading while lying down, Onanism or imperfect or suppressed intercourse in order to prevent conception, subjects of anger, grief or vexation, a passion for play, over-exertion of the mind or body, especially after meals, dwelling in marshy districts, damp rooms, penurious living, etc. All these things must be as far as possible avoided or removed, in order that the cure may not be obstructed or rendered impossible. Some of my disciples seem needlessly to increase the difficulties of the patient's dietary by forbidding the use of many more, tolerably indifferent things, which is not to be commended.

146.   This is, however, rare. Thus, for instance, in pure inflammatory diseases, where aconite is so indispensable, whose action would be destroyed by partaking of vegetable acids, the desire of the patient is almost always for pure cold water only.

147.   All crude animal and vegetable substances have a greater or less amount of medicinal power, and are capable of altering man's health, each in its own peculiar way. Those plants and animals used by the most enlightened nations as food have this advantage over all others, that they contain a larger amount of nutritious constituents; and they differ from the others in this that their medicinal powers in their raw state are either not very great in themselves, or are diminished by the culinary processes they are subjected to in cooking for domestic use, by the expression of the pernicious juice (like the cassava root of South America), by fermentation (of the rye-flour in the dough for making bread, sour-crout prepared without vinegar and pickled gherkins), by smoking and by the action of heat (in boiling, stewing, toasting, roasting, baking), whereby the medicinal parts of many of these substances are in part destroyed and dissipated. By the addition of salt (pickling) and vinegar (sauces, salads) animal and vegetable substances certainly lose much of their injurious medicinal qualities, but other disadvantages result from these additions. But even those plants that possess most medicinal power lose that in part or completely by such processes. By perfect desiccation all the roots of the various kinds of iris, of the horseradish, of the different species or arum and the peonies lose almost all their medicinal virtue. The juice of the most virulent plants often becomes inert, pitch-like mass, from the heat employed in preparing the ordinary extracts. By merely standing a long time, the expressed juice of the most deadly plants becomes quite powerless; even at moderate atmospheric temperature it rapidly takes on the vinous fermentation (and thereby loses much of its medicinal power), and immediately thereafter the acetous and putrid fermentation, whereby it is deprived of all peculiar medicinal properties; the fecula that is then deposited, if well washed, is quite innocuous, like ordinary starch. By the transudation that takes place when a number of green plants are laid one above the other, the greatest part of their medicinal properties is lost.

148. Buchholz (Taschenb. f. Scheidek. u. Apoth. a. d. J., 1815, Weimar, Abth. I, vi) assures his readers (and his reviewer in the Leipziger Literaturzeitung, 1816, No. 82, does not contradict him) that for this excellent mode of operating medicines we have to thank the campaign in Russia, whence it was (in 1812) imported into Germany. According to the noble practice of many Germans to be unjust towards their own countrymen, he conceals the fact that this discovery and those directions, which he quotes in my very words from the first edition of the Organon of Rational Medicine, 230 and note, proceed from me, and that I first published them to the world two years before the Russian campaign (the Organon appeared in 1810). Some folks would rather assign the origin of a discovery to the deserts of Asia than to a German to whom the honor belongs. O tempora! O mores! Alcohol has certainly been sometimes before this used for mixing with vegetable juices, e.g., to preserve them some time before making extracts of them, but never with the view of administering them in this form.

149. Although equal parts of alcohol and freshly expressed juice are usually the most suitable proportion for affecting the deposition of the fibrinous and albuminous matters, yet for plants that contain much thick mucus (e.g. Symphytum officinale, Viola tricolor, etc.), or an excess of albumen (e.g., Aethusa cynapium, Solanum nigrum, etc.), a double proportion of alcohol is generally required for this object. Plants that are very deficient in juice, as Oleander, Buxus, Taxus, Ledum, Sabina, etc., must first be pounded up alone into a moist, fine mass and the stirred up with a double quantity of alcohol, in order that the juice may combine with it, and being thus extracted by the alcohol, may be pressed out; these latter may also when dried be brought with milk-sugar to the millionfold trituration, and then be further diluted and potentized (v. 271)

150. In order to preserve them in the form of powder, a precaution is requisite that has hitherto been usually neglected by druggists, and hence powders, even of well-dried animal and vegetable substances could not be preserved uninjured even in well-corked bottles. The entire crude vegetable substances, though perfectly dry, yet contain, as an indispensable condition of the cohesion of their texture, a certain quantity of moisture, which dose not indeed prevent the unpulverized drug from remaining in as dry a state as is requisite to preserve it from corruption, but which is quite too much for the finely pulverized state. The animal or vegetable substance which in its entire state was perfectly dry, furnishes, therefore, when finely pulverized, a somewhat moist powder, which without rapidly becoming spoilt and mouldy, can yet not be preserved in corked bottles if not previously freed from this superfluous moisture. This is the best effected by spreading out the powder in a flat tin saucer with a raised edge, which floats in a vessel full of boiling water (i.e. a water-bath), and, by means of stirring it about, drying it to such a degree that all the small atoms of it (no longer stick together in lumps, but) like dry, fine sand, are easily separated from each other, and are readily converted into dust. In this dry state the fine powders may be kept forever uninjured in well-corked and sealed bottles, in all their original complete medicinal power, without ever being injured by mites or mould; and they are best preserved when the bottles are kept protected from the daylight (in covered boxes, chests, cases). If not shut up in air-tight vessels, and not preserved from the access of the light of the sun and day, all animal and vegetable substances in time gradually lose their medicinal power more and more, even in the entire state, but still more in the form of powder.

151. Long before this discovery of mine, experience had taught several changes which could be brought about in different natural substances by means of friction, for instance, warmth, heat, fire, development of odor in odorless bodies, magnetization of steel, and so forth. But all these properties produced by friction were related only to physical and inanimate things, whereas it is a law of nature according to which physiological

and pathogenic changes take place in the body's condition by means of forces capable of changing the crude material of drugs, even in such as had never shown any medicinal properties. This is brought about by trituration and succussion, but under the condition of employing an indifferent vehicle in certain proportions. this wonderful physical and especially physiological and pathogenic law of nature had not been discovered before my time. No wonder then, that the present students of nature and physicians (so for unknowing) cannot have faith in the magical curative powers of the minute doses of medicines prepared according to homoeopathic rules (dynamized).

152. The same thing is seen in a bar of iron and steel where a slumbering trace of latent magnetic force cannot but be recognized in their interior. Both, after their completion by means of the forge stand upright, repulse the north pole of a magnetic needle with the lower end and attract the south pole, while the upper end shows itself as the south pole of the magnetic needle. But this is only a latent force; not even the finest iron particles can be drawn magnetically or held on either end of such a bar. Only after this bar of steel is dynamized, rubbing it with a dull file in one direction, will it become a true active powerful magnet, one able to attract iron and steel to itself and impart to another bar of steel by mere contact and even some distance away, magnetic power and this in a higher degree the more it has been rubbed. In the same way will triturating a medicinal substance and shaking of its solution (dynamization, potentation) develop the medicinal powers hidden within and manifest them more and more or if one may say so, spiritualizes the material substance itself.

153. On this account it refers to the increase and stronger development of their power to cause changes in the health of animals and men if these natural substances in this improved state, are brought very near to the living sensitive fibre or come in contact with it (by means of intake or olfaction). Just as a magnetic bar especially if its magnetic force is increased (dynamized) can show magnetic power only in a needle of steel whose pole is near or touches it. The steel itself remains unchanged in the remaining chemical and physical properties and can bring about no changes in other metals (for instance, in brass), just as little as dynamized medicines can have any action upon lifeless things.

154. We hear daily how homoeopathic medicinal potencies are called mere dilutions, when they are the very opposite, i.e., a true opening up of the natural substances bringing to light and revealing the hidden specific medicinal powers contained within and brought forth by rubbing and shaking. The aid of a chosen, unmedicinal medium of attenuation is but a secondary condition. Simple dilution, for instance, the solution of a grain of salt will become water, the grain of salt will disappear in the dilution with much water and will never develop into medicinal salt which by means of our well prepared dynamization, is raised to most marvellous power.

155. One-third of one hundred grains sugar of milk is put in a glazed porcelain mortar, the bottom dulled previously by rubbing it with fine, moist sand. Upon this powder is put one grain of the powdered drug to be triturated (one drop of quicksilver, petroleum, etc.). The sugar of milk used for dynamization must be of that special pure quality that is crystallized on strings and comes to us in the shape of long bars. For a moment the medicines and powder are mixed with a porcelain spatula and triturated rather strongly, six to seven minutes, with the pestle rubbed dull, then the mass is scraped from the bottom of the mortar and from the pestle for three to four minutes, in order to make it homogeneous. This is followed by triturating it in the same way 6 – 7 minutes without adding anything more and again scraping 3 – 4 minutes from what adhered to the mortar and pestle. The second third of the sugar of milk is now added, mixed with the spatula and again triturated 6 – 7 minutes, followed by the scraping

for 3 – 4 minutes and trituration without further addition for 6 – 7 minutes. The last third of sugar of milk is then added, mixed with the spatula and triturated as before 6 -7 minutes with most careful scraping together. The powder thus prepared is put in a vial, well corked, protected from direct sunlight to which the name of the substance and the designation of the first product marked /100 is given. In order to raise this product to /10000, one grain of the powdered /100 is mixed with the third part of 100 grains of powdered sugar of milk and then proceed as before, but every third must be carefully triturated twice thoroughly each time for 6 -7 minutes and scraped together 3 -4 minutes before the second and last third of sugar of milk is added. After each third, the same procedure is taken. When all is finished, the powder is put in a well corked vial and labelled /10000, i.e., (I), each grain containing 1/1,000,000 the original substance. Accordingly, such a trituration of the three degrees requires six times six to seven minutes for triturating and six times 3 -4 minutes for scraping, thus one hour for every degree. After one hour such trituration of the first degree, each grain will contain 1/000; of the second 1/10,000; and in the third 1/1,000,000 of the drug used.* Mortar and spatula must be cleaned well before they are used for another medicine. Washed first with warm water and dried, both mortar and pestle, as well as spatula are then put in a kettle of boiling water for half an hour. precaution might be used to such an extent as to put these utensils on a coal fire exposed to a glowing heat. * These are the three degrees of the dry powder trituration, which if carried out correctly, will effect a good beginning for the dynamization of the medicinal substance.

156.   The vial used for potentizing is filled two-thirds full.

157.   Perhaps on a leather bound book.

158.   They are prepared under supervision by the confectioner from starch and sugar and the small globules freed from fine dusty parts by passing them through a sieve. Then they are put through a strainer that will permit only 100 to pass through weighing one grain, the most serviceable size for the needs of a homoeopathic physician.

159.   A small cylindrical vessel shaped like a thimble, made of glass, porcelain or silver, with a small opening at the bottom in which the globules are put to be medicated. They are moistened with some of the dynamized medicinal alcohol, stirred and poured out on blotting paper, in order to dry them quickly.

160.   According to first directions, one drop of the liquid of a lower potency was to be taken to 100 drops of alcohol for higher potentiation. This proportion of the medicine of attenuation to the medicine that is to be dynamized (100:1) was found altogether too limited to develop thoroughly and to a high degree the power of the medicine by means of a number of such successions without specially using great force of which wearisome experiments have convinced me.
But if only one such globule be taken, of which 100 weigh one grain, and dynamize it with 100 drops of alcohol, the proportion of 1 to 50,000 and even greater will be had, for 500 such globules can hardly absorb one drop, for their saturation. With this disproportionate higher ratio between medicine and diluting medium many successive strokes of the vial filled two-thirds with alcohol can produce a much greater development of power. But with so small a diluting medium as 100 to 1 of the medicine, if many successions by means of a powerful machine are forced into it, medicines are then developed which, especially in the higher degrees of dynamization, act almost immediately, but with furious, even dangerous violence, especially in weakly patients, without having a lasting, mild reaction of the vital principle. But the method described by me, on the contrary, produces medicines of highest development of power and mildest action, which, however, if well chosen, touches all suffering parts curatively.* In acute fevers, the small doses of the lowest dynamization degrees of these

thus perfected medicinal preparations, even of medicines of long continued action (for instance, belladonna) may be repeated in short intervals. In the treatment of chronic diseases, it is best to begin with the lowest degrees of dynamization and when necessary advance to higher, even more powerful but mildly acting degrees.
* In very rare cases, notwithstanding almost full recovery of health and with good vital strength, an old annoying local trouble continuing undisturbed it is wholly permitted and even indispensably necessary, to administer in increasing doses the homoeopathic remedy that has proved itself efficacious but potenized to a very high degree by means of many succussions by hand. Such a local disease will often then disappear in a wonderful way.

161.   This assertion will not appear improbable, if one considers that by means of this method of dynamization (the preparations thus produced, I have found after many laborious experiments and counter-experiments, to be the most powerful and at the same time mildest in action, i.e., as the most perfected) the material part of the medicine is lessened with each degree of dynamization 50,000 times yet incredibly increased in power, so that the further dynamization of 125 and 18 ciphers reaches only the third degree of dynamization. The thirtieth thus progressively prepared would give a fraction almost impossible to be expressed in numbers. It becomes uncommonly evident that the material part by means of such dynamization (development of its true, inner medicinal essence) will ultimately dissolve into its individual spirit-like, (conceptual) essence. In its crude state therefore, it may be considered to consist really only of this underdeveloped conceptual essence.

162.   Until the State, in the future, after having attained insight into the indispensability of perfectly prepared homoeopathic medicines, will have them manufactured by a competent impartial person, in order to give them free of charge to homoeopathic physicians trained in homoeopathic hospitals, who have been examined theoretically and practically, and thus legally qualified. The physician may then become convinced of these divine tools for purposes of healing, but also to give them free of charge to his patients – rich and poor.

163.   These globules (270) retain their medicinal virtue for many years, if protected against sunlight and heat.

164.   Two substances, opposite to each other, united into neutral Natrum and middle salts by chemical affinity in unchangeable proportions, as well as sulphurated metals found in the earth and those produced by technical art in constant combining proportions of sulphur and alkaline salts and earths, for instance (natrum sulph. and calcarea sulph.) as well as those ethers produced by distillation of alcohol and acids may together with phosphorus be considered as simple medicinal substances by the homoeopathic physician and used for patients. On the other hand, those extracts obtained by means of acids of the so-called alkaloids of plants, are exposed to great variety in their preparation (for instance, chinin, strychnine, morphine), and can, therefore, not be accepted by the homoeopathic physician as simple medicines, always the same, especially as he possesses, in the plants themselves, in their natural state (Peruvian bark, nux vomica, opium) every quality necessary for healing. Moreover, the alkaloids are not the only constituents of the plants.

165.   When the rational physician has chosen the perfectly homoeopathic medicine for the well-considered case of disease and administered it internally, he will leave to irrational allopathic routine the practice of giving drinks or fomentations of different plants, of injecting medicated glysters and of rubbing in this or the other ointment.

166.   The praise bestowed of late years by some homoeopathists on the larger doses is owing to this, either that they chose low dynamizations of the medicine to be administered (as I myself used to do twenty years ago, from nor knowing any better), or that the medicines selected were not homoeopathic and imperfectly prepared by their manufacturers.

167.   Thus, the continuous use of aggressive allopathic large doses of mercurials against syphilis develops almost incurable maladies, when yet one or several doses of a mild but active mercurial preparation would certainly have radically cured in a few days the whole venereal disease, together with the chancre, provided it had not been destroyed by external measures (as is always done by allopathy). In the same way, the allopath gives Peruvian bark and quinine in intermittent fever daily in very large doses, where they are correctly indicated and where one very small dose of a highly potentized China would unfailingly help (in marsh intermittents and even in persons who were not affected by any evident psoric disease). A chronic China malady (coupled at the same time with the development of psora) is produced, which, if it dose not gradually kill the patient by damaging the internal important vital organs, especially spleen and liver, will put him, nevertheless suffering for years in a sad state of health. A homoeopathic antidote for such a misfortune produced by abuse of large doses of homoeopathic remedies is hardly conceivable.

168.   The rule to commence the homoeopathic treatment if chronic diseases with the smallest possible doses and only gradually to augment them is subject to a notable exception in the treatment of the three great miasms while they still effloresce on the skin, i.e., recently erupted itch, the untouched chancre (on the sexual organs, labia, mouth or lips, and so forth), and the figwarts. These not only tolerate, but indeed require, from the very beginning large doses of their specific remedies of ever higher and higher degrees of dynamization daily (possibly also several times daily). If this course be pursued, there is no danger to be feared as is the case in the treatment of diseases hidden within, that the excessive dose while it extinguishes the disease, initiates and by continued usage possible produces a chronic medicinal disease. During external manifestations of these three miasms this is not the case; for from the daily progress of their treatment it can be observed and judged to what degree the large dose withdraws the sensation of the disease from the vital principle day by day; for none of these three can be cured without giving the physician the conviction through their disappearance that there is no longer any further need of these medicines.

Since diseases in general are but dynamic attacks upon the life principle and nothing material – no materia peccans – as their basis (as the old school in its delusion has fabulated for a thousand years and treated the sick accordingly to their ruin) there is also in these cases nothing material to take away, nothing to smear away, to burn or tie or cut away, without making the patient endlessly sicker and more incurable (Chron. Dis. Part 1), than he was before local treatment of these three miasms was instituted. The dynamic, inimical principle exerting its influence upon the vital energy is the essence of these external signs of the inner malignant miasms that can be extinguished solely by the action of a homoeopathic medicine upon the vital principle which affects it in a similar but stronger manner and thus extracts the sensation of internal and external spirit-like (conceptual) disease enemy in such a way that it no longer exists for the life principle (for the organism) and thus releases the patient of his illness and he is cured.

Experience, however, teaches that the itch, plus its external manifestations, as well as the chancre, together with the inner venereal miasm, can and must be cured only by means of specific medicines taken internally. But the figwarts, if they have existed for some time without treatment, have need for their perfect cure, the external application of their specific medicines as well as their internal use at the same time.

169. The power of medicines acting upon the infant through the milk of the mother or wet nurse is wonderfully helpful. Every disease in a child yields to the rightly chosen homoeopathic medicines given in moderate doses to the nursing mother and so administered, is more easily and certainly utilized by these new world-citizens than is possible in later years. Since most infants usually have imparted to them psora through the milk of the nurse, if they do not already possess it through heredity from the mother, they may be at the same time protected antipsorically by means of the milk of the nurse rendered medicinally in this manner. But the case of mothers in their (first) pregnancy by means of a mild antipsoric treatment, especially with sulphur dynamizations prepared according to the directions in this edition (270), is indispensable in order to destroy the psora – that producer of most chronic diseases – which is given them hereditarily; destroy it both within themselves and in the foetus, thereby protecting posterity in advance. This is true of pregnant women thus treated; they have given birth to children usually more healthy and stronger, to the astonishment of everybody. A new confirmation of the great truth of the psora theory discovered by me.

170. From this fact may be explained those marvellous cures, however infrequent, where chronic deformed patients, whose skin nevertheless was sound and clean, were cured quickly and permanently after a few baths whose medicinal constituents (by, chance) were homoeopathically related. On the other hand, the mineral baths very often brought on increased injury with patients, whose eruptions on the skin were suppressed. After a brief period of well-being, the life principle allowed the inner, uncured malady to appear elsewhere, more important for life and health.
At times, instead, the ocular nerve would become paralyzed and produce amaurosis, sometimes the crystalline lens would become clouded, hearing lost, mania or suffocating asthma would follow or an apoplexy would end the sufferings of the deluded patient.
A fundamental principle of the homoeopathic physician (which distinguishes him from every physician of all older schools) is this, that he never employs for any patient a medicine, whose effects on the healthy human has not previously been carefully proven and thus made known to him (20,21). To prescribe for the sick on mere conjecture of some possible usefulness for some similar disease or from hearsay "that a remedy has helped in such and such a disease" – such conscienceless venture the philanthropic homoeopathist will leave to the allopath. A genuine physician and practitioner or our art will therefore never send the sick to any of the numerous mineral baths, because almost all are unknown so far as their accurate, positive effects on the healthy human organism is concerned, and when misused, must be counted among the most violent and dangerous drugs. In this way, out of a thousand sent to the most celebrated of these baths by ignorant physicians allopathically uncured and blindly sent there perhaps one or two are cured by chance more often return only apparently cured and the miracle is proclaimed aloud. Hundreds, meanwhile sneak quietly away, more or less worse and the rest remain to prepare themselves for their eternal resting place, a fact that is verified by the presence of numerous well-filled graveyards surrounding the most celebrated of these spas.*
* A true homoeopathic physician, one who never acts without correct fundamental principles, never gambles with the life of the sick entrusted to him as in a lottery where the winner is in the ratio of 1 to 500 or 1000 (blanks here consisting of aggravation or death), will never expose any one of his patients to such danger and send

him for good luck to a mineral bath, as is done so frequently by allopaths in order to get rid of the sick in an acceptable manner spoiled by him or others.

171.   Especially of one of such persons, of whom there are not many, who, along with great kindness of disposition and perfect bodily powers, possesses but a very moderate desire for sexual intercourse, which it would give him very little trouble wholly to suppress, in whom, consequently, all the fine vital spirits that would otherwise be employed in the production of the semen, are ready to be communicated to others, by touching them and powerfully exerting the will. Some powerful mesmerisers, with whom I have become aquatinted, had all this peculiar character.

172.   When I here speak of the decided and certain curative power of positive mesmerism, I most assuredly do not mean that abuse of it, where, by repeated passes of this kind, continued for half an hour or a whole hour at a time, and, even day after day, performed on weak, nervous patients, that monstrous revolution of the whole human system is effected which is termed somnambulism, wherein the human being is ravished from the world of sense and seems to belong more to the world of spirits – a highly unnatural and dangerous state, by means of which it has not infrequently been attempted to cure chronic diseases.

173.   It is a well known rule that a person who is either to be positively or negatively mesmerised, should not wear silk on any part of the body.

174.   Hence a negative pass, especially if it be very rapid, is extremely injurious to a delicate person affected with a chronic ailment and deficient in vital force.

175.   A strong country lad, ten years of age, received in the morning, on account of slight indisposition, from a professed female mesmeriser, several very powerful passes with the points of both thumbs, from the pit of the stomach along the lower edge of the ribs, and he instantly grew deathly pale, and fell into such a state of unconsciousness and immobility that no effort could arouse him, and he was almost given up for dead. I made his eldest brother give him a very rapid negative pass from the crown of the head over the body to the feet, and in one instance he recovered his consciousness and became lively and well.

176.   Rubbing-in appears to favour the action of the medicines only in this way, that the friction makes the skin more sensitive, and the living fibres thereby more capable of feeling, as it were, the medicinal power and of communicating to the whole organism this health-affecting sensation. The previous employment of friction to the inside of the thigh makes the mere laying on the mercurial ointment afterwards quite as powerfully medicinal as if the ointment itself had been rubbed upon that part, a process which is termed rubbing-in, but it is very doubtful whether the mental itself can penetrate in substance into the interior of the body, or be taken up by the absorbent vessels by means of this so-called rubbing-in. Homoeopathy, however, hardly ever requires for its cures the rubbing-in of any medication, nor does it need any mercurial ointment.

177.   The smallest homoeopathic dose, which however, often effects wonders when used on proper occasions. Imperfect homoeopathists, who think themselves monstrously clever, not infrequently deluge their patients in difficult diseases with doses of different medicines, given rapidly one after the other, which, although they may have been homoeopathically selected and given in highly potentized attenuation, bring the patients into such an over-excited state that life and death are struggling for the mastery, and the least additional quantity of medicine would infallibly kill them. In such cases a mere gentle mesmeric pass and the frequent application, for a short time of the hand of a well-intentioned person to the part that is particularly affected, produce

the harmonious uniform distribution of the vital force throughout the organism, and therewith rest, sleep and recovery.

178.   Although by this restoration of the vital force, which ought to be repeated from time to time, no permanent cure can be effected in cases where, as has been taught above, a general internal dyscrasia lies at the root of the old local affection, as it always does, yet this positive strengthening and immediate saturation with the vital force (which no more belongs to the category of palliatives than does eating and drinking when hunger and thirst are present) is no mean auxiliary to the actual treatment of the whole disease by homoeopathic medicines.

179.   Especially of one of those persons, of whom there are not many who, along with great kindness of disposition and perfect bodily powers, possesses but a very moderate desire for sexual intercourse, which it would give him very little trouble to suppress, in whom, consequently, all the fine vital spirits that would otherwise be employed in the preparation of the semen, are ready to be communicated to others, by touching them and powerfully exerting the will. Some powerful mesmerisers, with whom I have become acquainted, has all this peculiar character.

180.   When I here speak of the decided and certain curative power of positive mesmerism, I most assuredly do not mean the abuse of it, where, by repeated passes of this kind, continued for half an hour or a whole hour at a time, and, even day after day, performed on weak, nervous patients, that monstrous revolution of the whole human system is effected which is termed somnambulism, wherein the human being is ravished from the world of sense and seems to belong more to the world of spirits – a highly unnatural and dangerous state, by means of which it has not infrequently been attempted to cure chronic diseases.

181.   It is a well known rule that a person who is either to be positively or negatively mesmerised, should not wear silk on any part of the body.

182.   Hence a negative pass, especially if it be very rapid, is extremely injurious to a delicate person affected with a chronic ailment and deficient in vital force.

183.   A strong country lad, ten years of age, received in the morning, on account of slight indisposition, from a professed female mesmeriser, several very powerful passes with the points of both thumbs, from the pit of the stomach along the lower edge of the ribs, and he instantly grew pale, and fell into such a state of unconsciousness and immobility that no effort could arouse him, and he was almost given up for dead. I made his eldest brother give him a very rapid negative pass from the crown of the head over the body to the feet, and in one instant he recovered his consciousness and became lively and well.

184.   Organon, xxxii.

185.   Op. cit. xxxi.

186.   Ibid. xxxiii.

187.   Op. cit. xxxviii.

188.   Organon, xl. This will be found to be the case in all diseases that are dissimilar; the stronger suspends the weaker, except in case of complication, which is a rare occurrence in acute diseases, but they never cure each other reciprocally.

189.   On Chronic Diseases. Translation of Begel, p. 107.

190.   Sir Gilbert Blane's Medical Logic.

191.   Organon, v.

192.   Ibid. vi.

193.   Sir G. Blane.